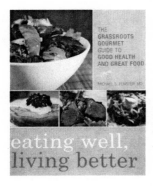

Dr. Mike's previous book:
Eating Well, Living Better

Everyone loves to eat. And everyone wants to be healthy. But how do we navigate between today's extremes—between those offering us gastronomic gluttony and the siren song of convenient junk food and those preaching salvation only through deprivation and boring food choices? Dr. Michael Fenster draws upon his expertise and training as an interventional cardiologist and as a chef to forge a path through this wilderness to offer readers a middle path that endorses both fine dining and health eating. As a chef and foodie, and someone who has battled the bulge himself, he knows that if the food doesn't taste great, no one will sustain any program for a lifetime. This is a culinary survival guide for every kitchen.

The Fallacy of The Calorie
by Dr. Mike Fenster

ISBN 978-1-94019-289-5

Published by
◤ köehlerbooks™

210 60th Street
Virginia Beach, VA 23451
212-574-7939
www.koehlerbooks.com

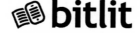

A **$1.99 (or less)** eBook is available
with the purchase of this print book.

CLEARLY PRINT YOUR NAME ABOVE IN UPPER CASE

Instructions to claim your eBook edition:
1. Download the BitLit app for Android or iOS
2. Write your name in UPPER CASE on the line
3. Use the BitLit app to submit a photo
4. Download your eBook to any device

Dedicated to Jennifer,
The Queen of The Stones

The Fallacy Of The Calorie

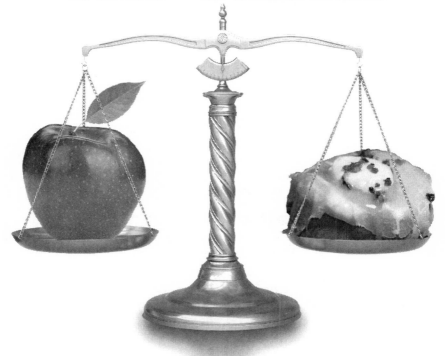

Why the Modern Western Diet is Killing Us and How to Stop It

Michael S. Fenster, MD

America's Culinary Interventionalist and Author of
*Eating Well, Living Better: A Grassroots Gourmet Approach
to Good Health and Great Food*

Table of Contents

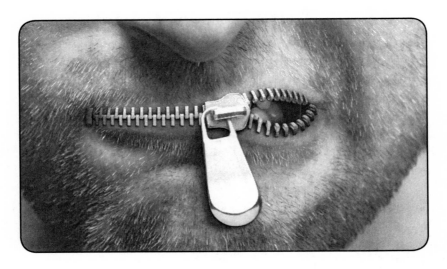

Shut the Hell Up!

"Everything should be made as simple as possible, but no simpler."
~Attributed to Albert Einstein

Many so-called food and health experts aren't. Our relationship with food is complex and most approaches are simply an oversimplification. Eat food high in cholesterol and it raises your blood cholesterol. High blood cholesterol leads to blockages in your heart arteries or coronary atherosclerosis. Blockages lead to heart attacks and death. Such lovely, simple, straightforward and linear observations are what led to the outcry against consuming eggs, and in particular, yolks. It is wonderful, unpretentious, and elegant—except that it's wrong. Your dietary cholesterol has little-to-no impact on what your blood cholesterol levels are let alone defining the complex relationship between *good* cholesterol (HDL cholesterol), *bad* cholesterol (LDL cholesterol) and a myriad of other lipoproteins.

Eggs from free-range chickens consuming their natural diet, *including the yolk,* are among nature's most healthful foods. After the initial front-page fire-and-brimstone damnation, no one bothers to read the official retraction on the back page. Commercials still abound and store shelves remain stacked with *healthy breakfast sandwich* options made with egg whites or synthetic pseudo-egg stuff and some sort of bread product loaded with preservatives, modern wheat, yoga mat ingredients, and sweeteners. The ingredients in the processed cheese food (whatever, by God, that actually is) and meat-like substance won't be found in Mother Nature's pantry. Parsimony is a great guide, but oversimplification and simple reduction can be more dangerous than exaggeration. You can end up using Occam's razor to slit your own throat.

Food is part necessity; we need food to live. We need proper nutrition. Our bond to food is part hardwired into our physiology and part subject to our psychology. We crave certain things at an instinctive, unconscious level; but what we choose to eat is a conscious decision. Food is part of our social fabric, part pleasure and experience. It is also big business. Without an understanding and appreciation for each of these aspects, the so-called experts are like the blind men in the room with the elephant. Each mistakes his limited experience for the entire animal. And the ones at the rectum always seem to preach loudest.

These days it seems as if everybody has an opinion about food and health. People watch Dr. Oz, tune in to the Food Network, or read some anecdotal diatribe on the Internet and all of a sudden they're full of expert opinions and analysis. A purported health and wellness network recently re-circulated an ongoing Internet meme about how people should eat bananas to prevent cancer because, according to the post, ripe bananas contain high levels of tumor necrosis factor (TNF). Firstly, the original study was performed in mice and the mice did not eat bananas, they had banana purée injected into their bellies.[1] The immune response of the mice was then observed. The study never actually evaluated whether there was any TNF in the bananas. Considering that TNF is produced by the human immune system, something lacking in a normal banana, the take-home message may be to avoid consuming Franken-nanas with human parts.

Elevated levels of TNF are associated with autoimmune disorders such as rheumatoid arthritis, ankylosing spondylitis, inflammatory bowel disease, psoriasis, hidradenitis suppurativa, refractory asthma, and congestive heart failure. So even if Mister Tallyman tallied you eight bunches of GMO bananas and they were stacked with TNF until the morning comes, eating them to excess may just make you terribly ill; BS comes and me wanna go home.

Chances are you have come across, or know, someone who claims to be an expert about food and health. Chances are most of these self-proclaimed experts have no training in food preparation or any kind of health-related or medical background. They have grandiose made-up titles like wellness enthusiast, lifestyle coach, the Duke of Diet, or something equally ridiculous.

The story about our relationship with food and our health is very intricate and continually evolves. And make no mistake, it *is* a story. It has a beginning, a history, and the tale to date. Many people do not take the time to get to the heart of the matter or evaluate data. But if you are calling yourself an expert and advising others about such intimate and powerful decisions as food and health, you need to. Stories like the banana and other unsubstantiated bits taken as conventional wisdom get circulated about long enough that they can become accepted as fact.

Many of the so-called experts lack the requisite training or experience in the realms of food and health—or any related training at all. Working out in a gym, starring in a movie or your own YouTube production doesn't make you qualified. It also doesn't mean these are bad people trying to run a scam—although many of them are. The road to bypass surgery is paved with good intentions. Less than seventy-five years ago, Lucky Strike cigarettes were "The Doctors' Choice." And "The Doctors' Choice" became "America's Choice." Women were advised that smoking Lucky Strikes would help them to stay slim, since they could "Reach for a Lucky instead of a sweet."[2] The road to bypass surgery is also paved with goodly profits.

There are many in the food industry who are excellent, professional chefs. They know food. But just because you know food and how to prepare it deliciously doesn't make you an expert on healthful eating. They tend to take the same tired misconceptions promulgated all over the Internet and blithely repost them.

There is a colleague who is an incredible chef. She is bright, charming, witty, and a lot of fun to hang out with. She posts on the Internet that "eating walnuts can reduce your chance of diabetes by 24 percent." She then proceeds to post a *great* recipe she developed using walnuts. The only problem is that when you candy the walnuts by encasing them in an armor of pure high fructose corn syrup (HFCS) you tend to lose the diabetic reduction benefits. She knows food, she knows how to make anything delicious, but she doesn't know diddly-squat about health. For all the professional chefs who think a 'genital heart defect' is something you are born with (it's congenital heart defect, by the way), when it comes to healthful eating, would you please just shut it!

Then there are the brain trusts that take anything you concoct and make it *healthier* by replacing any protein you have in a dish with vegetables. Yes, we all need to eat more fresh fruits and vegetables. We get it. But changing everything into a veggie tale does not necessarily contribute to a healthful, balanced diet. A french fry diet can be completely vegan but that does not make it a smart choice. A slice of apple embalmed with Clorox that smells like wet dog on a hot summer's day is not going to get any six-year-old on the vegetable and fruit bandwagon just because it is the *"healthy choice."* And, oh, by the way, Julia Child wanna-be, your tofu and zucchini faux *onglet* is not a tasty veggie variation of the red meat we were set to enjoy. It's not a delicious all-veggie alternative. It's a putrid abomination. If you're salivating for red meat like you're at a dinner party with Dr. Pavlov, there's a reason. And speaking of Julia Child, she and her husband both lived well into their nineties in good health on a diet of French cuisine. For all the Nutrition Nazis who want to turn every meal into a salad bar, would you please just shut it!

Then, of course there is the *chicken* approach. These people make everything *healthier* by substituting any form of red meat for poultry, usually chicken or turkey. They quote it as a leaner protein with fewer calories, although a four-ounce center-cut pork chop actually has less calories than half a chicken breast. Most of these experts can't even tell you what a calorie is, let alone comment about calories as a guide to better health. Industrially processed, tasteless ground ghetto birds do not have a superior nutritional profile compared to a delectable grass-fed, free-range piece of beef. You have to understand the consequences of where your food is sourced. For these self-described dietetic divas who take the fowl fat-reductive fallacy to the extreme: would you please just shut it!

And then there are all the celebrity chefs; all of them now experts on how to make *healthy cuisine.* They will do a take on some traditional recipe, maybe something that they have shown you how to make before that was absolutely scrumptious. They will then instruct you that they are going to make a *healthy* version by cutting out some or all of the fat. They say this because, you know "this ain't my mama's cooking." And because replacing the fat with something synthetic is the easiest way to shave off one hundred calories. What it does is take something that was an enjoyable, wonderful experience, and not necessarily bad for you depending on the fats used, and turn it into something that should be pooper scooped.

Replacing healthy fats with synthetic garbage is not necessarily a healthy approach. It is, in fact, a lazy and potentially deadly approach. Not all fats are bad. There are, in truth, essential fatty acids we cannot live without. Food groups are like people; some fats are good, some you can only take in small doses. Some carbohydrates are great and more is better, some are just bad news. So, the slandering of entire food groups is just palate profiling. Celebrity chefs, hot peppers cause your body to release endorphins, not *endolphins*. Stick to teaching us how to cook the mahi-mahi. When it comes to healthful eating commentary, would you please just shut it!

Then there are the fitness fadsters. They are attractive, svelte girls clad in as little skintight spandex as possible and buffed, invariably shirtless guys. They hawk the latest *super foods* with an audience full of testimonials so insincere they would cause a politician to blush. They proclaim from upon up high that you only have to drink this extract or eat this berry or suck this twig and you will magically shed pounds and live forever in good health. For the vast majority, these fitness experts seem to have gotten their healthful eating credentials from a magazine cut out in the waiting room between rounds of liposuction and Botox. It's about balance and common sense in your diet not a couple of magic beans. When it comes to healthful eating there, Buffy and Baxter, would you please just shut it!

The only thing worse than these fadsters are the celebrity superstar spokespeople. They tell you how some program of food shipped in a box each month transformed them. They lost weight and now they are feeling great! What they don't tell you is that they didn't pay for any food, they are receiving an obscene amount of money for promoting the product, and they spent eight hours a day in the gym with a personal trainer— which they also didn't pay for. These programs put you on the hook paying out a lot of your hard-earned money each month for some processed, powdered, and wretched-tasting slop out of a box. You still have to supply the expensive fresh vegetables and fruit. By the process of caloric restriction you will lose weight. You will not necessarily obtain health or wellness. You are then condemned to consume this diet, delivered in an unrefrigerated box to your home every thirty days—for the rest of your life.

There is something unholy about food that has a longer shelf life than a formaldehyde-infused Keith Richards. The world of celebrity is not the world for the rest of the 99.9 percent of us; would you please just shut it!

It is not just the celebrities who drop a turd every time they open their mouth. There are a number of medical professionals and people in health-related fields who know a lot about their respective specialties but know nothing about food. All of us know many colleagues, friends, and peers who are fantastic physicians, nurses, cardiologists, and other health professionals who work their butts off 24/7 to help people. They are remarkable, exceptionally dedicated people deserving of the highest praise. But the truth is a number of them can't boil water. Yet they spout off ultimatums like Nick Fury on a three-day crack bender. They tell you don't eat red meat because you will have a heart attack. Don't put salt on anything or you will die from hypertension. Only use vegetable oils and, oh, by the way, according to your body mass index (BMI) you should be twelve feet tall for your weight. They then give you a list of things in which you cannot partake. It is an approach of salvation through starvation, but there is no resurrection by deprivation. While they *No*, they do not know a thing about food; would you please just shut it!

This is a book for lost souls. For everyone confused by all the contradictory information out there regarding what you eat and how it affects your health; for all the people pissed off about all the nonsense that circulates as conventional wisdom; for all the people annoyed about being told that they can't have a shrimp or an egg because it's toxic with cholesterol, then finding that three years later that statement has been retracted because, "Oh geez, we guess we got that wrong. These things really are good for you. In fact they're so good for you that they are now the latest superfood. Sorry about the food substitute loaded with trans-fatty acids. Oops."

If you are easily offended, put this book down because you will be more annoyed than Jack Sparrow at an AA meeting. If you are a true believer in the conventional foodie wisdom, put this book down because it will rock that false foundation like Krakatoa. If you think the modern Western diet is a boon to mankind, put this book down because it will kick you right in your boons. If you are happy with the food you eat and how it makes you feel, your state of health and wellness, put this book down, put your hands in the air and walk away. This is not for you.

This book is for people who want to understand what has happened to our food and how it impacts our health. It is for people who want to enjoy a variety of the incredible, delicious bounty nature offers without restriction. It is for people who want to become empowered and understand the vast potential locked away in the correct balance and ratio of all the various foodstuffs we can partake of. It is for people who want some guidelines, a map upon which they can chart their own culinary journey. This book is about giving you the tools you need to understand the current state of the modern Western diet and why and what you need to change.

It is about giving you the knowledge to understand your own weaknesses to manipulation and subterfuge. That awareness gives you the power to eliminate those vulnerabilities. It is about giving you the ability to charter your own course based on solid principles founded in science; yet that can yield to your own taste and pleasure. It is written so you may enjoy both delicious, wholesome foods that bring you happiness and at the same time supply your body with the resources it needs for good health and wellness. It is about realizing that we truly are what we eat. We are a manifestation of the interaction between our genetics and our environment. The most powerful and intimate happening between these two forces occurs in our gut; mediated by a host of symbiotic bacteria.

This book is about food for nutrition, for health, for enjoyment and celebration and, perhaps most importantly, it is about food for the soul. It is about enabling you to spot the false prophets issuing a cacophony of misinformed nonsense. It is about giving you the facts to tell the shysters, self-anointed doyens and just plain ignorant know-it-all idiots to "Shut the hell up!"

Because in the deepest circles of Dante's Culinary Inferno await the most hellish health consequences.

Question everything.

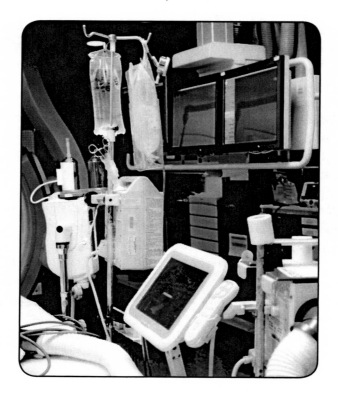

Discordance and Despair:
The Diseases of Modern Civilization

"Abandon all hope, ye who enter here!"
~DANTE ALIGHIERI, THE DIVINE COMEDY

The human brain is often compared to a computer. Sadly, for a number of the contemporary populace their model resembles a Commodore 64 or perhaps a Texas Instruments calculator. If you do not know what that means then ask someone who remembers when a Honey Boo Boo was simply an affectionate smack on the rump. Fortunately in many other cases, like obviously the readers of this book, it is not just your average PC that the brain resembles, but a supercomputer. Regardless, even in its most limited expression, the brain is an incredibly complex organ. The functioning of the brain is something we are just beginning to understand. Somewhere beyond the neurons and gray matter, the brain also contains our mind—the essence of who we are. And we know less about the functioning of our mind than we do of our brain, which is to say not very much at all.

To understand how totally clueless we are, one need only think about a thought. Where does it come from? Where, out of the ether, do thoughts come to us? Are they simply the result of some random neurochemical discharges? How are they organized? And with all the competing and contradicting thoughts, how do we ever prioritize, categorize, and undertake any meaningful action? Simply imagine Congress as the brain of government and you see how difficult it is to perform the tasks we customarily take for granted. Of course, if the government were a person and Congress were the brain, it would ride a short bus and wear a helmet. But unlike Congress, we deal with the reality of our lives, perform our jobs, and function in our 24/7/365 helter-skelter culture.

How amazing is this thing we routinely do every day?

The power of our minds is reflected in the accomplishments of our contemporary civilization. It is only through superior intellect that we have constructed the most complex social structure and technologically advanced civilization. We dominate our world with brain, not brawn. The dinosaurs, among the largest herbivores and carnivores ever to roam the earth, ruled for over a hundred and fifty million years before becoming extinct. Modern humans have dominated the scene for just about one-tenth of 1 percent of that time. In our two hundred thousand years of control we have remade the planet in our image. But these endeavors are not without cost; there are no free rides.

The brain may be the driver, but the driver needs a car, and that car needs energy. The body sustains the brain and our diet fuels the body. Our physiology makes us a hybrid model. It places us among the omnivores of this planet; although with our shortened long-intestine our gut construction is more akin to a carnivore than an herbivore—or at least an omnivore that prefers cooked food.[3] We cannot simply graze the plains and chew the leaves like an impala to fuel our body and our mind. With relatively weak jaws, no fangs or claws, and generally puny musculature, we are hardly the most physically impressive or intimidating hunters based on anatomy alone. No, our accomplishments most certainly have not been the result of our physical prowess. Nerds rule here.

But even supercomputers are subject to limitations. The conclusions that they reach are subject to both the quantity *and* the quality of the information; garbage in, garbage out. You want chicken salad, don't start with chicken shit. Not even Emeril can fix that.

In addition to the data, computers also require a proper power source. Human beings have changed the world and advanced civilization and technology to a point unimagined just mere centuries ago. But, have we done the same for ourselves? Has our superior intellect and technology improved *us*; have we transformed ourselves? And what price has been paid? Have we traded the famine and starvation of millennia ago for a slow poison and a shiny walker?

Are we healthier today than in times past or worse off?

Change can be a dangerous enterprise, and it's not always for the better. Change dressed as *progress* can be a fickle bitch; and even penicillin and Paxil may not cure all the misery that change can deliver. Beginning in the United States, what is now referred to worldwide as the modern Western diet has set in motion an irrevocable cascade of events. Some good, some not so good, and some literally heart-stopping. It is not without a degree of irony that the standard American diet is often referred to outside of the US by its acronym: SAD. Our diet has left us bland, without taste or texture and ill for our efforts. Unfettered, it is a harsh legacy. It is a woeful tale ending in chronic disability and disease.

These chronic disabilities and diseases are commonly referred to as the diseases of modern civilization. These are diseases that share a common inflammatory root. This state of chronic low-level inflammation links them together more tightly than the cast of Sister Wives. They are diseases and disabilities like obesity, diabetes, cardiovascular disease, autoimmune conditions and many cancers. The evidence is clear that our diets can contribute to the cause. It is also clear that they can also contribute to the cure. But our response to this crisis has been to execute more spasmodic gyrations than a twerking Miley Cyrus.

From a technological, societal, and cultural perspective we have rapidly evolved at a frantic pace. From a biologic and physiologic perspective, our bodies are not much changed from the first hairy hominins who wandered about the savannas of East Africa. The mechanisms and predispositions that drove us to seek out sugar, salt, and fat upon those African plains remain intact today. At that point in our evolution these were valuable and necessary foodstuffs.

The desire to seek them out is a hardwired survival instinct that has allowed us as individuals and as a species to survive and thrive. But in that success we have become out of balance with the world at many levels—including a deeply personal one.

In an environment where you can stuff your gob all day long, every day, the constant input of processed, adulterated, and excessive amounts of energy-dense and nutrient-poor *pseudo-phood* disrupts your body's natural balance. Nature is all about balance. Balance between eating and fasting, activity and rest, quality and quantity. It is important to remember that balance does not imply equality and equivalent amounts. Left to their own devices the impala and the lion exist in balance upon the plains of the Serengeti. But the natural order of things dictates that to remain in balance there are more impala than lions. They are in balance, but not in equal number.

Balance in Nature implies adherence to the inherent ratios and native rhythms.

These ratios and rhythms are all around us, reflected in the seasons and in our food. Our very health depends on this balance. We flourish at a balance point between building-up and tearing-down, between inflammation and quiescence, between anabolic and catabolic states. We call this point of balance *homeostasis*. It is a place where we exist in harmony with our gut microbiome; where we are metabolically healthy. It is our bodies' natural state, a position of comfort where we are at ease. Forced from this state we find ourselves suffering in an uncomfortable locus of *dis-ease*.

Many will argue this is not so. Many will say we may be a tad overweight, but just lose a few pounds and health and wellness is yours for the taking. Others will offer magic pills and plans to supplement your way to health without having to give up anything, other than a chunk of change. Still others will argue that there is no flaw to our food. They ask rhetorically, between bites of microwaved neon orange paste slathered over a link-shaped UFO (unidentified fried object): How can this modern diet be so detrimental to basic health if humankind is living longer than ever?

The average life expectancy (ALE) is often used as a surrogate for health. The argument is that we have obtained the highest ALE in recorded history, proof that we're the healthiest group of humans— ever. The problem with this perspective originates in its premise; just because you live longer, it does not mean you live better or healthier. The US ALE in 2010 for males was 76.1 years and for females 80.8

years, yielding an average life expectancy of 78.2 years. This is indeed the highest ALE ever recorded.

Yet these extra years are not the golden years we all dream of, they have become rusted and tarnished with chronic disability and disease. We have become the walking damn-near dead. These chronic afflictions are often referred to as the diseases of modern civilization: coronary artery disease, obesity, hypertension, diabetes, polycystic ovary syndrome, myopia, acne, gout, certain cancers, and many autoimmune disorders. In our modern obsession with numbers, we confuse quantity with value. What is important is not just the quantity of years that we have, but the *quality* of those years.

Taking those factors under consideration we can then reexamine the average life expectancy measurement. We can redefine our goal as a *healthy* average life expectancy, which the government has done for us at no small expense. A healthy average life expectancy (HALE) is one that is free from major disease and disability. If that is our goal—as it should be—then that value is only 68.1 years.[4] In other words, the average person will spend the last decade of his or her life suffering in misery from major chronic disability and lingering disease. What is perhaps most telling is that if we strive for excellence, meaning an existence totally free from any disability or disease, then our average life expectancy would be only 42.7 years. The bottom line is that the average person spends well over the last three decades of their life dealing with some form of significant chronic disability or disease.

Nearly half the financial fiasco that is health care costs in the US today is a result of such chronic disability and illness exacerbated by poor diet. Cardiovascular disease continues to be the leading cause of death and a major cause of morbidity. One in three Americans suffers from hypertension, with less than half ever achieving adequate control. According to body mass index measurements (BMI) almost two out of every three, almost 66 percent, of Americans are overweight or obese. In 2011 almost 10 percent of the population, more than twenty-five million Americans, suffered from diabetes. Worldwide it is estimated that three hundred and eighty-two million people are afflicted. Diabetes has climbed 4 percent over the past two years and is responsible for one person dying every six seconds. The number of people affected by the disease is expected to climb 55 percent to 592 million by 2035.[5]

In the elderly population hip fractures increase the risk of death and major injury. More than 7 percent of all women fifty and older have osteoporosis, with almost 40 percent suffering from osteopenia. In this group of women with such bone diseases, hip fractures carry an additional 20 percent excess mortality. Cancer is the second-leading cause of death in US, with cancers of the digestive system the number three killer.[6] These values pertain to the US, the country that spends more per capita on health care than any other country. The trends, though, are applicable across the globe to all Western and industrialized countries.

Why, if we are living longer, are we not living better?

For all the brouhaha from both sides of the health care debate still raging in the US, it is a little-appreciated fact that Americans spend twice as much on food than they do on health care. Even less appreciated is the impact of diet on our health. Experts conclude that approximately one third of all cancer deaths are the result of nutritional factors. The single largest risk factor for the number of years we spend with chronic disease and disability of any type is the composition of our diet. The dietary effects are so pervasive that they have supplanted tobacco, which now ranks second as a risk factor after diet.[7]

The danger does not just lie in the mass consumption of calories. The composition of your diet, the quality of your food, is more important than your BMI and whether you are obese or not. It's more than the calories.

To gauge the effects of the modern Western diet examine the incidence and prevalence of the disabilities and diseases of modern civilization in those populations with different diets. Several of the common measurements correlated with positive health benefits have been found in cultures deemed *primitive*. Yet, hunter-gatherer societies exhibit superior results when compared with our contemporary *advanced* Western societies. Compared to us, members of hunter-gatherer societies have lower resting blood pressures, a lack of age-related increases in hypertension and insulin resistance, lower fasting plasma insulin concentrations, lower fasting leptin (a hormone released by fat cells) levels, lower BMI, lower waist-to-height ratio, lower percent body fat, superior maximum oxygen consumption, preserved visual acuity, improved markers of bone health and lower fracture rates. Conditions as prevalent in our industrialized world as to be commonplace—metabolic syndrome, type 2 diabetes, cardiovascular disease, cancer, acne, and myopia—are hardly to be found in these societies. Where you don't find the SAD, people are glad.

Some may counter that these effects are genetics—not diet related. However, the Kuna Indians of Central America illustrate why this is simply not so. Within their indigenous lands, the Kuna Indians consume much more salt than the average American (along with a lot more cocoa). Yet, they have lower blood pressure, preserved kidney function into old age, and less diabetes and cancer than the average citizen of the United States or the average Central American. Even though they consume way more salt than the average American, they have fewer of the diseases and disabilities we attribute to excessive sodium consumption. Are they genetically superior?

Heil no!

There are members of the tribe who leave their native lands and settle on the Central American mainland. There, they adopt a modern Western lifestyle and diet. And there, they reap the rewards of said lifestyle and diet—rates of disease and disability similar to the average Central American.

If these individuals return to their native society and reengage native customs, lifestyle, and diet, their markers of health improve to their previous, more favorable values.[8,9,10] Other studies have examined dietary and nutritional interventions based on such a preindustrial diet as that of the Kuna Indians. These studies have confirmed positive, healthful outcomes utilizing less processed and minimally or completely unadulterated foods. These types of findings hint at the import of the environmental and dietary determinants on the quantity and the quality of our golden years; HALE yes!

Our ancient forebears battled non-dietary afflictions such as childhood diseases, accidents, warfare, infection, and exposure. These also affect modern hunter-gatherer societies. These are trials and tribulations that have been well dealt with within modern Western civilizations. If the ancients could survive these threats to existence and make it to middle-age, their likelihood of living well into their seventies and eighties was the same as it is today.[11] The average life expectancy is exactly that; an average of everyone in the population. It is not that the absolute life expectancy, or longevity, of human beings has increased. Our expiration date has not changed even if the average lifespan has. There are simply fewer of us dying in childhood, in pregnancy and delivery, from accidents, trauma, infection, and the like. Since more of us live longer, the average increases.

It is basic math and sanitation that is predominantly responsible for the increased ALE, not some form of genetic superiority.

Likewise, if a member of a modern hunter-gatherer society can survive these same perils and reach middle age, their average life expectancy is in the sixty-eight to seventy-eight year range. This is completely comparable to the most modern and advanced Western civilizations. More importantly, they enjoy these years free of the burden of chronic disease and disability seen in the more modern and so-called advanced Western countries. Their average health, if they survive into their autumn years, is comparatively superior to that of the average American.

How did we get here?

Like despots of old we have removed ourselves from the environs we have mastered. We shout, "Let them eat cake" between bites of Cinnabons big enough to wear as a hat. But we do not exist in isolation from our environment. We are constructed of parts derived from our habitat according to our genetic master plan. This genetic design is what is known as your individual genotype. It is the DNA blueprint that makes you, well, *you*. The parts of us built according to these designs are constantly being replaced with raw materials from our surroundings. That means the bits our body recycles, the air we breathe, the food we eat, and the products produced by our symbiotic gut microbiome. Our bodies and our internal gut microbiome are also modified in response to the environment. We shed our skin, our hair and nails grow, cuts heal, bones mend, and the entire lining of our gut from pie hole to poop shoot is replaced within short order.[12]

There are modifications to our parts that can occur in response to our environment. Just like your car, parts wear out and need to be replaced. Your DNA, your genotype is the architectural blueprint. The building that actually results from that blueprint is your phenotype. This is what makes you *uniquely* you. It is what makes identical twins with the same genetic blueprints ultimately singular. It is what allows each of them to be different individuals. Sometimes initially, but invariably over the years, as a result of our interaction with the environment, there are modifications and repairs that occur. Sometimes that NAPA car replacement part is better than the original. Sometimes it does not exactly fit the same way. And the software upgrade (invariably to repair the last security breach) can screw the operating system up more often than it seems to deliver any tangible improvement. Fortunately, our DNA is more reliable than Microsoft.

This simple truth of existence highlights the fact that we cannot isolate ourselves from our environment—whether you are a car, computer, building, or person. It is conventional wisdom, that for the average person, if you don't exercise, if you smoke cigarettes and make poor food choices, then you increase your likelihood of suffering disability and disease that result from cardiovascular causes. Every action has a consequence, intended or unintended. The bill will get paid in the end, whether it is due immediately or is deferred in nature and shows up years later. Karma is like the cosmic IRS; she will find you eventually. And when she does, there's always interest and penalties.

Your karma depends on your choices. Some choices have greater ramifications than others. The importance of dietary choices is rapidly becoming more apparent, although sometimes through surprising mechanisms. Every day it seems we learn something new about how what we eat transforms within us and how that ultimately transforms us. You see, we are not alone; even when we think we are alone.

It is estimated that each of us has more than one hundred trillion bacteria living within our guts. That is more bacteria than there are cells of your entire body by a factor of almost ten times.[13] We are a symbiotic creation, in some ways more alien than human. But unlike the technologically superior extraterrestrials of film and fantasy that impose their will upon us, in this case we ultimately have the control. That is because what we eat helps determine the composition of our gut bacteria, what is known as our gut microbiome. There is a reason toxic areas polluted by manufacturing waste look like a postcard from Mordor. Why would you expect anything different in your gut if you ingest industrial sludge? It too becomes "a barren wasteland, riddled with fire and ash and dust, the very air … a poisonous fume."[14] Not even a unicorn can shit glitter and rainbows after a Big McMordor.

We are ultimately the product of this interaction between our genetics and our environment, for better or for worse. How, what, when, where, and why we eat is our utmost expression of that interaction. There is no more intimate interface between our genetics and our environment than what we choose to consume, and its definitive expression through the interplay of our individual genome and our particular gut microbiome. Although it is so overused that it has become a bit cliché, it remains true that what we eat is who we are.

Any modification to a system can invoke the law of unintended consequences. Rapid and drastic changes, such as those occurring to our food and food pathways since the Industrial Revolution, do not allow time for physiological adaption. From the Industrial Revolution to the present is approximately 0.009 percent of the total time of human evolution. It is clearly an insufficient time frame for us to react from a biological perspective. When our bodies are confronted with such radical alterations to our basic diet, a conflict can arise. The previous strategies for individual survival, and survival as a species, that conferred success, can suddenly find themselves at odds with this new reality. This phenomenon is known as evolutionary discordance. This is exactly the position we find ourselves in today with respect to the modern Western diet.

One result of evolutionary discordance is that this conflict can manifest as disability and disease. The disability and disease in this situation may not manifest until middle age and can particularly vex the elderly. Again, this is exactly the situation we are encountering today. Evolutionary success, including successful responses to disability and disease, are generally geared to the young. From Nature's viewpoint the goal of our individual survival is to reach the reproductive years and achieve successful procreation. Only this ultimately matters; just poll any male member of the species for confirmation.

Therefore, our biology is not well equipped to deal with chronic diseases and disabilities that challenge survival into old age, once we are past our reproductive prime. The end result of evolutionary discordance is increasing morbidity and mortality as we get older, an increase in disability and disease as we age. These are precisely the challenges we confront today. Such biological consequences are particularly important when the cause of such affliction is the result of our own industry.

Triggered from within the gastrointestinal tract, these inflammatory effects produce increased oxidative stress, pro-inflammatory cytokine production, protein glycation and a disposition toward a pro-coagulant milieu throughout the entire body. These changes move us from our comfort point of natural balance. They drive us from homeostasis and metabolic health. We stew in a pot of chronic, low-grade inflammation like a frog on a slow boil.

Inflammation is the mechanism by which atherosclerosis, or hardening of the arteries, is believed to develop. Inflammation also plays an integral role in the pathophysiology associated with diabetes. Chronic elevation of glucose and insulin levels can lead to insulin resistance and metabolic syndrome—a precursor of diabetes and other diseases of modern civilization. Many of these diseases of modern civilization are either exceedingly rare or entirely absent in contemporary cultures that do not consume the foods commonly found in a modern Western diet. Many, if not most, of these types of foods have only come into existence with the last two hundred and fifty years.

At the end of the day it all comes down to a gut check. This complex and exceedingly multifaceted interplay of environmental factors, genetic factors, and complex nutritional factors begins and ends at this intimate interface between us and our environment—between what we eat and who we are. That arbitrator that runs interference between what we eat and what we become—that intermediary is the human gut microbiotica, or simply the gut microbiome.

This interface is a razor-thin microscopic margin composed of our symbiotic bacterial charge. It is a varied population of well over a thousand different species of bacteria that live inside us. It is estimated that of the over one hundred trillion bacteria in the gut, upwards of 80 percent of the intestinal species remain unknown because we cannot culture them. This means that over 70 percent of the cells within your body are actually intestinal bacteria that remain unidentified. We are composed of UFOs, unidentified fermenting organisms.

The composition of these UFOs is extremely important; are they friend or foe? As anyone who has ever suffered from food poisoning is well aware, changes in the diet can have significant ramifications to intestinal flora. This in turn can dramatically impact us resulting in immediate death from food poisoning or a slow death from chronic disability and disease. It is simply a matter of degrees.

Less fatal but still detrimental changes can lead to increased intestinal permeability and the potential for ongoing, low-grade chronic inflammation. Increased intestinal permeability is a condition in which the gut becomes leaky. The normally tight seals between the cells that line the gut wall no longer seal well. It is like a castle that has had its walls breached. Normally there is one way in or out across the guarded and well-manned drawbridge. Imagine huge holes in the castle walls. There is no longer an orderly controlled precession in or out. The exchange now resembles the US-Mexico border.

This type of chaos exposes the bloodstream to all sorts of compounds, including toxins that can potentially enter the circulation. Increased intestinal permeability is a known consequence of such diseases as gluten enteropathy or celiac sprue. This condition is the commonly quoted reason to avoid wheat products. This chronic low-grade, pro-inflammatory state is a common thread among many of the different disabilities and diseases of civilization. These include cardiovascular disease, type 2 diabetes, various forms of malignancy, autoimmune diseases, depression, schizophrenia, autism, Alzheimer-type dementia, and Parkinson disease, to name but a few.

In the following chapters we are going to get to the heart of the matter. We will see that the source of so many of our modern health issues is related to what we eat. We will examine how a diet that allowed us to develop a superior brain and become the most successful species on the planet, a diet that has sustained us for thousands of years, has completely changed over just the last two hundred years or so. Since the Industrial Revolution the quantity and quality of our food and the distribution of it through various food pathways has changed into something that has never before been seen. We will review how we have transformed a natural diet of sustenance and pleasure into the modern Western diet. And we will see how that diet is killing us from the inside out.

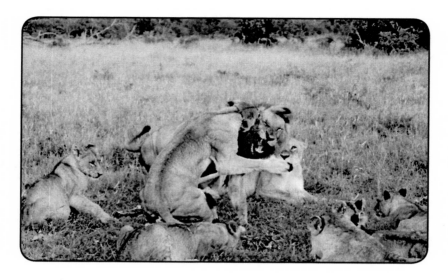

Survival of the Fittest: How the Greed for Sugar, Salt, and Fat Allowed Us to Conquer the World

"Greed, for lack of a better word, is good."
~GORDON GEKKO, WALL STREET (1987)[15]

Our modern society provides access to the components of the modern Western diet every hour of every day. We are gobsmacked with goodies, whatever we want, whenever we want it. The exponential pace of cultural and technological advancement has produced an unprecedented all-you-can-eat buffet open twenty-four hours a day. To make sure that you return to the trough diving in headfirst with snorkel at the ready, the buffet is crafted upon layer after layer of sugar, salt, and fat.

But this was not always so. A long, long time ago on a continent far, far away things were very different. Food itself could be a rare commodity. You often were not sure what you would find to eat and you were never sure exactly when you might find it. The human civilization has come a long way from those dark days as barely bipedal hairy hominins wandering about the Dark Continent. But our physiology hasn't. From a biological perspective, we are not much changed from our distant bearded brethren that wandered about the

African plains hundreds of thousands, if not millions, of years ago.

Like any child of nature at the time, our earliest ancestors sought out food. Then, as now, some types of food were preferred. Those foods that provide the greatest opportunity for an individual's survival are desired above others. A desired action is reinforced by making it pleasurable. Like all creatures, we seek pleasure and move to avoid suffering. As we repeat each enjoyable experience the action associated with it eventually becomes hardwired into our operating system after thousands and millions of years of evolution.

Such biological imperatives for individual and species survival have molded basic psychological drivers into our brains. The seeking and consumption of certain foods is inextricably linked to our pleasure and reward centers. While it has helped us survive as individuals and made us arguably the most successful species in the history of the world, it has left us vulnerable. It has left us with more security breaches in our operating system than Windows ME. We are, to some extent, the victims of our own technological cleverness.

The Physiologic Drive for Sugar: Come to The Dark Side, We Has Sugar Cookies

Sugar has the potential to be one of the great weapons of mass consumption used against humanity. Yet, for all the images and emotions it conjures, the word also breeds confusion. What do we mean when we refer to sugar? If it is so toxic, why did nature generate it in such abundance for us, and make it so darn yummy? Are pastry chefs wicked witches for creating those delectable desserts and sweet treats that continually tempt us? Are we nothing but helpless and innocent modern-day Hänsels und Gretels?

Part of the answer lies in understanding what is meant by the term sugar. There are several types of sweetness to be found in Nature; and all these forms are carbohydrates. All sugars are carbohydrates. But not all carbohydrates are sugars. Starches like those found in refined wheat products are a great example of compounds that are carbohydrates, but not sugars. Sugars, like people, can be further classified into simple or complex.

Complex sugars are often referred to as disaccharides or polysaccharides. But when it comes to processing complex sugars, we are a physiological Forrest Gump. We can only appropriate the simple.

Our bodies cannot utilize complex sugars directly; but they can be broken down to yield simple sugars. You don't stuff a whole sandwich in your pie hole at once; to consume it properly and avoid a side order of the Heimlich maneuver you consume it in reasonably sized, fairly uniform bites. Your body does the same thing to carbohydrates and sugars at a much tinier level. It simply breaks them down into manageable bits. Those manageable bits are called simple sugars.

Sucrose is a great example of a complex sugar that we break down into its simpler constituents. It is what most people think of when the term *sugar* is used. Pure sucrose is the common white table sugar most everyone is familiar with upon the grocery shelf, restaurant table, or in the cupboard. It is a disaccharide because it is made of two simpler sugars put together. A polysaccharide is merely any compound made from more than two simple sugar chunks. When you eat sucrose your body breaks it down into the simple sugars it is made from. That would be one molecule of glucose and one molecule of fructose for every molecule of the sucrose that you ingest.

Pure sucrose is derived naturally from sources such as sugar cane and sugar beets. The raw materials from sugar beets or sugar cane are refined to the highest degree to yield nothing but the recognizable white powdery, undiluted crystalline sucrose. Pure sucrose is pure sucrose, whatever the original source. But that is where refinement can take its toll. Molasses comes from unrefined sugar cane. Molasses is not only sweet but has a very distinctive flavor depending on its origin. In addition to the sucrose, however, it contains a number of healthful nutrients. Molasses is a great source of iron, copper, calcium and manganese—all vital and important minerals.

Pure refined sucrose from maple syrup is likewise no different from pure refined sugar from sugar cane or sugar beets. Pure sucrose is sucrose. It delivers sweetness and calories but nothing else. But maple syrup, another way that nature packages sucrose, is nutrient dense like molasses. It provides a great source of zinc and manganese, as well as a number of other important nutrients. All of these raw natural forms of sucrose have some nutritionally redeeming characteristics.

Consuming the raw forms of sugar such as molasses, honey, or maple syrup allows you to have a relationship with your food. These raw sources of sucrose also provide many other important nutrients and compounds that the body uses. In addition to the calories and the energy, your body is getting a nutritional bang for its buck. You get some nutritional benefit and that sensation quite literally hits that pleasure sweet spot. It is like, as Jimmy Buffett once noted, "getting a smart woman in a real short skirt."[16]

Refinement eliminates redemption. Pure sucrose is a cold, white, nutritional whore. There is no relationship. There is pleasure, but there is no redemption. And for your troubles she gives you empty calories, calories devoid of any nutritional value and thus devoid of meaning. Empty calories are the STDs of nutrition.

In addition to sucrose, there are other disaccharides that give us sweetness and simple sugars. Maltose, which is found in beer, cereal, pasta, potatoes, and many other products is a disaccharide sugar composed of two glucose molecules. Lactose is the sugar that is found in milk. Humans produce a specific enzyme, lactase, which cleaves the lactose into its respective simple sugar components: one molecule of glucose and one molecule of galactose.

Lactose intolerance is a genetic condition in which an individual loses the ability to digest lactose, usually after the age of seven or eight. Lactose intolerance is the norm for most of the world. Only about 35 percent of adults can digest lactose.[17] Persistent consumption of lactose in susceptible individuals can lead to the development of gastrointestinal conditions like inflammatory bowel disease (IBD).[18]

Regardless of the source, what matter are the simple sugars. In the modern Western diet the vast majority of these simple sugars are glucose and fructose. Glucose is often referred to as dextrose—for the primary reason that it seems to confuse people who actually try to read nutritional and ingredient labels, where it is listed as required by law but under an alias no one recognizes as sugar. It is also known as *blood sugar*. When people or medical personnel refer to the *blood sugar level* they are referring to a measurement of glucose in the blood.

The level of glucose in the blood is a vital source of energy for all living things. There is a reason that it is one of the most abundant organic molecules found in the natural world.[19] Without this sugar, life as we know it would not exist. If you do not get enough of it you cannot cogitate correctly (and as an example if you're struggling here you either need a Wonka bar or a thesaurus). While the average person's brain only counts for about 2 percent of total body weight, it uses about 25 percent of the body's glucose.[20] So important to proper cerebral function is glucose, that the brain will only use a few other fuels and only in extreme circumstances of deprivation and starvation. To be human is to be built to run on sugar.

Or more specifically, glucose.

It is important to understand that in this context the term sugar is referring to blood sugar or glucose, not sucrose or high fructose corn syrup (HFCS). Unscrupulous advertisers like to promote the body's need for glucose by using the term *sugar* or *natural sugar* in their marketing to the public. The product they are selling is usually some form of sucrose or HFCS. Although they do not directly make the claim, they imply a biological equivalence with glucose—*caveat emptor*. High fructose corn syrup is produced from industrially processing corn. The corn syrup undergoes a process to convert some of the glucose into varying percentages of fructose. The result is a sweet syrup that is a glucose-fructose blend.

Consumption of foods that can rapidly raise our blood sugar levels can provide a source of instant energy. In the ancient past, this could be the difference between life and death. Imagine your great, great ancestor over five hundred times removed—Grum the knuckle dragger. Grum, like all the other hairy dudes, has been foraging around the savanna all day looking for a decent grub to eat. Being a little sharper than the average hominin, Grum looks up and espies some delicious, low-hanging fruit. He has just finished devouring the delectable treat when his tribesman, Dum, crashes through the tall grass. Dum, being somewhat denser than the average hominin, has managed to attract the full attention of Smiley, the local, huge, and at this point very hungry saber tooth tiger. With readily available fuel for his heart and muscles, Grum makes a dash at a record pace and scurries up a nearby tree like Popeye after a can of spinach, remaining well out of Smiley's reach. Dum becomes dinner.

Any excess sugar Grum may have left after eating the fruit and escaping Smiley is efficiently utilized. It is transformed by his body into fat for storage and later use. In addition to the advantages of immediate increases in blood glucose for instant energy, the ability to store fat was also an additional survival advantage. In this prehistoric world and for millions of years afterward, meals would remain hard to come by. Food choices have always had Darwinian implications.

These factors combine to form a powerful biological narrative to seek out sweets. The consequence is that we are endowed with a sensory preference for sweets at birth.[21] Animal studies have demonstrated that this biological drive to consume sugars is ingrained at the most basic and instinctual level. It is so strong that animals, like people, will seek out sweets whether they are hungry or not. They will seek out sweets whether or not it requires extra work, which is why the candy bars sit within arm's reach at the checkout line.

In a more natural environment than our contemporary world, our access to sugar-containing foods would likely wax and wane with the seasons. Before the Industrial Revolution, it was extremely expensive and difficult to consume extraordinary amounts of sucrose. Most of the sugar in the diet would have come in the form of fruits and been supplemented by sweeteners such as honey. Today, sugar is unnaturally cheap and all too readily available.

But as the modern Western diet continues to prove, more is not always better. Nature is all about balance. Constant high levels of glucose circulating about are the hallmark of diabetes. In association with high levels of cortisol (a stress hormone) it has been shown to impair memory. High levels of glucose alone may likewise initiate an immune response that may result in conditions like Alzheimer disease.[22] These types of inflammatory effects along with the renal and cardiovascular complications are among the well-documented pathologies associated with diabetes.

While the ingestion of sucrose will rapidly raise blood glucose levels, since it is composed of glucose and fructose it also raises fructose levels. Fructose is commonly found in fruits and in honey where it is packaged with soluble fiber and other remnants of redemption. The way that nature packages her sweetness significantly impacts its absorption and metabolic processing. Eating fresh fruit won't fruc you up.

While comestibles such as naturally fresh fruits are sweet and gentle, there are some things that appear very sweet but can be potentially very dangerous—like the Terminator in drag. There is none of the natural packaging that occurs in fruits and other unadulterated sources when HFCS is added to processed, pre-prepared, and prepackaged foods as a cheap sweetener.

HFCS generally is utilized in two forms within the production of consumer foodstuffs. The form HFCS-42 is 42 percent fructose and 53 percent glucose with about 5 percent being other sugars. It is generally used in processed foods and baked goods. The other main form of high fructose corn syrup that is utilized is HFCS-55. It is 55 percent fructose and 41 percent glucose, with about 4 percent being other sugars. This is the form most often added to sweetened beverages. Unlike the buffering that occurs in naturally packaged products like fruit, the fructose that is available in these sweetened beverages is often rapidly absorbed into the bloodstream; it will fruc you up.

A study published in the *Journal of Clinical Endocrinology and Metabolism*[23] examined the cardiovascular risk in people consuming large amounts of sweetened beverages. The study looked at forty-eight volunteers ages eighteen to forty. The researchers examined an intake of 25 percent of total calories comprised of glucose, fructose, or HFCS. They measured such known cardiovascular risk factors as triglycerides, LDL (bad) cholesterol, and apolipoprotein B (apolipoprotein B is a type of protein associated with increased risk of cardiovascular disease) after just two weeks on the various sugars. They concluded that these risk factors for coronary heart disease would increase significantly with consumption of fructose or HFCS that supplies at least 25 percent of daily calories in just two weeks. Well "Holy Lipitor, Batman!" Simply drinking sugary sodas alone can increase risk factors for cardiovascular disease. Just one twelve-ounce soda a day can increase your risk of cardiovascular disease by 30 percent.[24] Put down the pop and perhaps you need not pop the pill.

Other studies looking at other cardiovascular risk factors show the same result. A study examined 810 men and women ages twenty-five to seventy who had hypertension.[25] All of them consumed sugary soft drinks. The study had them reduce their intake by just one twelve-ounce sugar-sweetened beverage per day. Over the ensuing eighteen months the group lost weight and reduced their blood pressure. This is important because it is not just correlative. The intervention, in this case decreasing the ingestion of sweetened soft drinks, led to a measurable positive health outcome. Since repetition is the mother of all learning: put down the pop and perhaps you need not pop the pill.

Another study looked to see if the risk of developing hypertension was increased if you consumed a lot of fructose.[26] The short answer is yes. The conclusion, which is consistent with many other studies, is that "those who ate and drank more fructose from added sugars (as opposed to healthy sources like fresh fruit) had higher blood pressure than those who didn't (p. 1543)."[27] Consuming more than 74 g of fructose per day resulted in a 77 percent higher risk for blood pressure greater than or equal to 160/100 mmHg. That value will win you medication for life, if you don't stroke first. Considering that the average 20-oz. HFCS-55 sweetened cola beverage has about 65 g of sugar,[28] that value of fructose can be achieved with a little over two beverages a day. Supersize your soft drink and you supersize your risk for hypertension—all for only sixty-nine cents more!

While the current Health and Human Services/United States Department of Agriculture (HHS/USDA) recommendations allow for up to 25 percent of daily calories from such sources as HFCS sweetened beverages, discretion might dictate consuming considerably less. While a teaspoon of sugar can help the medicine go down, if that teaspoon of sugar is HFCS it may be the reason you need medication in the first place.

These findings are particularly vexing because it does not seem to be the consumption of glucose or fructose *per se* that is the issue. Rather, it seems to have more to do with the current practice of processing and packaging. This is because other studies have demonstrated that eating a diet rich in natural sources of sugars, even fruits high in sugars such as blueberries and grapes (and many others including apples, pears, plums, etc.) can actually generate positive health effects. Blueberries have a plethora of health benefits including reducing the risk of certain cancers, heart attacks, and Alzheimer-type dementia; lowering blood pressure; and improving glycemic control.[29]

Grapes have been shown to lower blood pressure, improve heart function, and reduce other risk factors for metabolic syndrome and heart disease.[30] Metabolic syndrome is a pre-diabetic condition associated with impaired blood sugar regulation and the development of complications also associated with diabetes. It is thought that the benefits of blueberries, grapes, and other fruits could be due to phytochemicals and antioxidants; yet how all these compounds interact with each other, sugars, and other constituents is poorly understood. It seems the benefits of grapes are preserved in alcohol, correlating very well with human studies documenting the beneficial effects associated with moderate wine consumption.

However Nature packages her sweet treats, they are a beautiful food full of quality and value. It is a testament to the intricate complexity and the nonlinear relationship we have with our foodstuffs that fruits we consider high in sugar can actually help us regulate our own. Employing Nature's paradox can be a much healthier and less costly experience than depending upon your own pair of docs. Go have a grape day; be it fresh or fermented.

Behaviors like enjoying something sweet, which are pleasurable, can become subject to repetition. Experience enough pleasure and the behavior can become habit-forming and addictive. Addiction can be defined as the "state of being enslaved to a habit or practice which is something that is psychologically or physically habit-forming, as narcotics, to such an extent that its cessation causes severe trauma."[31] Among all the five senses, only taste is directly hardwired into our pleasure center. That is the very same pleasure center that responds to opioid narcotics like morphine and heroin. A taste of honey can light us up from the inside out through direct experience without conscious interference. This is where sugar can be damaging and addictive. And here's the rub. It need not be natural sugars that initiate the vicious cycle of sweet cravings. Artificial sweeteners can tap those same spots. [32]

The commonly preached gospel is that to avoid the horrors associated with excessive sucrose and HFCS consumption, simply switch to an artificial sweetener. That logic dictates that if it has no calories, it cannot be energy dense. True enough. These acolytes to the artificial also contend that if it also has no nutritive value and is both a caloric and nutritional zero, it can't be bad for you, right? Well, cyanide is calorie free. Simply switching to non-caloric artificial sweeteners may not lead to health benefits. While they reduce the energy density (by supplying less calories per serving) compared to naturally sweetened foodstuffs, it is not clear that this results in an overall reduction in total caloric intake, a more preferred body-weight, or overall better health.

In both the US and Australia, consumption of artificially sweetened beverages mirrors the increase in the percentage of the population defined as overweight and obese as measured by BMI. In other words, the more diet drinks consumed, the fatter the people, in direct proportion. Recent studies have found that the risk of significant weight gain and subsequent obesity were significantly greater in those consuming artificially sweetened beverages, compared to those who did not.[33,34] Something along the lines of "I'll have a quadruple bypass burger, a pound of flat-line fries and supersize me a Coke Zero" may explain some of these observations.

But there may be an even darker reason. Diets, like the modern Western diet, that are high in artificial sweeteners or fructose may confound the normal pathways for fat storage and utilization. In this case it may not be the calories alone you consume. The traffic jam is not always due to too many cars on the road; sometimes it's an accident and sometimes it's construction.

The risk of both metabolic syndrome and type 2 diabetes is significantly increased in those who consume artificially sweetened beverages to the same extent as it is for those who consume sugar sweetened beverages.[35] Consuming just one artificially sweetened beverage each day increased the risk of developing hypertension or cardiovascular events by the same magnitude as consuming traditionally sugar sweetened beverages.[36,37] Two or more diet beverages a day in postmenopausal women increased their risk of cardiovascular disease by 30 percent and made them 50 percent more likely to die from related causes.[38] Given about 20 percent of the US population consumes diet drinks on any given day, that's a helluva traffic jam. When it's both accidents and construction, it's time for alternate route planning.

Another reason to avoid the artificially sweetened highway is that animal studies have suggested that while artificially sweetened comestibles are indeed less energy dense than those sweetened with sucrose or glucose, there are other unwanted effects. Artificial sweeteners can alter normal physiologic responses. These aberrations can result in a reduction of energy expenditure and a decreased ability to regulate the intake of normal sweet-tasting foods.[39]

A reduction in energy expenditure equates with a decrease in your total basal metabolism. People go to the gym and exercise like the dickens to increase their energy expenditure and keep the basal metabolic rate cranked up to eleven. Artificial sweeteners can act to hit the mute button on your energy burning volume knob.

Consumption of artificial sweeteners can also impair the ability of your stomach to tell your brain you are full and that you need to shut your pie hole. Over time, the actual brain response patterns can be altered. While there is some overlap, when someone who does not routinely consume artificially sweetened beverages is given saccharine (an artificial sweetener) the general patterns of brain activation are very different from their response to a natural sugar like sucrose. In contrast, for those who regularly consume artificially sweetened beverages, there is no difference in their brain response between sucrose and saccharine.[40] Their brain can no longer tell the difference between what is real and what is artificial. That psychological state is the very definition of delusional.

But this mind freak can have physiological consequences. This altered brain activation may be associated with the deviations in post-prandial hormone release. The brain thinks it's getting sugar, but it is not. The brain is fooled, but the stomach is not.

Normally, when glucose or sucrose is delivered into the stomach or intestines it elicits changes in levels of insulin, glucagon-like peptide-1 (GLP-1), peptide YY (PYY), glucose-dependent insulinotropic peptide (GIP), and ghrelin. When you eat something sweet, your stomach knows it and responds as it's been trained to do over the course of millions of years.

This does not occur with artificial sweeteners. While this is an area of active investigation and much research still needs to be done, the data do appear to suggest that in comparison with naturally derived caloric sweeteners, artificial sweeteners engender a muted, nonexistent, or different biological response. It is the physiologic equivalent of the online dating bait and switch. The online bombshell photo is quite different from the in-person reality. The expectation of the brain sets in motion one series of responses and the body sets in motion potentially contradictory responses. It is a metabolic NASCAR wreck.

The promise of these popularly proselytized stratagems that sell the idea that by consuming artificially sweetened beverages, one can avoid the effects of overconsumption of natural sweeteners such as sucrose, glucose, fructose, and others is flawed. The data suggest that people who regularly consume artificially sweetened beverages are at an increased risk for potential weight gain and the development of the diseases of civilization such as metabolic syndrome, type 2 diabetes and cardiovascular disease.[41] In the long term, they are no better off than someone who spends too much time indulging sweet flights of fancy; in some ways they are perhaps worse off. Excessive sugar consumption changes the bacterial milieu of the mouth. The bacteria that flourish in this environment cause cavities. There is no telling the effects that artificial sweeteners have on the entire gut microbiome.

Sugar was once a treasured prize. Primarily in the form of fruits it lent a survival advantage to individuals and to us as a species. The Agricultural Revolution obviated that advantage. The Industrial Revolution exploited our basic programming based on the seasonal rhythms and natural order. Access to all forms of sugars is no longer subject to cyclical availabilities, regional access, or economic constraints. These refined forms of sugar and all their synthetic brethren are cheaper and more ubiquitous than at any other point in history. They chain us, bind us, and direct our food choices without us even recognizing that we are no longer masters of our own fate. We dance to their tunes of disability and disease.

The Physiologic Need for Salt: It's the Ratio!

It is possible, at least in theory, to live without carbohydrates.[42] You cannot live without salt. Given that our bodies consist of roughly 70 percent salt water, this is not surprising. But what is this compound we call *salt*?

From a chemical perspective, a salt is any ionic compound produced from the neutralization reaction of an acid with a base. A salt consists of a cation (positively charged particle) combined with an anion (negatively charged particle) such that the resulting compound is electrically neutral. A salt is like an unhappy, old married couple. The opposites, each full of flash and fire initially attract and then come together. Only to find that that once together any semblance of a spark is gone. Each particle waits, longing for the union to dissolve so that they may recapture their former sparkle. It is Brad Pitt and Angelina Jolie in *Mr. and Mrs. Smith.*

When we refer to salt in its physiologic sense, we are most often referring to the salt compound sodium chloride, also known as common table salt. Common table salt is of course anything but common; it is in fact quite amazing. As individual components, sodium is an explosive metal that can burst into flame when exposed to water, much like Angelina Jolie. Chlorine exists as a highly poisonous gas. However, put them together and what you have is as exciting as a rock; because it is a rock. Albeit, it is the rock of all life. Both sodium and chloride are necessary for the proper physiologic functioning of any animal. However when speaking about salt ingestion, it is the sodium we are most often concerned about.

Sodium is all about your bodily fluids. It is incredibly important in maintaining an adequate fluid status of the body; it plays an integral role in assuring the proper intracellular and extracellular volumes. Adequate amounts of sodium are necessary for your heart to beat. The nervous system could not properly transmit impulses without the proper ratio of sodium, chloride, and other ions. Many other organ and cellular functions also depend on the adequate regulation of sodium. Under normal circumstances, the proper sodium balance is managed primarily by the kidneys through hemodynamic, neural, and hormonal inputs that work in close concert with the cardiovascular and respiratory systems.

None of this is unique to human beings. It is something common to all terrestrial life forms. Life began in the sea, surrounded by salt water. As evolution progressed and animals made the transition from sea to shore they carried the remnants of their humble beginnings with them: salt water. The salinity of our blood approximates the salinity of the oceans from whence our most distant forebears first wriggled out into the mud. The seas have gotten a lot saltier since then, but we still carry this umbilical tie to Mother Ocean in every cell of our body. Marine creatures can get all the salt they need from their immediate environment. On land, carnivores can get all the salt they require from the flesh they consume. For herbivores, they must seek it out from other sources like plants and salt licks. But what of hominins?

Despite what PETA and radical vegans would have you believe, our prehistoric cuisine was not an episode of Veggie Tales. Our most ancient relatives were omnivores, like modern day chimpanzees. Also like modern day chimpanzees, they probably sought out sodium sources like the sodium rich pith of the Raphia palm tree that modern-day chimps utilize as a source of sodium. As our ancestors evolved and transitioned into hunter-gatherers more of their salt needs could be met from the energy and nutrient dense animal flesh they consumed.

Many contemporary hunter-gatherer societies derive a significant portion of their daily total energy and nutrient needs from such animal products. They expend little, if any, time and effort in the pursuit of other exogenous salt sources. The modern pursuit of salt likely originated thousands of years ago with the onset of agriculture. The domestication of herbivores that required salt to thrive and the dietary changes accompanying the introduction of grains as a significant portion of the daily diet were likely powerful initial motivators in seeking out salt. And we haven't stopped seeking since.

In 1912 Ernest Jones, a Welsh psychologist, observed that "In all ages salt has been invested with a significance far exceeding that inherent in its natural properties, interesting and important as these are. Homer calls it a divine substance, Plato describes it as especially

dear to the Gods, and we shall presently note the importance attached to it in religious ceremonies, covenants, and magical charms.
That this should have been so in all parts of the world and in all times
shows that we are dealing with a general human tendency and not
with any local custom, circumstance or notion" (pp. 2–3).[43]

Salt gives life and preserves food. It is also inextricably wound
into our history, religion, customs, and our very fate. The ancient
Egyptians used it not only to preserve food but also used it to preserve people, in the form of mummies. To the ancient Jews, the
covenant between God and Israel was represented by salt. In Islam,
an agreement is sealed in salt because of its immutable nature. The
ancient Egyptians, Greeks, and Romans included salt in their sacri-
fices to the gods, a tradition carried on in Christianity with the dis-
pensing of *Sal Sapientia*, the holy salt of wisdom. In ancient Japanese
theater, salt was sprinkled on the stage prior to each performance to
protect against evil spirits. The Chinese were gathering salt at least
eight thousand years ago in the northern reaches of the province of
Shanxi, by the shores of Lake Yuncheng.[44] And as every modern-day
zombie apocalypse prepper is aware, salt is the only way to break the
curse of the zombie and bring peace to the dead (p. 132).[45] That, of
course, and disconnecting head from torso.

With the pursuit of salt so ingrained into our physiology and our
history, there is a touch of irony in the exchange of contemporary
salty language. The discussion is no longer about how to acquire
salt. In the current debate we discourse, not always very politely, as
to whether we ingest too much sodium. The warning cries about the
dangers of our current levels of salt consumption have resounded
from the ivory towers of the medical community and from public
health advocates everywhere. Self-anointed *experts* cadge, coax,
and cajole while celebrity (and not so celebrity) chefs prepare an
improved low salt/no salt, healthy cuisine. All this is done in the
laudable pursuit of improving our personal health and promoting
the greater public interest.

The argument goes as follows. Salt acts to make us retain fluid.
When we retain more fluid it increases our blood pressure, which
is true although the effect is just temporary. Increased blood pressure is hypertension. Hypertension is a risk factor for cardiovascular
disease like heart attacks and stroke. Heart attacks and strokes are
bad. Therefore, salt is bad. Reduce sodium intake and you will reduce
blood pressure and thus reduce the incidence of stroke and heart

attack. This is the so-called *salt hypothesis*.[46] A perfectly logical and sound hypothesis, except that one thing is missing—the data.

The search for this holy shaker of knowledge has been going on quite a while. For over half a century, starting in the 1960s, there has been a vehement and saliferous exchange just out of public earshot. It involves respected scientists on both sides of this line drawn in the salt. The public policy on salt first got shaken up almost forty years ago in 1977 when US Sen. George McGovern released a report entitled *Dietary Goals for the United States*. This report introduced the first national salt consumption recommendations. The guidelines at that time were set at 3 g per day.[47] These recommendations were based on studies performed in rats that were genetically bred to become hypertensive in response to salt.[48] While many people may be considered dirty rats, rats are not people.

The aforementioned salt hypothesis quickly became science fact or wickedly deceptive urban legend, depending on your take on the information, or lack of it. A report from the Surgeon General issued over a decade later highlighted this disagreement. It acknowledged that the policy to restrict salt consumption had been implemented in the absence of studies that proved that a low-salt diet might prevent increases in blood pressure.[49] Throughout the decade of the eighties we waited on the definitive answer. It continued to remain as elusive as a follow up to Dexys Midnight Runners' eighties mega-hit, "Come on Eileen."

The Framingham study was a seminal trial following a cohort of Americans from Framingham, Massachusetts since 1948. It has yielded many landmark insights into cardiovascular risk, morbidity, and mortality, including one of the earliest multifactorial tools for cardiovascular risk assessment. However, the Framingham study failed to find any correlation between sodium and blood pressure.[50]

Another study in 1985 of over eight thousand men of Japanese descent found no relationship between sodium consumption and stroke.[51] Halfway around the globe over seven thousand Scottish men were studied and it was found that the "association between sodium and blood pressure is extremely weak."[52] By the end of that decade, in 1990, the then Director of Nutrition at the FDA remarked in a newspaper article that "there is no conclusive evidence that salt consumption causes hypertension, it's only a hypothesis."[53] Dexys Midnight Runners are *still* making albums and we are *still* waiting on the definitive answer.

Despite the lack of a clearly defined benefit, under Mayor Bloomberg in 2008, "the New York City Department of Health coordinated the launch of the national salt reduction initiative, a public-private partnership of more than 85 state and local health authorities and national health organizations that has set voluntary targets to lower salt levels in packaged and restaurant food."[54] In 2010, the Institute of Medicine (IOM) recommended methods of sodium reduction in its report, *Strategies to Reduce Sodium Intake in the United States*. The group had been asked to develop strategies *for* sodium reduction, not to evaluate *whether* sodium reduction was of any benefit. Garbage in, garbage out; you have to ask the right questions to get the right answers, Perry Mason.

The IOM plan was based on the presupposition that increased salt consumption caused significant harm.[55] Thomas Frieden, Director of the Centers for Disease Control and Prevention, along with other professional organizations like the American Heart Association have moved forward with national campaigns like the million hearts initiative aimed at reducing sodium consumption, initiating strategies based on this report. Programs like this, paid in part with tax dollars, aim to reduce sodium consumption by 20 percent despite any solid evidence for a return on that investment.

In 2011, experts involved in a rigorous scientific review of the salt studies to date concluded that it "is surprising that many countries have uncritically adopted sodium restriction, which probably is the largest delusion in the history of preventive medicine."[56] Despite this call for critical evaluation based on actual data, "public health recommendations at global, national, and local levels have been nearly unanimous in asserting that the evidence is incontrovertible that salt consumption should be reduced."[57]

At the crux of the argument there are fundamentally two questions: Do low-sodium diets prevent hypertension? Would a population-level decrease in salt consumption save lives?[58]

Answering these questions requires an evidence-based approach. That means you actually look at the facts objectively before reaching a conclusion. That is something about as common in the political problem-solving approach these days as the word *bipartisan*.

Those who feel the current level of evidence is sufficient argue that more data collection will take too much time, cost lives, and that such studies may simply be too expensive. When reputations, careers, and a whole lot of money are at stake people have a tendency to avoid allowing the facts to get in the way of their arguments. It becomes a *buy-partisan* solution. However, it should be noted that over the last forty-five years while sodium intake has gone up and alarmists continue to warn of an ever-impending cardiovascular apocalypse, death from heart disease has continued to decrease.[59] Advocates for salt reduction believe, as Sir Michael Rawlins, Chair of the National Institute for Health and Clinical Excellence in the United Kingdom notes, that "guidance is based on the best available evidence. The evidence may not, however, be very good and is rarely complete."[60]

The key tools for the successful implementation of evidence-based approaches include meta-analyses to identify effects that may not be apparent in individual smaller studies, and the use of randomized clinical trials (RCTs) to help eliminate bias. Meta-analyses combine the results of many smaller studies to tease out subtle effects that may not be apparent from any singular, smaller individual trial. It is a bit like looking at the difference between your score from the SAT exam that almost every high school senior takes versus your high school GPA. If you're the smartest kid in a herd of goats, it doesn't make you Einstein. When your SAT score reveals you to be somewhere between Lindsay Lohan and a small pebble, the truth is revealed. That is the power of numbers.

The first meta-analysis involving salt was performed in 1986. It found that lowering sodium intake may reduce blood pressure, particularly in people with pre-existing hypertension, but that the effect was extremely small.[61] Subsequent meta-analyses delivered similar results.[62]

These proponents for salt reduction also assume there is no consequence to a low-sodium diet. This may not hold true; everyone agrees that some amount of sodium is necessary for life. A low-sodium diet has some known negative effects. Significantly decreasing the salt in the diet increases renin secretion by the kidneys. Renin is associated with the development of hypertension and can contribute to the development of cardiovascular morbidities and mortality.

Decreasing salt intake also increases aldosterone secretion by the adrenal gland. Increasing aldosterone makes our body retain more sodium. This, paradoxically, can act to increase the blood pressure. Lowering the salt ingested also increases sympathetic nerve activity and increases insulin resistance (the condition associated with type 2 diabetes). Unilaterally reducing the absolute amount of salt we consume each day could actually have some very adverse health consequences.

These concerns are not all theoretical, either. In 2011, in a European study performed by the European Project on Genes in Hypertension (EPOGH), investigators looked to see if a reduction in salt intake would reduce the number of cardiovascular events. They looked at over 3,500 participants who were followed for almost eight years. Those who ate less salt had the highest risk of dying; those who ate the most salt had the lowest mortality rate.[63]

An even larger study was done by Dr. Yusef and his group out of McMaster University in Canada and published in *The Journal of the American Medical Association*, again in 2011. Over thirty thousand people were studied for about four years. They examined low sodium intake (less than 2.3 g), moderate intake (2.3 to 7 g) and high (more than 7 g). The moderate sodium intake group reflects the daily sodium consumption of the average American at 3.4 g. This group had the lowest risk of cardiovascular morbidity and mortality[64]. The group with the lowest level of sodium intake had an increased risk of cardiovascular death and an increased risk of hospitalization for heart failure. In addition, the low sodium group had a 2.5 percent increase in their cholesterol and a 7 percent increase in their triglyceride levels, changes not seen in the other groups.

These are not just isolated, anomalous, outlier studies from somewhere south of Hobbiton. Yet another meta-analysis examining one hundred sixty-seven smaller studies drew similar conclusions.[65] The study author, Niels Graudal of Copenhagen University Hospital in Denmark, concluded, "I can't really see, if you look at the total evidence, that there is any reason to believe there is a net benefit of decreasing sodium intake in the general population." Other leading authorities like Dr. Yusef agree and assert that the link between sodium reduction and benefit is, at best, "weak and inconclusive."[66]

Finally, in 2011 two Cochrane reports were released that seemed to rub even more salt in the "I want less salt for better health" wound. Cochrane reports generally consist of meta-analyses and RCTs and are considered a gold standard in delivering reviews of the available data. The first Cochrane review focused on people without hypertension. It found "no strong evidence" that sodium reduction reduced all-cause mortality.[67] The second review also examined persons without hypertension. The report concluded that all available evidence did not permit a determination as to whether a low-salt diet improved or worsened health. However, the authors concluded that "after more than 150 RCTs and 13 population studies without an obvious signal in favor of sodium reduction, another position could be to accept that such a signal may not exist."[68]

A study published in 2014 examined over 100,000 adults from the general population of seventeen countries. They found "an estimated sodium intake between 3 g per day and 6 g per day was associated with a lower risk of death and cardiovascular events than with either a higher or lower estimated level of intake.[69]" Such findings have led experts in the field to conclude that such "results argue against reductions of dietary sodium as an isolated public health recommendation.[70]"

If it is not as simple as more salt is bad, eat less salt and be healthy, wealthy and wise, an A+B type linear relationship, is there any relationship at all? What we are learning is that the key may not lie in any absolute amounts, but in the ratios between sodium and potassium. The previously mentioned study not only found the lowest risk for death and cardiovascular morbidity associated at a sodium intake between 3 g and 6 g per day, but a risk of death and cardiovascular events associated with the intake of potassium and the relationship between absolute amounts of sodium and potassium.[71] The goal of that relationship would be to maintain a ratio of ≤ 1. The diet of many ancient peoples and contemporary hunter-gatherer societies often consists of significant quantities of vegetables. Unprocessed, unadulterated vegetables are a premier source for adding significant amounts of potassium to the diet. Potassium is something sorely lacking in the modern Western diet.

Potassium is another element that is necessary for proper bodily functioning and is especially important from a cardiovascular perspective. The current recommendations are for about 4,700 mg of potassium per day. The average daily potassium intake for the average American is about 3,200 mg for men and 2,400 mg for women.[72] The potassium intake in ancient diets may have been over 10,000 mg per day.[73]

This creates an interesting alternative to the hypothesis that any health benefit is a result of isolated sodium reduction. Any positive findings from the hundreds of studies done may arise because of increased potassium consumption and a restoration of a sodium-to-potassium ratio less than or equal to 1. Sodium and potassium exist in the body in a natural balance. Potassium is often a component of salt substitutes, fresh fruit, vegetables, legumes, salmon, and chicken. Many of the studies performed over the years reduced the sodium in the diet by using the potassium salt substitute or by adding fresh fruit and vegetables to the diet to reduce the consumption of salt-infested modern processed offerings.

This is because modern processing affects the sodium-to-potassium ratio. For example, a 100 g (about 3.5 oz.) serving of fresh pork contains roughly 60 mg of sodium and about 340 mg of potassium. That is a sodium-to-potassium ratio of 0.18. But if you industrially process that into the average deli ham you end up with 920 mg of sodium and only 240 mg of potassium. The sodium-to-potassium ratio is now 3.8. You don't have to be Stephen Hawking to do the math.

A study out of Sweden scrutinized ten previous trials looking at data from almost two hundred and seventy thousand people and examining those who suffered strokes. They found that the higher the potassium intake, the less the risk of stroke.[74] Another study examined more than twelve thousand people for all cause and cardiovascular risk as part of the Third National Health and Nutritional Examination Survey (NHANES III). What they found over fifteen years was that the highest risk group had a very high ratio of sodium to potassium in their diet.[75] It is not the absolute amount of sodium in the diet; it's the ratio.

For most normotensive people, sodium intake can vary tremendously from day-to-day without significant problems. Even quintupling the amount of sodium ingested does not affect blood pressure adversely. The longest lived people on earth, and by some accounts the healthiest. are the Japanese. These are the same Japanese who routinely consume two to three times as much salt as the average American.

Despite a continuing rise in the diseases of modern civilization, Americans' salt consumption has been stable over the last several decades.[76] However, due to the continuing consumption of highly processed and adulterated foods and the displacement of fresh fruits and vegetables from the diet, the sodium-to-potassium ratio has continued to climb. The effect of isolated dietary sodium restriction, if any, on blood pressure, appears extremely modest and significant sodium reduction may have potentially negative health consequences.

The continuing rise of the diseases of modern civilization also exhibits an opposing trend from salt consumption when examined in a larger historical context. In most areas of the world, salt consumption is actually decreasing. The advent of modern techniques such as freezing, refrigeration, canning, and vacuum sealing combined with modern transportation has all but eliminated the dependency on salt for the preservation of foods. The average twentieth-century European consumed half as much salt as the average nineteenth-century European.[77] While the 18 g of salt per day consumed in nineteenth-century Europe may seem high, there are some suggestions that salt intake was as high as 100 g per day in sixteenth-century Sweden.[78]

By comparison, the average American currently consumes around 8 g of salt (sodium chloride) or about 3.4 g of sodium per day.[79] This value has not changed significantly over the last several decades, despite the increase in the incidence and prevalence of hypertension and other cardiovascular disease during the same time.[80] The government asserts that since "consuming less salt or sodium is not harmful, it is understandable why the Federal Government recommends that healthy normal individuals moderate their salt and sodium intake" (p. 2).[81] The only problem here is that many studies, some briefly previously discussed here and others acknowledged in the government's own position paper, have questioned the safety of too much sodium restriction—or even the need for any restriction at all. Based on the aforementioned data, for an otherwise healthy active person, a daily sodium consumption of between 3,000 mg and less than 6,000 mg or between 1.5 teaspoons to about a tablespoon of salt per day seems reasonable for optimum health.

While the debate rages regarding the absolute amount of sodium consumption and the question of deleterious health effects, there is no debate as to where the bulk of daily sodium consumption comes from. Approximately 77 percent of the daily sodium intake comes from processed, pre-packaged and pre-prepared foods. Only about 5 percent of daily sodium intake comes from salt added to properly season food that is freshly cooked. Even if you add salt at the table, this makes up only about 6 percent of daily intake. Another roughly 10 percent is inherent in food itself. The remaining sodium consumed comes from other sources such as pharmaceuticals.

The call to arms for decreased sodium consumption is predicated on the assumption that the taste for sodium is acquired and can be modified.[82] But can it be? Salt is so necessary that it constitutes one of our basic tastes. We are built to recognize it and seek it out. It is hardly an acquired taste like caviar or country music. And therein lays the danger of its incorporation into the displacing, processed foods of the modern Western diet.

Our psychological dependence on salt is only a mirror to our basic physiologic dependence upon it. For any mammal, and man is no exception, the loss of sodium, or hyponatremia, has profound physiologic and neurologic consequences. Animals raised on a low sodium diet can exhibit abnormalities of fat, bone, and muscle tissue. They tend to have smaller brains and are less likely to survive than those given access to normal amounts of salt.[83] It is for this very reason there are built-in hemodynamic, hormonal. and neural safeguards. These can act and be reinforced at the highest levels of the central nervous system. These can ultimately affect our behavior.

Unfortunately, these behaviors toward consuming saltier foods can be manipulated and become addictive. Native populations with low salt intake, like the New Guinea Highlanders whose average daily salt intake is about 0.5 g per day, often have an initially adverse response toward very salty foods. However, with repeated exposure they exhibit a repetitive consumptive pattern and addictive behavior with respect to the salty foods they once disdained.[84,85] It is why, after a while, you would sell your firstborn for another bag of those salty chips.

The areas of the brain that are involved with sodium homeostasis are overlapped by areas associated with motivation, reward, mood, and other cerebral processes.[86] Salt gives pleasure; and salty food is the saltiest of wenches. Patients who suffer from adrenal insufficiency are not able to secrete the sodium-regulating hormone aldosterone. They suffer from low sodium. or hyponatremia. What they reportedly crave is not salt, but a deep desire for salty foods. The body's mechanism for increasing sodium is not a direct salt–seeking behavior, but a behavior directed toward consuming salt-rich foods.[87] Patients treated for hypertension with long-term sodium deprivation likewise exhibit increased pleasure with the consumption of saltier foods.[88] When we crave salt at an instinctive level, it is not salt we seek. It is salty food.

Certain areas of the brain such as the nucleus accumbens and the areas that use dopaminergic pathways are associated with pleasure and reward. Virtually all addictive drugs increase the extracellular levels of dopamine in the brain.[89] Following the consumption of pleasurable foods, like salty foods, the nucleus accumbens is activated and dopamine released. There is some suggestion, that the consumption of sodium may also activate the brains endogenous opioidergic systems.[90] In other words, pleasurable salty foods give you a natural high. There are some suggestions that this innate salt-seeking behavior is the origin of *all* addictive behaviors.

While our ability to taste salty foods and the pleasurable reinforcement from their consumption once aided survival in an environment where salt was hard to come by, it is now subverted against us. Adding salt to food is like adding Scarlett Johansson to any crap movie. We don't like it; we don't want it; but the next thing you know we're sitting there with the popcorn watching *Don Jon*.

It is such an inherent psychobiology of sodium intake that leaves us vulnerable. Drugs are often combined because the effects in tandem can be more dramatic than their individual performances. And the effect of adding salt to sugar or fat is like adding the *vi* to *agra*. Adding salt along with sugar and fat to processed foods increases their palatability. We like them more and seek them out. The danger of the foods that make up the modern Western diet is not in the absolute amount of sodium they deliver. It is in the fact that their highly processed and adulterated nature disrupts the natural sodium-to-potassium balance. This is compounded by the fact that natural sources of potassium like fresh fruits and vegetables are displaced out of the modern Western diet. The resultant high levels of sodium help form an addictive pattern of consumption for foods that no rational human being would otherwise consume.

The Physiologic Need for Fat: Grease, for Lack of a Better Word, is Good

Fats are PHAT: pretty, hot, and tempting. They tempt us because they impart to food delicious flavors and textures. But like the sexy librarian they not only tempt us, they impart goodness. They are essential for life. We cannot survive without fat. But fats have lousy PR. They suffer from an undeserved big bum rap. That is partly because they are victim of their own provocative energy density.

Fats play a crucial role from an energy perspective. At approximately 9 kcal per gram, they are the most potent and efficient source of fuel for the body. Both protein and carbohydrates check in at roughly 4 kcal per gram, less than half of that found per weight in fats. In terms of fuel, fats are the most energy-dense source we have. When fats are broken down into free fatty acids (FFAs), they can also serve as a direct source of energy. Free fatty acids along with glucose are the major fuel source for cardiac muscle.[91] In a word, the heart grooves to one fat beat, you dig?

However, it is more than their desirability as fuel that makes fat, PHAT. Fats are also important in the production of the body's signaling mechanisms, hormones, and messenger molecules such as prostaglandins, thromboxanes, leukotrienes, resolvins, and protectins. Fats are a critical component of lipoproteins, which are molecules made from fats and proteins together. Fats also assure the proper functioning of the cellular membrane, receptors, transporters, ion channels, and enzymes for every cell in the human body. Without them, cells cannot communicate and genes cannot be correctly expressed.[92] Without fats, there is not life as we know it.

Fats are also vital to our brains. We are all *fatheads*; our brain is composed of 60 percent fat. The acquisition of such a huge cranium to accommodate a larger brain size was not metabolically cheap. Fats were the coinage that allowed us to purchase the Ferrari of brains. And like a Ferrari, the cost of ownership can be as expensive as the purchase price. To meet the increased energy demands of a large brain, humans must consume a diet that is much more energy dense compared to other primates.[93] The high cost of maintenance for the adult human brain can be seen in the human brain accounting for about 25 percent of the resting metabolic rate (RMR). In other primates, the brain accounts for only about 10 percent of RMR and only about 4 percent for non-primate mammals[94] and members of Congress.

The human digestive system has evolved to meet these challenges. Unlike herbivores or other omnivores, even other primates, the human gastrointestinal tract has an expanded small intestinal length and a reduced colonic length. This construction is primed for an energy-dense diet with large amounts of animal matter.[95] It is particularly primed for a diet rich in cooked foods and flesh.[96] On a number of levels the human gastrointestinal tract more resembles that of a carnivore than an herbivore given its predilection to a diet that is energy dense and rich in fat.

PETA has been around forever; people have been eating tasty animals (PETA) since people began eating. Human beings have consumed animal products for most, if not all of our two and a half million years of existence.[97,98,99] Human evolutionary genetics suggest the selection of *meat-adaptive* genes was a critical step in our dietary evolution, which allowed us to utilize fat-rich and energy-dense diets to develop superior intellect.[100]

The first significant evolutionary change toward a larger brain occurred somewhere around two million years ago. Other significant physical changes that also occurred during this period included a reduction in the facial size, jaw muscles, and grinding teeth. These changes are the exact opposite of what you would expect if you spent the day eating roots and berries.

These physical changes were accompanied by increasing tool sophistication and the utilization of fire.[101] This time frame also correlates with significant dietary and energetic changes. All these developments point toward the putative consumption of energy-dense foods such as cooked foods and animal foods rich in fats. The consumptive changes of this period were also accompanied by the direct dietary acquisition of such long chain polyunsaturated fatty acids (LCPUFA) as docosahexaenoic acid (DHA) and arachidonic acid (AA).[102] We ate seafood and eggs—great sources of DHA and AA. These are critical building blocks in the assembly of the modern human brain.

The indispensable nature of the LCPUFAs can be attested to by their absence. You don't appreciate how important something is until it's not around. An *in utero* deficit of fats such as may occur during a famine, extreme dieting, or modeling, is associated with terrible sequelae for the offspring. The children of mothers who do not consume enough of the proper fats while pregnant are cursed at birth. They will spend the rest of their years with both an increased inclination for fat-rich foods and a decreased ability to properly metabolize these fats later in life.

Fats are like love. Deprived of access during their formative years children will spend the rest of their adult lives innately seeking it out. Once found, they will be unable to properly process it. For children who were denied proper access to fats in the womb this is expressed as being underweight at birth and an undesirable serum lipid profile as an adult.[103] It is Sisyphus with a doughnut. Low birth weight babies suffer from a notorious litany of other complications later in life, as well. Among those complications is the risk for an increased level of chronic inflammation.[104]

Fats are where it's at for us as newbies. The brain that gave rise to our modern civilization starts life in overdrive. The phenomenal growth of the infant brain is evidenced by the fact that it may utilize upwards of 60 percent of the resting metabolic rate (RMR), almost three times that of an adult human brain.[105] Babies may babble incoherently, drool on themselves, need to be waited on hand and foot, not infrequently need their diapers changed, or otherwise act like the judges on *American Idol*; but unlike such their brains are moving at warp speed.

The internal dilithium crystals supplying the energy for such neural gymnastics are fat. This need for speed is why human infants, at 15 percent to 16 percent total body fat, have the highest body fat level of any mammalian species. During the first year, a period of rapid brain growth, this can increase to 25 percent body fat. This incredibly rapid brain development is also a potential vulnerability.

The infant body will act to preserve fat stores and reserves for the brain at the expense of the development and function of other organs and structures. Current American Heart Association (AHA) recommendations reflect the developmental effects of the quality and quantity of fat in our diet. Human breast milk is loaded with fat, saturated fat, and other goodies. The AHA currently recommends breast-feeding for at least four to six months and up to a year if possible because the positive effects on the prevention of adult obesity and hypertension, and the relationship with a positive lipid profile in adulthood. A lack of breast-feeding correlates with increased chronic inflammation as an adult.[106] We always knew boobies rocked.

To meet these increased metabolic demands that begin before infancy, humans evolved to consume diets dense in both energy and nutrients. Modern hunter-gatherers typically derive over half of their energy requirements from animal sources.[107] Anywhere from 28 percent to 58 percent of their daily energy requirements are derived from dietary fat.[108] When foods are energy and nutrient dense, such as the naturally derived animal sources consumed by hunter-gatherers, less volume is required to deliver needed amounts of energy and nutrients. A fatal flaw in the modern Western diet is that while it may remain energy dense, it is now nutrient poor.

In nature form often follows function, thus the need for such energy-rich foods has in turn shaped our basic hardwiring. The culmination of our evolutionarily derived distinct molecular pathways and hardwired survival mechanisms is a unique ability within the animal kingdom. Human beings have the uncanny capacity to quickly and accurately assess the energy content of potential food via smell, taste, and texture. Unlike many animals, even most mammals, the human brain is able to process with remarkable speed and accuracy the energy content of a variety of foods.[109] This allows us to be remarkably adept at picking out the fatty goodness we prefer to eat. But we can't distinguish between nutrient rich fatty foods and nutrient poor fatty foods, presumably because the latter have not existed until the most recent times.

Our love affair with fats is '60s style, no discrimination or segregation. We just love fat in whatever form it shows up: saturated, monounsaturated, or polyunsaturated. Saturated fats are fats in which the triglyceride fatty acids have no double bonds between the carbon atoms; the fatty acid is *saturated* with hydrogen. These are often solid at room temperature and associated with animal fats, although most foods are mixtures of the different types of fatty acids.

Monounsaturated fats have one carbon double bond and polyunsaturated fats have more than one. Polyunsaturated fats are also known as polyunsaturated fatty acids (PUFAs). Many of the diets associated with health benefits are particularly rich in PUFAs. This group of fats also contains the omega-3 and omega-6 polyunsaturated fatty acids. The omega-3 and omega-6 groups contain the essential fatty acids (EFAs) linoleic acid (LA) and alpha-linolenic acid (ALA).

LA is an omega-6 fatty acid, which means the first of the two carbon double bonds is at the sixth carbon counting from the tail, or omega, end of the molecule. ALA is an omega-3 fatty acid, which means the first of its three carbon double bonds occurs at the third carbon counting from the tail, or omega, end. These fats are known as essential fatty acids because human beings cannot synthesize them.

Despite the fact that human beings cannot synthesize them, they are fundamental in the assembly of a number of important biological compounds that are required for proper physiologic function and the maintenance of good health. These products include, but are not limited to: modulators of inflammation, mood, behavior, cellular signaling, and hormones, and effectors of the transcription of DNA at the cellular level. EFAs are like cell phones—you can't make one but just try to survive without them.

Deficiencies of EFAs have been associated with excessive thirst and urination, skin changes, hair and nail malformations, poor wound healing, asthma, allergies, cardiovascular problems, and poor vision. EFAs play a particularly important role in proper brain development and function. Deficiencies have also been correlated with the development of ADD, dyslexia, depression, fatigue, poor memory, autism, and sleep disturbances.[110,111] In infants and small children deficiencies may manifest as decreased growth and failure to thrive.[112] In addition to the many other roles they play, the EFAs are further synthesized by the human body into derivatives known as long chain polyunsaturated fatty acids. In terms of human development as previously discussed, the long chain polyunsaturated fatty acids (LCPUFAs) are critical.[113]

The omega-3 LCPUFAs such as eicosapentaenoic acid (EPA) and DHA are also critical for the proper functioning of adults. They have important effects on endothelial function, blood pressure, triglyceride levels and have anti-thrombotic, anti-atherosclerotic, and anti-inflammatory effects.[114,115,116] These are of paramount importance in preventing against cardiovascular disease and other conditions that are rooted in a pro-inflammatory foundation. Fats such as these may reduce the development of abdominal obesity, type 2 diabetes, and other inflammatory conditions including the neurodegenerative disorders such as Alzheimer-type dementia, Parkinson disease, ALS, multiple sclerosis, and depression.[117,118] It is about ratios and proper balance, not exclusion of entire classes. Without fats you may be thin, but without the right fats you will not be healthy. Every single prisoner at Dachau was skinny.

To be a championship football team you need the right ratio and the proper balance of players. You need an offense that can score. That means you need a star quarterback and a star running back. That also means that you need a good offensive line that can block. For these two star players you need five or six offensive linemen to do the grunt work. To balance your offense you also need a defense to prevent the other team from scoring. A good defense requires the right combination of powerful defensive linemen and quick and nimble defensive backs. The right ratio and the proper balance of different types of fats is what your body needs to be in championship form.

From an evolutionary perspective, it is likely that a significant contribution to brain growth is attributable in part to a diet rich in fatty acids, particularly omega-3 PUFAs. The East African environment where *Homo sapiens* became the smartest ape on the savanna was a likely source of marine foods and other foods that provided access to omega-3 PUFAs. The byproducts of these essential fatty acids, the LCPUFAs are also critical in the maintenance of proper homeostasis and health. Some of these important derivatives like DHA, however, may also need to be supplemented directly through the diet when there is increased demand, a condition known as conditionally essential.

DHA is derived from ALA, which we can get from plants. But we can also get DHA directly from the diet by eating fish and other marine creatures. The levels of DHA in vegans are significantly lower compared with people who eat meat and fish. Supplementing vegans with ALA does not increase their DHA levels. Supplementing their diet with animals that are vegan does; of course, that pretty much makes them the opposite of vegan.

It appears that the capability to synthesize DHA is rate limited in the liver.[119] This suggests that in part higher DHA levels need to be acquired through dietary means.[120] It is this particular scenario during periods of higher DHA demand that makes DHA a conditionally essential fatty acid. This means that a dietary source is required under circumstances in which demand exceeds synthetic capabilities.

Such circumstances are not just theoretical. Essential fatty acids and their associated long chain derivatives are the foundation for the membranes of every cell in the body. The membranes of cells not only act to ensure cellular integrity but hold the channels, receptors, transporters, binding sites, and information that allow each cell to function properly.

They are especially important in the brain, where the essential fatty acids alone make up 20 percent of the dry weight of the brain. Here they play not only a role in the construction and maintenance of neural membranes but also protect neurological integrity by functioning as neuroprotectins. Because of metabolism, on a daily basis the brain requires replacement of approximately 5 percent of its stores of arachidonic acid (AA) and DHA. AA is an omega-6 PUFA derived product, and DHA utilized is derived from both diet and ALA.[121] Like the Doormouse told Alice, you've got to feed your head, literally.

ALA does more than supply your brain with DHA. Within the brain a critical deficiency of the essential fatty acid ALA decreases dopamine in the areas of higher cortical function such as the frontal cortex. This leads to hyperfunction in more reptilian areas of the brain such as the nucleus accumbens.[122] You don't feel happy, you can't think clearly, and you react instinctively like an animal; in other words, you become a teenager.

The ALA-derived metabolite, DHA, affects not only the dopaminergic but also the serotonergic and cholinergic systems within the brain as well. Deficiencies can result in the dysfunction of such critical areas as the frontal cortex and hippocampus. It is interesting to note the observational correlation between low levels of the omega-3 PUFAs EPA and DHA and the high incidence of depression associated with the adherence to a modern Western diet.[123] The SAD diet can really make you sad—sad but true.

In other areas of the body EFAs and their LCPUFA derivatives function as stop signals called lipoxins and resolvins. Lipoxins and resolvins act to reduce inflammation. By reducing chronic inflammation lipoxins may help prevent conditions like colon cancer.[124] It is through resolvins that aspirin exerts its beneficial anti-inflammatory effect.[125]

The LCPUFAs also play a key role in gene expression. They are involved in the proper function of a class of nuclear receptor proteins responsible for the expression of genes known as peroxisome proliferator-activated receptor (PPAR). These receptors are important because they form a link between lipids, glucose and inflammation.[126] PPAR-γ, for example, stimulates fat storage in the liver and adipose tissue.[127] LCPUFAs are among the most powerful naturally occurring ligands for PPARs.[128]

A ligand is a compound that binds to a site on a target protein and sets it to task. This complex then serves as a signal-triggering molecule. Without the ligand, the target molecules have about as much get-up-and-go as the DMV at lunchtime. With the ligand these molecules work like a NASCAR pit crew. These fat-derived ligands influence how and when our bodies store fat and impact how our bodies handle glucose. Pathways such as this help explain how a condition like diabetes with its abnormalities of glucose is tied to fat abnormalities and how fat and sugar are connected to inflammation.

Such inflammation is the hallmark of diseases of modern civilization like diabetes, which is often associated with unfavorable lipid profiles that involve protein and fat molecules containing cholesterol.

Cholesterol itself is hardly evil. Cholesterol is ubiquitous and required for proper health. Our bodies require about 1,000 mg of cholesterol daily.

Cholesterol is a critical component of every cell in your body. It is essential for the proper integrity and function of cell membranes. It is imperative in the pathways and production of many different hormones such as estrogen, testosterone, and vitamin D. No cholesterol ... no sex hormones ... no sex hormones ... and not even a Cialis bath is going to freshen up that wilted flower.

Cholesterol is also a key component of the bile salts that are required for adequate digestion of dietary fats. Cholesterol plays a major role in our nervous system as well by serving as an intrinsic building block of the myelin sheaths for the nerve cells. These myelin sheaths act as an insulating cable for proper nerve transmission, much like the insulation around the wires in your home allows the electrical system to function without shorting out. Cholesterol is not the bad guy.

How does *dietary* cholesterol impact all this? Most cholesterol that is consumed is esterified, which means it is poorly absorbed from the gastrointestinal tract. It must first be hydrolyzed by intestinal pancreatic enzymes to yield fatty acids and non-esterified cholesterol. Depending on genetics, unless outrageous amounts of cholesterol are consumed, dietary cholesterol does not play a major role in determining blood cholesterol levels.[129] That's one reason why drugs to lower cholesterol levels are such big business.

Thinking that tossing out that stick of butter along with the statue of St. Paula will magically drop your cholesterol? Forget it. A study replaced 50 percent of the intake of regular butter with a cholesterol-free substitute. This reduction of butter intake resulted in a 0.3 percent decrease in total blood cholesterol levels. That is fifteen times less than the physiological weekly variation.[130] Removing the cholesterol from butter has no impact on your resulting blood cholesterol level.

Removing butter from your diet is not necessarily a better choice. Butter is the real deal. Butter from cows that eat grass is rich in the fat soluble vitamins A, D, E, and K. About 30 percent of the fats in such butter are monounsaturated; that's the same type of fat that is believed to be responsible for the beneficial health effects of olive oil. These fats also have valuable antimicrobial activity. There is evidence that some of the short and medium chain fatty acids found in butter can actually act to help us burn storage fat. Fat from grass-fed cows also contains significant levels of omega-3 fatty acids. Grass-fed cows produce butter that is rich in conjugated linoleic acid (CLA), which has been shown to have anticancer properties. A pat of butter is a simple example of the complex relationship that exists between real nutrient dense foods and us. It is an edible ode to St. Paula, Dean of Butter. There are plenty reasons to toss out that statue, but real butter isn't one of them.

If butter is not cholesterol dense enough for you, examine the incredible, edible, and much maligned egg. It is one of the most cholesterol rich foods found in nature at approximately 250 mg of cholesterol per egg, located primarily in the yolk. If we take *a priori* that consumption of eggs is a reasonable substitute for cholesterol consumption, then greater egg consumption should reasonably lead to higher blood cholesterol levels. However, multiple studies have shown that this assumption does not bear out under scientific investigation.[131]

Eggs are one of the best sources of protein available. They also contain the essential nutrient, choline, which must be acquired through the diet and is indispensable for health. It is the basis of the critical neurotransmitter, acetylcholine. Choline interacts with certain fats and can help prevent the development of atherosclerosis. Choline, like cholesterol, is found in the yolk of the egg. Eggs also contain lutein and zeaxanthin. These are carotenoids that help preserve vision and may prevent certain cancers. They are also found in the yolks.[132] The yolk is the part you are not getting on your drive-through "healthy option" egg white only or totally syntho-egg McDonkadonk.

Eggs are also a great source of fifteen different vitamins and vital minerals. The eggs produced by happy chickens, like the butter produced by happy cows, are rich in the important omega-3 fatty acids. Despite all the hoopla and expert marketing labeling foods "low cholesterol" or "cholesterol free," the fact remains that our cholesterol levels are not primarily determined by the amount of cholesterol we ingest. And the natural foods containing cholesterol like eggs and butter are not only nutritious, but also delicious. They are soul food.

Of greater impact on blood cholesterol levels are the consumption of certain saturated fats and in particular the consumption of trans-fatty acids (TFAs).[133] The consumption of TFAs has been shown to unequivocally contribute to higher blood levels of LDL ("bad") cholesterol and to accelerate and facilitate the initiation of the atherosclerotic process.[134] TFAs lodge themselves in the arterial walls like some improvised explosive device. When they go off in the arteries they wreck immense inflammatory havoc and accelerate the atherosclerotic process.

The other source of cholesterol absorption is not from the food we eat. It is from the bile that is released into the intestine during the digestive process. Biliary cholesterol is already non-esterified and therefore ready for reabsorption. Because cholesterol is so valuable to the body, it acts to recycle what it can. Any cholesterol that is absorbed is subsequently delivered to the liver. Once received at this *hub*, the absorbed cholesterol from all sources is recorded as incoming deliveries. The liver takes these incoming deliveries into account as it strives to meet the body's daily need of around 1,000 mg per day.

If the amount of cholesterol received is short of the daily requirement, and it almost always is, the additional cholesterol needed is manufactured in the liver. The amount of cholesterol produced by the liver is adjusted so that the amount shipped out for distribution and delivery to the body remains fairly constant. Our bodies make cholesterol, and the amount and the type of packaging is to some extent genetically determined.

From the liver, cholesterol must be transported via the bloodstream throughout the rest of the body. Since the blood is primarily saltwater and cholesterol is a lipid, the two do not mix, much like oil and water do not mix. The transport of cholesterol from the liver to the rest of the entire body where it is utilized by different cells and organs is accomplished by packaging it in molecules called lipoproteins. Think of cholesterol as a package and the lipoproteins as UPS trucks. The UPS trucks come in all shapes and sizes. LDL and HDL are two of the cholesterol carriers; they are two different kinds of trucks.

The package distribution hub is the liver. This hub is responsible for making sure that all the packages are delivered each day. That means the liver must deliver about one thousand cholesterol packages each day. The LDL (and some other molecules) are the delivery trucks dropping off cholesterol packages. The HDL are the pickup trucks collecting unclaimed or extra cholesterol packages and returning them to the distribution hub: the liver. The liver monitors the amount of return cholesterol that is dropped off by the HDL trucks. The liver then acts to increase or decrease the production of the cholesterol so that the body's order for roughly one thousand cholesterol packages are promptly delivered each day.

The problems of atherosclerosis do not arise from the delivery of the cholesterol packages by itself. Certain types of LDL delivery trucks known as small dense LDL are not as reliable as other types. It's like Lindsay Lohan driving for UPS. These small dense LDL lipoproteins act like they're drunk. They wind up leaving the bloodstream and wrecking in the walls of the arteries.

Even here, the cholesterol does not become a problem until it becomes oxidized. Once these small dense LDL trucks get stuck in the arterial walls they can spill out their cholesterol "packages." Once these packages are exposed in the arterial wall they can spoil or become oxidized. It is this oxidized cholesterol that is believed to attract the attention of macrophages.

Macrophages are infection-fighting white blood cells. They are the cops on the scene of this cholesterol wreck. The macrophages start trying to clean up the spoiled cholesterol that is scattered about the arterial wall. Like highway workers on the side of the road, they keep filling up bags full of trash. But no one ever comes to remove the bags. These macrophages full of trashed and spoiled cholesterol become known as foam cells. And so it goes on and on. This is the start of the inflammatory reaction that ultimately manifests as atherosclerosis, or blockages and plaques.

Some recent studies suggest that local proliferation of the macrophages in these plaques may also be a contributor to the development of atherosclerotic blockages.[135] In other words, the macrophages don't keep arriving via the bloodstream like a scene from *Cops*. They proliferate on site, faster than boppers at a Bieber sighting.

Other evidence suggests that LDL cholesterol may not even be involved in the inflammatory process; that the inflammatory aspect of CAD may be caused by remnant cholesterol. Remnant cholesterol is not LDL cholesterol, but cholesterol found in other lipoproteins like very low density lipoproteins (vLDL), intermediate LDL (iLDL) and chylomicrons.[136] These are different types of delivery trucks, although Lohan would still be the driver. The truth is that the exact details, like LiLo's memory, are still a wee bit fuzzy. What is clear is that it is not just the quantity of cholesterol, but the type of cholesterol and the lipoprotein that has a significant impact on the initiation of inflammation and the growth of arterial blockages.

To further complicate the equation, like many other systems in the body, it appears that one of the keys to health resides not in any absolute numbers, but in maintaining proper ratios and balance. For example, a LDL-to-HDL ratio ≤ 7.0 is associated with a decreased risk of cardiovascular disease. This is a ratio and therefore independent of the absolute LDL value. The most recent guidelines have abandoned treating people by their absolute cholesterol values.

Rather the new guidelines suggest four categories of patients who would receive statin therapy. They are those with known cardiovascular disease; those with a LDL greater than 190; diabetics; and those without these three conditions but who have a ten-year cardiovascular risk of > 7.5 percent. The initial dosage is determined not by LDL level, but by condition. The goal is a percentage reduction, not an absolute LDL number.[137]

The new guidelines focus specifically on the use of medications called statins. Other pharmacologic agents such as fibrates, niacin, and fish oils are not recommended unless statins cannot be tolerated. This is mainly because outcomes data for these agents are limited or negative. Even though these other drugs lower cholesterol, they do not result in a robust clinical benefit.[138] The results they produce are like kissing your sibling. One of the major effects of statins appears to be a result of their anti-inflammatory properties. These properties may or may not be related to their LDL-lowering effect.

We learned to love fats eons ago because they give us even more than calories and a few essential molecules. Imagine our great, great ancestor Grum as he finally climbs out of the tree having had to bear witness to Dum's unfortunate fate. Heading in the opposite direction of Smiley, Grum wanders alone upon the African plains. After two days with nothing but sparse berries and a few raggedy greens to eat he happens upon a relatively fresh carcass. Meat is back on the menu! Meat means protein and fat. Already ravenous and unsure when and where his next meal may be, his instincts kick in. He intuitively and quickly devours the fat-rich delicacies. Within twenty minutes, his engorged abdomen resembles the potbelly shapes destined to be the twenty-first century norm.

Grum's savvy actions enable him to recover his energy and store adequate reserves to make his way back to the village. A feat a less rapt-for-fat hominin may not have been able to accomplish. Once back among the tribe, he recounts his now somewhat exaggerated tales of derring-do; the risks to life and limb in an effort to save Dum, the hand-to-claw combat with Smiley, the near-death starvation and exposure suffered wandering in the inhospitable outlands, and so on. Each tale an episode holding the lowbrow masses spellbound. Grum becomes the world's first reality celebrity. He immediately takes to calling himself Grum the Dashing or Grumdashian. He never works another day in his life.

Although he didn't know it at the time, Grum not only acquired the energy and essential fatty acids he needed when feasting on fats. He also acquired other essential nutrients and vitamins like A, D, E, and K.

Vitamins A, D, E, and K are what are known as the fat-soluble vitamins. They are required in small amounts and often stored in the liver and fat tissue, which means that they need not be consumed every day. However, their presence is indispensable for proper health. Being fat soluble, we can only ingest them by eating them along with fats.

Vitamin A is important for proper vision, bone and tooth health, proper cellular function, healthy skin, and immune function. Vitamin D is critical in the body's handling of phosphorus and calcium. It is necessary for proper immune function as well as bone and tooth health. A vitamin D deficiency in our modern civilization has been found to be a blight of near epidemic portions. The Vitamin D receptor has been found to be expressed in virtually all the cells in the body. It is clearly implicated in the pathways that are involved in the development of chronic metabolic, cardiovascular, and neoplastic diseases.[139]

Cholesterol is not only necessary for all the aforementioned reasons, but it is also related to vitamin D. The vitamin D level correlates positively with the total cholesterol level—low total cholesterol, low vitamin D.[140] The molecule 7-dehydrocholesterol is intimately associated with cholesterol production. It derives from the same cholesterol pathway and may be derived directly from cholesterol through its oxidation in the intestine.[141] The 7-dehydrocholesterol particle is also known as pro-vitamin D_3.

This molecule is then photolyzed, which means it is activated by the exposure to ultraviolet light of sunlight in the skin to form pre-vitamin D_3. The pre-vitamin D_3 spontaneously isomerizes to form vitamin D_3. Vitamin D_3, or cholecalciferol, is then converted into calcitriol, or 1,25-dihydroxycholecalciferol. This final conversion to the active hormone occurs by hydroxylation reactions in the liver and kidneys. There is some suggestion that statins may exert their beneficial anti-inflammatory effect through increasing endogenous levels of vitamin D.[142,143] Although supplementation with exogenous vitamin D has not demonstrated mortality benefits or reductions in cardiovascular or other disease morbidity.

Vitamin E is a powerful antioxidant and may play a role in reducing the risk of cardiovascular disease and certain types of cancers.

Vitamin K is also necessary for proper bone health, proper kidney function, and for normal blood clotting.[144] All of these are required for our bodies to function properly and all of these require that we eat some fat.

It is for reasons like this that animals prefer high-fat foods. As animals, we too prefer high-fat foods. It is hardwired into us, for all the motivating forces previously discussed. And the intensity of desire increases with increasing fat concentration.[145] Sir Mix-a-Lot was right; we like big butts, we cannot deny.

Even mice, when offered the choice between boiled potatoes and fried potatoes will always prefer the fried option.[146] Phenomenon such as this begs the question, "Do we have a taste for fat?" To answer that, we must first understand our peripheral gustatory system, what it is and what purpose it serves us. It has two principal functions: the appetitive property and the aversive system.

The function of the appetitive property is to allow us to identify essential nutrients. We identify those with such properties as sweet, salty, and umami. If it tastes yummy we think it has some redeeming value and we want to eat. The aversive system functions to guide us away from potentially harmful components. We generally identify those as bitter. Bitter food, like bitter people are best avoided. Sour, however, is not easily classified into either system;[147] perhaps because we can always make lemonade ... or sangria.

To guide us as to whether a food should be consumed or avoided, taste buds are distributed throughout the tongue. However, they are also located in the soft palate, the epiglottis, the larynx, and the nasopharynx. There is a particularly concentrated region of taste buds between the hard and soft palate; this is referred to as the *geschmackstreifen*, or taste stripe. Our entire gob is one big tasting machine.

Each of the individual taste buds, and perhaps even the individual cells, may respond to multiple taste sensations. It is not, as it was once thought, that there are only certain regions of the tongue that respond to unique taste. Taste occurs everywhere throughout the oral cavity and throughout we appreciate not only the taste of food but its texture as well. Food, like love, is a multisensory experience. The beauty catches our eye and draws us nigh. The scent intoxicates and texture at times is soft and yielding, at times firm and hard. The contrast is accompanied by a supple simmering rhapsody that boils to a climax. And dinner is served.

It is the textural aspect of fat that contributes significantly to its perception. Every chef knows that a little fat added to the dish contributes to a pleasant mouth feel. However, it also seems that the free fatty acids present could potentially generate a genuine taste for fat. It has been well described that they serve as specific input and extracellular messengers in a number of other body systems including cardiac, smooth and skeletal muscle.[148] The tongue, after all, is but another muscle.

Specifically, there is evidence that the essential fatty acids may elicit a taste response. As they are required for proper health, it makes teleological sense that there should have evolved an adaptive mechanism for identification and ingestion. Dietary oils are over 90 percent triacylglycerols. These little fat blobs are critical for life. They are found in all animals, plants, mycobacteria, and yeasts.

When we eat some fat the lingual lipase from Ebner's glands cleave the triacylglycerols and release free fatty acids. Digestion starts before the first bite, with that first bit of drool. Ingestion of free fatty acids not attached to triacylglycerols can be perceived as unpalatable and bitter.[149] Since free fatty acids that are not attached to triacylglycerols are involved in food spoilage, the ability to detect them was likely an important evolutionary survival mechanism. For this reason, they are often removed from processed food. This makes the sniff test for processed foods a lot less reliable.

At the same time fats are beginning to undergo digestion in the mouth there is stimulation of the pancreas to begin enzymatic release. There are even taste receptors in the intestine, and these may play a role in glucose homeostasis.[150] Your body carries out a whole series of automatic responses based on the expectation of what you have consumed. Once within the body, free fatty acids can undergo beta-oxidation and be used as an energy source. After fat is consumed, there are a number of post-ingestive effects that increase the desire to consume more fats.[151] The long-term ramifications, if any, of trying to trick yourself with artificial sweeteners and fake fats is unknown. The act of eating is more than the simple absorption of calories. It involves us from brain to butt.

This automatic cascade of gustatory reactions can begin simply with the smell of food. The olfactory system is important in the recognition, detection, and desire for fatty foods.[152] While some areas of the brain are tuned to recognize that characteristic as odor, other areas like the amygdala appear to be tuned to recognize such characteristics as texture.[153] Food of love literally affects our brains in a manner not unlike that most complex of emotions.

An innocuous whiff of a certain perfume or cologne can unleash a multisensory deluge; memories, experiences and sensations can rush in upon us as quickly and as violently as the day we experienced them. A passing scent of perfume can take you back to a torrid night of intense pleasure without conscious interference. That may be so even though it was many years ago. The fragrance of food can strike just as suddenly and deeply.

Our choice and preference of foods is derived not only from the oral pharyngeal experience, but also from the experience throughout the gastrointestinal tract that is relayed back to different areas of the brain. Eating lights our brains up like the Griswold's house at Christmas.

Once identification of fats is confirmed by the gustatory system, the brain then inputs this information and uses it to coordinate patterns of food intake and dietary preference. Although this is still an area of active research, the evidence does seem to indicate that there are receptors that respond specifically to essential fatty acids and medium chain fatty acids. In other words, fat does not just add texture to the other tastes, but in human beings there is actually a specific taste for fat.

There exists a positive relationship between this taste for fat and dietary intake. The pleasurable experience of the fat taste is directed to the central nervous system where it is translated into behavioral patterns.[154] These behavioral patterns involve areas of the brain sensitive to neurotransmitters such as dopamine.

Dopamine is found throughout the central nervous system and many addictive drugs are mediated via these pathways. Dopamine D_1 and D_2 receptors appear to be involved in the central nervous system response to food. Specific responses to fat may be mediated through the D_2 receptors. The D_1 receptors may contribute to the central nervous system reward process.[155] Eating fat is a hardwired reward. That pint of Ben & Jerry's really does make you feel better.

Dopamine also seems to be involved in the food addictions associated with sweet and high-fat foods.[156] If for some reason our natural levels of dopamine are at the low end, it can make us feel a little low. We may then pursue activities that make the dopamine levels, and us, higher. Low levels of brain dopamine predict overeating and obesity in women.[157] Some people really do eat more of sweet and high-fat foods because they feel depressed. Eating these foods can really make them feel happier. However, like any drug the effect is temporary, subject to habituation, and is ultimately a vicious, negative cycle.

It also appears the natural endogenous opioid system of the central nervous system (CNS) is related to food reinforcement, particularly as it applies to fats.[158] Eating fat gives us the reward in the form of a natural high. This is the same reward process involved in a runner's high. And let's face it, when you can get the same high from running twenty miles or a pint of double fudge gelato, who in their right mind is going to lace up? The most palatable foods, and thus those that deliver the greatest reward, tend to be those that are energy dense and high in fat content.[159]

But eating natural fats is not infinitely addicting like watching the never-ending buffet of social misfit sister-brothers on the Jerry Springer show. Natural fats come with their own off-switch. Being energy dense, the ingestion of lipids can act to induce satiety and suppress later food intake.[160,161,162] One reason a diet with regular chocolate consumption is associated with lower weight may be that a regular *small* chocolate treat acts to turn off the hunger pangs. Trying to reduce your craving by using artificially produced fat substitutes does not usually work. The strategy of using fat substitutes does not seem to reduce the total energy intake in the end.[163] A study found that women who consumed the most diet beverages had the highest BMI.[164]

The positive effect of real fat on satiety appears to regulate appetite through several mechanisms including the regulation of appetite hormones and inhibition of gastric emptying and intestinal transit.[165] However, the types of fat consumed can make a difference. Not all fats are equivalent in their magnitude and effect of making us feel happy and full.

Medium chain triacylglycerols (MCTs) have a carbon length of eight to twelve. They are more effective in initiating satiety than are long chain triacylglycerols (LCTs).[166] LCTs have a carbon length greater than twelve. MCTs are also metabolized differently, being rapidly taken up and oxidized by the liver. The metabolism of LCT favors their deposition as adipose tissue. The LCTs are also able to induce the secretion of cholecystokinin, gastric inhibitory peptide, neurotensin, and pancreatic polypeptide. These differences in metabolism may be associated with the more effective inducement of satiation associated with MCT. Combining fat with fiber leads to a synergistic increase in the satiating potential.[167] It is not just the quantity of fat you eat, but the quality or different types of fats and what you eat them with that are important.

Other factors also contribute to feeling full and satisfied after eating a meal. Bile is composed of bile acids, cholesterol, and various phospholipids that are produced in the liver. They are stored in the gallbladder and released into the intestine when you eat something that contains fat. Bile and particularly the bile acids derived from cholesterol are important in the feedback systems regulating hunger and satiety.[168]

Properly seasoning the food, vibrant flavors and judicious spicing also leave an impression as to how we perceive a meal. This ultimately can also affect how much we eat. A meal that successfully combines favorable smell, taste, and taste sensations increases satiety compared with a bland version of the same meal.[169] Subtly complex quality cuisine, like a paramour, can leave you a lot more satisfied with a lot less. The foodie equivalent of bimbo limbo is just as disappointing.

Within the brain the areas that control taste, satiety, and emotion all overlap. The same areas that respond to the mouth feel, viscosity, odor, texture, and the pleasantness of fat are also associated with satiety and other important physiologic signals.[170,171] For all the blabbering about blubber, the engine of our modern civilization has been greased with good old fashioned fat. In the right ratios and in the right combinations fats are truly phat; protective, heart healthy, anti-inflammatory and tumor fighting; not to mention pretty, hot, and tempting.

Greed: The Driving Force Toward Civilization

The desires for sugar, salt, and fat are hardwired survival instincts. They reflect the time when our physiology and our technology were more on par with each other. But the ancient desire for sugar, salt, and fat was not just some flimsy passing fancy. It was a deep-rooted burning desire. It was a lust for life. It was greed.

Let us examine the concept of greed. It is a simple proposition for an individual; the more resources the better the chances for individual survival. This competition for resources is as old as life itself. A strangler fig will kill other trees in a quest to obtain more nutrients and sunlight. Animals will fight for access to the greatest number of the choicest morsels. Like all animals, we intuitively know we need food, and thus desire the most food in order to ensure our own survival. It is so hardwired into our brains that, as the character Gordon Gekko noted in *Wall Street*, "Greed, for lack of a better word, is good."[172]

This is especially true as it relates to food. Until the most recent of times, food had a habit of becoming scarce. Hundreds of thousands of years ago food was extremely scarce. Each day was spent foraging for sustenance. Our ancestors were never sure when times might get extremely lean.

Coming across some fresh meat, it behooved them to be able to gorge themselves. It takes about twenty minutes for our stomach to start to signal our brain that we are full. That is plenty of time to pack in some extra mastodon before Smiley comes back to claim the rest. The modern consequence is that we chow down those extra portions heaped upon our plate as we hustle and bustle about in a modern 24/7 world. But our next meal awaits right around the corner deli, not days away.

We don't just eat greedily, we order greedily. We are built to seek out sugar, salt, and fat. We are built to consume as much as possible. In the days of Grum, all the food was organic, free range, and grass fed. As long as it was not spoiled, there was little difference in the meat from mastodon to mastodon. If the quality of the food is all the same, then its value is simply determined by its quantity.

Every US dollar has the same quality; it is worth a dollar. The value lay in how many dollars you have. It is the quantity of dollars by which we measure value. We innately place a value on food in the same way. For most of our history a chicken was a chicken. The value was not the types of chicken, but the number of chickens you had. The more chickens on the plate, the greater the value; just having more on the plate makes for an adult happy meal.

But today a chicken is not a chicken. We choose from organic, free-range birds to reassembled nuggets in a bucket. Our intuitive, hardwired measure of value, however, is still stuck on the quantity set before us. That occurs, even when the copious quantity of consumables offered is a toxic collection of energy dense, nutrient poor, modern rubbish. But this is why we love to super-size; deep down it is the sheer volume that gives us greedy unconscious pleasure. And while repetition is the mother of all learning; pleasure is the mother of repetition. In the following chapter we shall examine the pleasure principle.

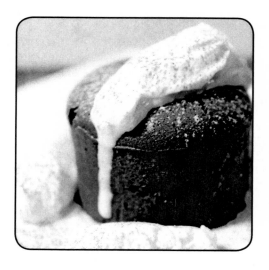

The Pleasure Principle: Why We Love Sugar, Salt, and Fat

"Do not bite at the bait of pleasure,
till you know there is no hook beneath it."
~THOMAS JEFFERSON

What weighs more, a pound of feathers or a pound of bricks?

"Aha!" you cry. They are equal; a pound is a pound. Well, yes and ... no.

They are equivalent in terms of weight; a pound *is* a pound. Sixteen ounces is a pint and is also a pound, which is why a pint is a pound the world around. That is also why you can reliably order a pint of beer anywhere in the world and know exactly how much you're getting. The same cannot be said for simply ordering a glass of beer. God Save the Queen.

But how many bricks, using an average red clay brick, would be needed to make a pound? Since the average red clay brick weighs about 5 pounds[173], you would only need about 20 percent, or one-fifth of one brick. And how many feathers, using an average feather weight, would be needed to make a pound? Since the average feather weighs just 0.00125 of a pound[174] it would take eight hundred feathers to make a pound. While they are equal with respect to weight, they are clearly not equal with respect to quantity. It is why the bag of goodies that says "sold by weight not by volume" always looks annoyingly half empty.

The definition of *equal* defines equality in terms of some specific variable or parameter; "Equal: of the same measure, quantity, amount, or number as another; identical in mathematical value or logical denotation; like in quality, nature, or status; like for each member of a group, class, or society."[175]

If things are equal in all respects then they are identical; "Identical: being the same; having such close resemblance as to be essentially the same; having the same cause or origin."[176] Identical things are equivalent, but not all equivalent things are identical. Kristen Stewart and Scarlett Johansson may be equivalent as defined by leading ladies in Hollywood, but if you think they're identical then you just qualified for that handicapped parking permit.

If things are equivalent with respect to their fundamental nature we tend to label them as similar; "Similar: having characteristics in common; alike in substance or essentials; not differing in shape but only in size or position."[177] Kristen Stewart and Scarlett Johansson are not similar. K-Stew and Stewie Griffen are.

Many people believe that all human beings are equal based on ideas like those expressed in the preamble to the Declaration of Independence: "We hold these truths to be self-evident, that all men are created equal, that they are endowed by their Creator with certain inalienable rights, that among these are life, liberty and the pursuit of happiness."[178] This and other documents express equality with respect to the ability and opportunity to pursue innate rights and identical protection under the law. No argument here.

But it only takes a quick look around to clearly demonstrate that we are not equal in all respects. If we as a species were categorized in some extraterrestrial guidebook our description would read like something straight out of the imagination of Dr. Seuss: wide person tall person, thin person small person, fit person fat person, dog person cat person, poor person rich person, nice person snitch person, smart person dumb person, beer person rum person, and so on.

As a consequence we are not identical. But while it is clear that we are abundantly different on the outside, we do share a common physical and social evolution, biology, and physiology. The commonality that makes us all human also makes us similarly vulnerable.

But where and how are we vulnerable, particularly when it comes to food?

Being human, we are susceptible at both a psychological and biological level. While individual psychological and psychosocial forces have molded us for thousands of years, the imperatives at the biological level have existed for millions. Under duress, the basic instincts for survival and procreation buried deep within our reptilian brains can crack the veneer of more recent social constructs; just look at *The Hangover 1, 2* or *3*.

On a good day we keep the beasts caged and go about our business. We are able to function in our crazy balls-to-the-wall modern society because we have both a conscious mind and an unconscious mind. The conscious mind controls our everyday awareness. It allows us to function in our daily world by processing the pertinent information, sensory and intellectual, in a rational way. It incorporates this logical information with perceptions, memories, feelings, and fantasies.[179] The conscious mind contains everything that you are aware of, which is of course why it is your conscious mind.

The unconscious or subconscious mind is composed of those feelings, thoughts, urges, and memories that lie just outside of conscious perception. Although you are not consciously aware of them they can have a tremendous influence on how you perceive, decide, act, and ultimately on what you choose to eat.[180]

The subconscious mind exerts its influence by way of instincts and learned responses. Instincts are hardwired into the base of the most primal parts of our brain. They are the result of millions of years of evolution. When you respond by instinct you are generating an immediate physical reaction and bypassing conscious control. Instinct is how a spider builds a web and a bird builds a nest, and why your cat keeps dropping dead things on your doorstep.

Our subconscious mind operates on such an instinctive level. These preprogrammed instincts are how baby geese avoid being eaten. Goslings execute an escape response when confronted by a silhouette cast by a cardboard hawk, even though they have not had any previous exposure to a hawk. When the silhouette resembles a goose, there is no such reaction.[181] Powerful stimuli elicit such potent reaction from modern humans as well. It's why we intuitively cower at the Batman but ask Aquaman for an order of fish tacos.

When we respond to such a stimulus by instinct it generates some immediate physical reaction. It is an action that bypasses any intellectual control. Anyone who has gone out for a night to remember, only to find the next morning they can't, has had an experience bypassing frontal cortex inhibition. There is a reason Viagra is not to be combined with alcohol.

These selfsame actions operate on the basis of principles fundamental to all living things. It is a natural inclination of all living things to seek happiness and avoid suffering. Instincts and behaviors that increase an organism's likelihood for continued existence are instincts and behaviors that bear repetition. This is accomplished through the production of pleasure. Since organisms seek that which gives them pleasure and makes them happy, these instincts and behaviors are repeated. These become hardwired over the eons.

Human beings, as animals, have the same basic hardwiring. We seek happiness and avoid suffering. One of the most potent of these instincts is the impulse for survival. Since we are defined in part by our social constructs, it is reasonable to extend the application of the self-preservation instinct to other people like family members.

That is, except when you have to eat them to stay alive. The breakdown of societal and personal taboos in the case of the Donner party, and those in the *Alive* story who engaged in cannibalism of friends and family to survive, highlight just how powerful individual survival instincts can be, particularly in severe circumstances. However, the survival instinct does not only operate in extreme situations. It operates all the time. Albeit at times in the background and much more subtly than forcing us to eat like zombies. That same instinct for survival, when actually faced with zombies, may compel us to merely flee instead of joining them for dinner.

This survival instinct is often executed with a light touch of influence by our subconscious. It may manifest as a subtle urge to avoid a dark alley or to pick up some flowers on your anniversary. Every organism will avoid those situations or elements which it feels threatens its survival.

Conversely, it will actively seek out those situations or elements that enhance survival. The survival instinct includes the opportunity to pass one's genes forward—to procreate. The result is that we are hardwired to move toward anything that augments or increases access to obtaining adequate oxygenation, hydration, rest, food, and sex. And in the history of mankind, as long as he is breathing, he has been obsessed with dreaming, drinking, feasting, and fornicating, and not necessarily in that order.

In addition to instinctive responses, the unconscious mind also operates by learned responses. A learned response is simply a modified instinctive reaction. It is a programmed response that becomes automatic. These modified urges are more than instincts but less than feelings. They are as, Capt. Jack Sparrow revealed while conversing with Master Gibbs:

"I may have had ... briefly, mind you ... stirrings."

"Stirrings?"

"Stirrings."

"What, like feelings, you mean?"

"No, no, no, no, not quite all the way to feelings."[182]

Eventually, at least in some of us, the *stirrings* progress to feelings. These feelings come not from our intellect, but from deep within our core and give birth to emotion. It is exemplified by the common expression of a *gut* feeling. It is the non-conscious sentiment about something that influences your conscious decision-making. Choices made on such hunches are the result of subconscious or unconscious direction. More often than not, they turn out better than the purely logical alternative. But they can be dangerous. Intuition got many a woman burned at the stake as a witch. That, and turning people into newts.

Upon graduating to feelings, human emotions may spring forth as the result of our interaction with our environment. Feelings form the basis of human emotions. These emotions result from how the unconscious mind reacts to the external environment. The subconscious mind can affect the conscious mind by projecting feelings. We know we feel a certain way about a person or situation, although we may not consciously know *why* we feel that way. It is that occasion when you meet someone that just "rubs you the wrong way."

It is through such emotions that the subconscious mind colors our conscious perception of reality. Our subconscious mind sets the emotional tone for conscious action. If you have ever been in a bad mood and weren't really sure why, if you ever just woke up on the wrong side of the bed, if you're just feeling blue for no particular reason, then you have experienced your subconscious mind affecting your present conscious reality. Or you have not taken your medication.

As emotion emerges, it causes changes to our physiology. When that long anticipated romantic date finally arrives, respiratory rate increases, blood pressure increases, heart rate increases, and pupils dilate; hormones are released and we are not even out the door. This huge change to our physiology happens without our awareness. And these are only a few examples of the involuntary responses to emotion. We combine our feelings and emotion with our conscious mind—not always in equal measure—and fuse them into action. In this way the subconscious affects our behavior, cognition, and subjective experience.[183] It is precisely why we do anything in the name of love, and why men do stupid things in the name of their penises. It is also precisely why eating food in our modern society can never be an objective experience. The time of human consumption purely for nutritive subsistence is long gone.

We are not lab rats. The interaction of the survival instinct with learned responses to form behavior patterns increases in complexity with the increasing complexity of the organism. A praying mantis hunts purely by instinct. While a lion is born to hunt, many aspects and complex social interactions that occur when a pride seeks prey are learned. When a man hunts it can result in fervent social discourse.

Humans differ from even the higher mammals by consciously altering their innate responses. If you have ever been publicly dressed down by your boss in the workplace and kept your job, you consciously altered your fight-or-flight response. Intuitively (and you know you did) you wanted to either smack your boss upside the head or flee. But you held it together, likely thinking impure thoughts the entire time, because you needed your job. You consciously overrode your instinct to strangle your boss.

As human beings we have behavioral drivers beyond biological imperatives and logical deduction. We exist in perhaps the most complex social structure on earth. It is this combination of biology and society that ultimately makes us who we are and makes us do what we do. Our reptilian brain instinctively responds to stimuli based on millions of years of genetic hardwiring. Our subconscious modifies those instinctive reactions through learned responses and nudges our conscious rational decision-making apparatus forward. This is filtered through the lens of our social structure and action is birthed. We are ... complicated.

This complex process is performed thousands of times each day by all of us. It is commonplace because we live in an extremely multifaceted society. Human beings overrule instincts on a daily basis because our social relationships are so intricate. Yet while our culture has rapidly evolved over the last several thousand (and particularly the last several hundred) years from a technological and societal perspective, biologically we remain not far removed from our most ancient ancestors upon the African plains. It explains our penchant for sugar, salt, and fat and our susceptibility for large portions and supersizing. These are vulnerabilities ripe for exploitation.

For all organisms, among the most desirable resources that enhance our chance for survival, is food. For an individual human, in terms of resources, sugar, salt, and fat were the power triple that let you steal home and procreate. And for all items of that trifecta, the more the better. For our ancestors, food was indeed scarce. That their individual survival depended—to some degree—on the ability to be greedy in the acquisition of comestibles is a fact.[184] Some things never change; men still use dinner, drinks, and dessert as a chance to procreate.

The results of the implementation of such instincts and actions can have other effects. It can make us smarter. If the hairy paleo-forefather of Gordon Gekko were to execute his "greed is good" philosophy, how would he do so? Well, he could try secretly hoarding some nuts and berries. He would have to hope that they weren't discovered and that they didn't spoil. And of course, he would have to remember where they were. By engaging in tasks requiring a bit of brainpower, by using our brain because we are greedy, we become smarter. These tasks became particularly challenging if the lifestyle became the least bit nomadic. It takes even more brainpower to secure the most of the best when you are constantly on the go. That's why gypsies are so crafty.

Modern human beings are not beyond the basic blueprint that allowed our ancestors to evolve. This greed-is-good spirit has allowed us to create such showcases to our civilization as the annual Nathan's Fourth of July "stuff as much meat-like goo in tubular form into your gob as possible" competition. But this exhibition reveals the biological adjunct of greed. Competitive eaters and Adam Richman, of *Man Versus Food* fame, often talk about *The Wall*. It takes about twenty minutes for the stomach to start to signal the brain that it is full. That gives you about twenty minutes to stuff your trap before, if you continue to eat, you will lose it. Why can we, and do we, eat more than we need?

After a kill, a pride of lions can so gorge themselves that they appear distressed, with their bellies tremendously distended. This ability to pack away the protein and fat is critical to their survival.

It may be days or even weeks before the next meal. The ability to consume as much food as possible at one sitting was an important survival mechanism for our early human ancestors struggling for existence in a violent, Pleistocene world. In the industrialized modern Western world, food is a liability that appeals to our baser instincts, quite literally. The more we can stuff in our skull cave, the better we feel, and we don't even know why. We don't even think about it. And that is the problem; we don't consciously think.

Yet despite such everyday evidence on display in Washington to the contrary, humans *can* think. Humans have the ability to remember the past, relate it to the present, and project into the future. Humans can analyze data and reason. We can manipulate the environment. Our modern society and technological advancements have allowed us near-instant communication across vast distances. This has allowed the formation of large civilizations and cultures within cultures.

We can recognize from a societal perspective that too much individual greed can be detrimental. Too many resources or too much power concentrated in the hands of a few can cause suffering for the many. It is the societal and intellectual constraints upon our instinctive reactions that allow us to modulate our behaviors and function in our modern, highly social and interdependent civilization. While our instincts may influence our behaviors at an unconscious level, human beings have the ability to consciously override such drives and alter our behaviors. This can be achieved, although not always easily, even when such behaviors have become so ingrained as to become habits.

Habits are behaviors that tend to be regularly repeated. Very often, they are repeated at the subconscious level, although they may start with a conscious decision.[185] Take the case of Average Joe. Average Joe is driving to work when he sees a billboard announcing a special at the local fast food restaurant. For a limited time only, the purchase of the McMortum breakfast sandwich comes with a free supersized deep fried potato slab and extra-large soft drink. Average Joe stops by every morning for the next week during the special. He feels pretty good about himself. He's getting an increased quantity at no extra charge; he's a pretty smart shopper. He pays no mind to the slow damage to his body from what he is ingesting.

The next week, even though the offer has expired, he finds himself shelling out several dollars extra for the sandwich, slab, and coffee. He can't even remember driving there. The initially conscious decision resulted in an action reinforced at the subconscious level. The positive reinforcement led to the repetition of the behavior until it became an unconscious habit. If this sounds hauntingly familiar, it should.

How Joe responds to the advertising and to the offer can vary significantly. It can vary by the season, the month, the day, the time of day, who he is with, if he is alone, his mood, his schedule, and an infinite number of other variables. There are genetic, psychological, and behavioral factors that interact with physiological and metabolic systems and impact directly upon our food behavior. The bottom line is that there is not only significant variation between persons, but tremendous intra-individual variation depending on the flavor of the moment.

We even change with what we eat and even with simply the act of eating. With the ingestion of food, insulin peaks and the body shifts to an anabolic state. During the fasting state, glucagon and epinephrine peak and the body shifts to a catabolic, oxidative state. This balancing act is partly mediated by insulin sensitivity, leptin action, and the hypothalamic response within the brain.[186] Constant change makes predictions difficult, especially regarding the future. That is why people and companies who are so successful at getting people to buy someone else's crap make so much money.

This is especially true with regards to what we put in our yapper. In the US and in many industrialized countries we cram ourselves full of the overly processed, artificially preserved, prepackaged, and pre-prepared foods of the modern Western diet. The modern Western diet, while well advertised and marketed, is no more nutritious than a *scheiße* sandwich.

We know it. We know how it makes us feel. So why do we eat it? Why do we go back time after time? Why is this siren song so irresistible?

The short answer is *addiction*.

The eating experience is directly hardwired into our pleasure center. The cerebral response to the ubiquitous ingredients of the modern Western diet, such as sugar, is to tweak on those areas that respond to other refined white powders—of the illegal variety. And like Walter White there are those who work to make foodie crack. They are not just *Breaking Bad*; they are cranking SAD.

Individuals have what is commonly referred to in the food industry as a *bliss point* or breakpoint with respect to sugar, salt, and fat.[187] On a graph of pleasure versus quantity, the bliss point sits at the top of an arc. For these ingredients there is generally increasing pleasure with increasing quantity, to a point. After that point there is decreasing pleasure with increasing quantity. The breakpoint is that point between these experiences. It is the point after which a dessert becomes too sweet or a chip too salty.

It is somewhat analogous to the dose response curve of any drug. If the dose of the drug is too small, it does not have the desired effect. At too high a dose there can be significant toxicity. The area between these two regions is known as the therapeutic window. The highest point within the therapeutic window, where there is the highest benefit and the least amount of toxicity, is the optimal dose. The bliss point is the food industry's optimum dose of sugar, salt, or fat. It is the dose at which there is the greatest opportunity to subconsciously affect and modify your behavior. And by modify, we mean *buy* their stuff.

Drug effectiveness can vary by individual and depend upon the conditions in which they are administered; for example whether the drug is taken on an empty stomach or taken with food. In a similar manner the exact percentage of saltiness or sweetness that delivers the most pleasure varies not only with the individual but also with the food. You enjoy a sweet doughnut or a salty potato chip. With sweet treats such as sweetened beverages, the average bliss point is around 10 percent sucrose.[188] Sweetening above that level puts you on the downside of the arc and is often perceived as too sweet. Below that level maximum pleasure is not delivered.

In the food industry, not hitting the bliss point can mean that a competitor's product is preferred. The result is a loss of sales and customer loyalty. That could translate into the loss of tens of millions of dollars or more. By adding sweetening agents at a barely perceptible or even an unconscious level, the pleasure centers can be stimulated. Sweetened food delivers pleasure even if the perception of the food remains savory without any noticeable hint of sweetness. It is why sweeteners can be found added to the bread or buns of so many fast food and take-out establishments.[189]

It is not just sweets that ring our pleasure bells. The areas of the brain that are involved with sodium homeostasis overlap areas associated with motivation, reward, mood, and other higher cerebral processes. These areas associated with pleasure and reward are also involved in the response to addictive drugs. Combine this salty approach with a little sweet and you have an enticing combination— like a caramel and sea salt topping. Add in some fat in the form of chocolate and it becomes nigh irresistible.

All animals, humans included, have a deep-fried desire for fat.[190] One role of the sense of taste is to allow us to identify foods that contain the essential nutrients like essential fatty acids that we need for life. This appetitive aspect of the gustatory system is the crave monster.

One way fats stimulate our appetite is through the textures they supply—something often referred to as the fifth taste, or umami. But there also exists evidence for a more direct and multisensory response to fat. In addition to taste and texture, the odor of foods plays an important part in the recognition, detection, and ultimately the desire for fatty foods. There is its distinct and purposeful reason you can smell the deep fryer at work when you walk into a modern fast food restaurant. Pleasant smells can make you pay for something you don't need or want. Cheap perfume has often exacted a heavy price.

The tastes, textures, and odors of the experience are relayed directly back to the brain. Like the effects of many addictive drugs, specific cerebral responses to sugar, salt, and fat appear to be involved with the central nervous system's reward and behavior process. Eating the right combination of sugar, salt, and fats makes us feel good. That is why good hangover food is always heavy on the salt, sweet, and grease. The brain uses information like experience and pleasure to coordinate patterns of food intake and dietary preference. This biological imperative, this fancy for sugar, salt, and fat, directly impacts our food choices and subsequent behavior.

The ability to exploit sugar, salt, and fat in combination enhances the response in a manner greater than would be expected of the individual components. The effect of a Snickers bar is greater than the sum of its individual components. Unlike sugar and salt, there does not appear to be a breakpoint for fat.[191] This means that when you combine sugar or salt with fat, you can deliver a greater quantity of sugar and salt and the food will still be considered quite delicious. In fact, because you are delivering a greater dose of pleasure the item will be perceived as even more desirable than what could be accomplished by salt or sugar alone. That is why french fries, with the addition of fat, are more desirable than boiled, salted potatoes, even if both are perfectly seasoned.

Our biological imperatives that drove us to unconsciously and consciously seek out sugar, salt, and fat allowed us not only to survive as a species; they also helped us develop the intellect to change the world and construct our modern civilization. With the onset of the Industrial Revolution there were changes to our food and food pathways that we had never before encountered in the history of human kind. Our weaknesses were exposed. With the rise of agribusiness and the modern food industry those weaknesses have been exploited. Like an outdated operating system we have serious security vulnerabilities. Like evil programmers, the modern food industry pulls the strings from these backdoors. They chain us, bind us, and direct our food choices without us even recognizing that we are no longer masters of our own fate. We have been hacked.

We are surrounded by and offered nonstop availability of highly palatable foods. This can activate the hedonic system and cause addictive behavior like any pleasure-producing drug. It can overwhelm the normal homeostatic appetite regulatory mechanisms. It is ScarJo in 3-D triplicate and we can't turn it off, even if we wanted, which we don't. This situation can lead to mental mastication and chronic overconsumption. [192] It can also result in habituation.

Habituation has nothing to do with habits. Habituation is a decrease in response to a stimulus after repeated presentations.[193] It is why many married men can no longer get their wives to have sex with them. Habituation promotes the consumption of even more fatty food to experience the same pleasure you used to get with less. It is why after a bit, you *need* to supersize that value meal. Ultimately this results in even more excessive energy intake.[194]

By combining sugar and salt with fat, people will consume more food. When combined, our awareness of the fat is very dependent upon the texture of the food.[195] If the mouth-feel is right, if it is crafted surreptitiously enough, tremendous amounts of sugar, salt, and fat can be delivered. That translates into a whole lot of pleasure. For the food industry, like the world's oldest profession, pleasure translates into customer loyalty and lots of cash. Unfortunately for us, this combination is associated with a predilection for overconsumption; whether due to increased palatability or a decreased satiety response or some element of both is unclear.

It may be so powerful because there is a link between the ingestion of sweet, salty and high-fat foods and the production of endogenous opioids. Sweet, salty, and fatty foods can take us to a special place. This may be one of the reasons that sweet, high-fat foods are the ones most likely to be desired and consumed under chronic stress.[196] While the original preferences for energy-dense sweet and high-fat foods may have provided an evolutionary survival advantage, the current hedonistic response with the production of endogenous opioids to this combination allows subtle manipulation and control of food preferences and eating behaviors. You are yanked about, your pockets emptied and you dumbly smile, all the while, comfortably numb. Whoever does the yanking and whatever the reason, the end result is the same—people eat more of what they should consume less of, if not avoid entirely.

In our daily lives we struggle as we try to navigate between biological imperatives and social necessity. Human beings are animals. At the very core of our brain lie our animal instincts, which respond to our environmental stimuli. The desire for food and survival are among our most powerful motivators. As members of the most complex social network on the planet, these instincts can be manipulated at the unconscious level by consciously affecting our self-esteem, personal enjoyment, constructiveness, destructiveness, curiosity, imitation, and altruism.[197] Our subconscious will always react to our perceptions.

As long as there is something to perceive the subconscious mind will perceive it and react to it. Agribusiness, the food industry, and Madison Avenue all know this very well. Their job is to translate your reaction into profit. Our ancient instinct for survival can cause us to show up at the drive-through, order, pay for, and blindly ruminate pseudo-food before we have consciously even perceived what we have done.

An ancient hardwired instinct for survival, forged long ago in a challenging, ferocious environment, can be made to betray us. The renowned scientist Carl Sagan remarked that "(s)urely there is something in us deeply seated, self-propelled, and on occasion able to evade our conscious control" (p. 405).[198] That something has been beguiled. The natural inclinations for balance, homeostasis, have been overwhelmed by abundance, accessibility, and the tweaking of our pleasure knobs. We have been massaged with subtle control and misdirection about the content of what we eat.

Quantity substitutes for value, and does a poor job. It is an addictive black hole at the center of the hot, sugar-glazed donut. It is a vicious cycle; the deeper you descend the harder it is to get out. Our weakness has been exposed and exploited. We stand stripped of our ability to taste anything at all. Worse, we no longer even seem to care; we wander unaware. Amid the machinations and maneuverings, in the cold confusion of The Borg Agribusiness and Food Conglomerate, we feel resistance is futile. But if we know our weakness, we can fight back.

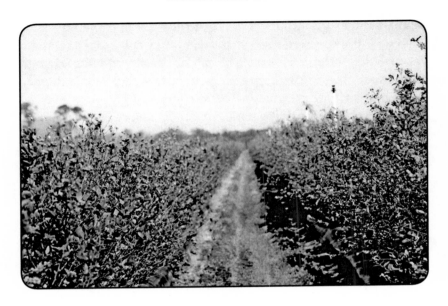

A Weakness Exposed: The Agricultural to the Industrial Revolution

"He who learns but does not think, is lost! He who thinks but does not learn is in great danger."

~CONFUCIUS[199]

According to Zooey Deschanel, "To be a gluten-free vegan is, like, the most difficult thing you can possibly be."[200] Considering that in the history of human kind being a gluten-free vegan ranks right up there with, like, riding unicorns, she may be right. Outside the world of pixie dust and Hollywood, human beings have always been omnivores. We still remain so. Our biology and physiology and thus our health and wellness remain predominantly determined by the combination of genetic and evolutionary forces. In the saga of our diet, there have only been two events of sweeping, historical proportions. The first of those was the Agricultural Revolution. The second was not Zooey Deschanel.

For hundreds of thousands of years during the early part of our evolution, mankind engaged in the world's oldest profession—hunting and gathering. Our ancestors spent their time doing what all animals and college students still do, which is wander about to find food and drink. At least ten to thirteen thousand years ago, if not much earlier during the Mesolithic period, there was a huge change. Humans domesticated animals and started farming. People stopped chasing their food around and took control of it. Human beings now had some authority to determine their source of energy. They introduced natural approaches to preservation such as smoking, salting, brining, pickling, fermenting, and many other methods. For approximately the next three hundred and fifty generations of *Homo sapiens* to follow, with respect to food and food pathways, things would remain essentially unchanged.

One of the major outcomes of the Agricultural Revolution was the growing and harvesting of crops. Increasingly, cereals and grains became a substantial portion of the human diet. While the consumption of cereals and grains was nothing new—ancient humans may have consumed grains as far back as over forty-five thousand years ago during the Upper Paleolithic[201]—their new role as a dietary mainstay was unprecedented. Prior to the Agricultural Revolution, the consumption of cereals and grains likely resembled what is observed in contemporary hunter-gatherer societies. Within these groups, those that consume some forms of cereals or grains tend to do so seasonally and in limited amounts.[202]

Among the crops cultivated, wheat became a staple. It has sustained populations, civilizations, and empires for thousands of years. But that wheat was very different from our modern variety. Modern wheat has undergone more transformations than Megatron. But all the modern varieties can trace their lineage to earlier landraces. The earliest known cultivated form of wheat was einkorn, *Triticum monococcum*.

Einkorn is what is known as a diploid wheat. That means it has a genome that consists of two parts and is commonly notated AA. Each letter represents specific genomes of seven chromosomes each. That gives einkorn wheat a total of fourteen chromosomes. This wheat is still cultivated, although in limited quantities.

Other ancient forms of wheat are several varieties known as the tetraploid group. This group contains both emmer and durum wheat. Their genome is notated AABB. This reflects the four genomes of seven chromosomes each. Each of these varieties has a total of twenty-eight chromosomes. Durum wheat, *Triticum durum*, was the original pasta wheat and is still cultivated for this purpose.

Dried Italian pasta, by law, can only be made from this wheat. Semolina durum wheat refers to the grind of the durum wheat flour, not the variety. Semolina is a term derived from the Latin word *simila*, meaning flour. Emmer wheat, *Triticum dicoccum*, is also cultivated in limited quantities.

The modern variety of wheat, *Triticum aestivum*, first appeared approximately nine thousand years ago. It contains six genomes of seven chromosomes each for a total of forty-two chromosomes. This makes it what is known as a hexaploid cultivar.[203] This variety of wheat is generally notated AABBDD. This variety known as bread wheat has undergone intensive selection and breeding. It has seen more makeovers than a casting call for *The Bachelor*. Spelt, or *Triticum spelta*, is another early hexaploid variety of wheat that remains much less intensively propagated.

Kamut, *Triticum turanicum* or khorasan wheat, is another variety of tetraploid wheat which shares a relationship to durum. A study was performed examining twenty-two otherwise healthy subjects who consumed various wheat products made from either kamut or modern semi–whole grain wheat. Modern semi–whole grain wheat is made from modern bread wheat, *Triticum aestivum*. A diet utilizing this ancient grain as compared to its more modern counterpart showed a significant reduction in total cholesterol, LDL ("bad") cholesterol, and baseline blood glucose levels.[204]

Grains like kamut produce carbohydrates that are not as rapidly assimilated into the bloodstream as more modern varieties; they have a lower glycemic index (GI). These more ancient grains still produce wheat-derived carbohydrates and proteins just like modern wheat. The nutrition label may read exactly the same between the two varieties, although obviously there can be dramatic differences in the biologic effect.

That is because these older species produce carbohydrates and protein that are qualitatively different from what is produced by the modern wheat varietal. Labeling in broad terms like proteins and carbohydrates is like having a discussion about flowers. There are over four hundred thousand different types of flowers.[205] Even a rose by any other name is not identical; there are over a hundred different kinds of roses. If you think there's no difference try sending your lover a dozen black roses instead of a dozen red ones.

In much the same way, wheat carbohydrates and proteins from different varietals can have very different biological effects. The results of studies like the kamut study suggest that the carbohydrates of earlier varieties may demonstrate even more than just a lower glycemic index. There are also increases in the levels of the essential minerals potassium and magnesium when kamut is compared to the modern variety of wheat. Other markers of endovascular and overall health, such as a reduction in the pro-inflammatory cytokines, interleukin-6, interleukin-12, tumor necrosis factor alpha, and vascular endothelial growth factor, were observed after participants consumed the khorasan wheat diet.[206]

Older strains of wheat may contribute positively to our health and reduce inflammation compared to the more modern version. These historic forms of wheat were sources of necessary vitamins and nutrients as well as sources of dietary energy up until very recently. That energy is supplied primarily in the form of both carbohydrates and protein.

Wheat has relatively low protein content at between 8 and 15 percent. However, because of the sheer amount of wheat consumed, it became an important source of protein for both humans and livestock. Ancient Egyptians who built the pyramids were paid in beer and bread, both of which were produced from wheat. The ancient Egyptians made a sophisticated malted beer and over forty different kinds of bread. And you thought the pyramids were just about the monuments; their living legacy can be found in every pub and tavern. Today, the descendants of that wheat continue to feed much of the world. While modern wheat may have its roots in such early varietals, it is as far removed from its forebears as we are from the pharaohs.

Our modern methods of processing cereals and grains are likewise far removed. From thirteen thousand years ago in the Levant up until the mid-1700s, the majority of all grains were stone ground. This method produces very little heat and does not oxidize and destroy the important phytonutrients. The stone-ground meal was then sieved to produce various flours. The wheat flours produced in this way contained not only the starchy endosperm, but bits of the bran and germ as well.

The germ is the innermost portion; it is the embryo that germinates to grow into the plant. The cereal germ is a concentrated source of important nutrients such as vitamin E, folate, phosphorus, thiamine, zinc, and magnesium. The germ also contains essential fatty acids and fiber. Like the germ, the bran also contains essential fatty acids, proteins, vitamins, and minerals. The bran is the outer layer of the grain. This is the portion that is particularly rich in dietary fiber, so important for the maintenance of intestinal health.

Fiber at one time was considered unessential by the medical community because it was not broken down by our bodies nor did it supply any energy. File that one along with "11,105 doctors say Lucky Strikes prevent throat irritation."[207] We now know fiber is a key determinant for metabolic and overall health.

A deficiency of fiber is associated with constipation, appendicitis, hemorrhoids, deep vein thrombosis, varicose veins, diverticulitis, hiatal hernia, and gastroesophageal reflux. According to Forbes magazine, Nexium, which is a drug used to treat gastroesophageal reflux disease, is one of the top twenty best-selling pharma drugs of all time. It generated over five billion dollars in sales during its peak year; and those numbers are for this one drug alone.[208] Fiber is cheap, but you can't patent it.

Prior to the Industrial Revolution, the US diet was high in vegetables and fruits. Fresh fruit contains twice the amount of fiber found in whole grains, while fresh vegetables contain almost eight times as much when measured on an energy basis. Additionally, fruit and vegetables typically contain soluble fiber, in contrast to the fiber found in cereal grains, which is often insoluble.[209] Soluble fiber is very beneficial. It helps to fill you up, aids in controlling blood sugar levels, and is important for proper intestinal health.[210,211] The diets of contemporary hunter-gatherers do not usually contain a lot of grains. But because of the vegetable and fruit consumption it does tend to contain dietary fiber that is in excess of current US dietary recommendations.[212]

A diet high in fiber has been shown to reduce total cholesterol, reduce LDL (bad) cholesterol, and help reduce caloric intake.[213] Fiber is critical for the proper health and balance of our gut microbiology. It seems that gut bacteria, like most people, enjoy the end products of the fermentation process. When dietary fiber undergoes fermentation by our intestinal residents it produces short chain fatty acids, like butyric acid. Butyric acid, which is also found in butter, has been shown to be anti-inflammatory, anti-bacterial, and helps prevent intestinal permeability. Short chain fatty acids such as these have many healthful benefits including maintenance of gut integrity and a potential reduction in the likelihood of developing colorectal cancer.[214]

Intestinal permeability is a condition also associated with celiac disease (CD) or gluten enteropathy. It is a disorder where the lining of the intestine becomes leaky. Normally, the lining of the gut is an impenetrable citadel on the order of Fort Knox. The only way in or out is through well-guarded and maintained passageways. When this boundary becomes leaky, it generates more holes than a Casey Anthony alibi. Untreated over time, intestinal permeability can lead to a number of pathologic gastric and inflammatory conditions.

Today, everyone seems to suffer from gluten enteropathy or some adverse reaction to gluten. This popular desire to be gluten-free has spawned an entire food specialty industry—cookbooks, videos, classes and an entire subculture of vegans. What is a little odd about this story is that gluten has been a mainstay of the human diet for at least the last ten thousand to thirteen thousand years, if not much longer.

Gluten is a protein found in wheat, and to a lesser extent in rye and barley. There is evidence that people have been consuming grains, which likely contained gluten, at least as far back as the Upper Paleolithic. Wheat and bread have been so important in the history of human kind that it has been at the forefront of many cultural and religious traditions throughout the world. It is an icon and a symbol unto itself.

Three of the world's major religions all recognize the importance of bread. The Jews recite *"Baruch ata Adonai, Eloheinu Melech ha'olam, hamotzi lechem, min ha aretz;* Blessed are You, O Lord our God, King of the Universe, Who has brought forth bread from the earth."[215] Jesus himself "... took bread and gave thanks and broke it, and gave it to them and said, 'This is my body, which is given for your sake; this do in remembrance of me (Luke 22:19)."[216] For Muslims, bread represents all food.[217] For civilizations, empires, and beyond recorded time, it was quite literally the stuff, if not the staff, of life.

One has to wonder: Why after thousands of years of consumption and thousands of years as the dietary staple does it seem that within the last several decades every other person on the planet now has an allergy or intolerance to gluten? To be gluten free is the new foodie chic.

While it may seem incredibly hipster cool to deride gluten as passé as Disco Stu, the biology simply doesn't work that way. Something that people have consumed for millennia does not all of a sudden garner immunologic reactions in 99 percent of the population. In fact, the data suggests the opposite. Since its identification in the modern era, true gluten enteropathy has been estimated to occur in only about 0.4 to 1 percent of the population.[218,219]

Even at that paltry rate it is still significantly more common than the true IgE mediated allergic reactions. CD is an immunologic disease, but not a true allergy. True gluten enteropathy is most prevalent in Europeans, Americans, and Australians. Some studies suggest that the incidence of gluten enteropathy may have increased slightly over the last several decades, yet it still remains at most around the 1 percent mark.[220] However, it is difficult to ascertain whether that is due totally to a true increase in the disease, improved surveillance and detection, or a combination of both.

Regardless, over the last half a century there have been several increasing trends of modern wheat consumption. These include an increase in consumption, an increase in the use of gluten in the processing of a variety of foods, an increase in the incidence, prevalence, and diagnostic intensity of celiac disease and related gluten enteropathies.

Gluten is commonly added to many processed foods as a binder. It is widely used in the production of soups; sauces; snacks like potato chips; candies; ice cream; various meat products; and even vitamin supplements; not only is it increasingly added to processed foods, but it is even found in some medicines.[221,222] It does appear that the initiation of celiac disease is related not only to the amount of gluten exposure, but the duration.[223] It's not the singular question, "Are we there yet?" that is the problem. It is the incessant thirty-second cycle of high-pitched whiny exposure to the question over hours that drive one to the brink of Homer Simpson-esque filicide. Likewise, unremitting gluten exposure in susceptible individuals can set their immune system completely awry.

The most recent studies of the most susceptible populations in the US and Scandinavia suggest similar prevalence to what has been observed historically, around 1 percent. The findings confirm that at the most, only about one out of a hundred people truly suffer from gluten enteropathy or celiac disease. For the rest of us, for the 99-plus percent, we do not suffer from true celiac sprue. Although you would never know that from the marketing.

Nonetheless, there are those people who do not have celiac disease but have a true allergy to wheat proteins, just as there are people who have allergies to other dietary staples such as nuts, peanuts— which are a legume and not a true nut—dairy, shellfish, and others. The fact that some of us can consume what makes others feel ill is a window into the diverse origins and capabilities of humans.

True wheat allergies come in a variety of forms, but they all involve an immunoglobulin response. Activation of the immune system and the production of autoantibodies are also involved in true celiac disease, but this mechanism is different from a true allergic reaction. True gluten enteropathy is often confused with a gluten intolerance, which is often mislabeled as a true gluten allergy. There are also respiratory allergies and other true allergic reactions to wheat, which tend to be far less common than CD. Lumping everything together as a gluten allergy makes things simpler and more confused. The distinctions are important.

Many wheat allergies have been known for thousands of years prior to the discovery of the gluten component. The Romans required slaves handling flour to wear masks. Today that food allergy is known as baker's asthma and is classified as an occupational allergy. It is a true immunoglobulin E (IgE) mediated allergy. This is the same type of allergic reaction people can have to a bee sting.

A number of different wheat proteins have been implicated in this type of allergy. However, there is a single class of wheat proteins that seem to be the predominant causative agents. These proteins belong to a class of α-amylase inhibitors known as CM proteins.[224] However, many other allergens have also been identified which cause baker's asthma including additives, molds, and even insect parts.[225] Baker's asthma is not generally considered a gluten allergy.

Another immunoglobulin E mediated reaction is wheat dependent exercise-induced anaphylaxis (WDEIA). This allergic reaction seems to be associated with a group of ω-gliadins, specifically the ω5-gliadins. In this syndrome, eating something containing wheat followed by significant physical exertion or exercise can result in anaphylaxis. It is not the wheat, but the exercise that follows that can kill you. When your mother told you that you couldn't run around after eating she was, as always, right. Other truly allergic reactions have also been well described including skin reactions like urticaria and dermatitis herpetiformis. This allergy produces itchy welts or painful blisters on the skin. These are mediated by immunoglobulin A, not IgE.

Despite their graphic effects, the incidence of these true immunoglobulin mediated wheat allergies fortunately remains rare.

Other conditions that have been reported to be associated with wheat proteins include schizophrenia, sporadic idiopathic ataxia, migraines, psychoses, and autism. The exact mechanism and degree of association remains unclear.

It is hypothesized that other metabolic products from the breakdown of gluten may be involved in these pathologic conditions. Such breakdown products include exorphins, which are opioid peptides. That means they have the potential to act like morphine and heroin. The wheat peptides that have this potential are referred to as gliadomorphins. Still other metabolic breakdown products include inhibitors of angiotensin I converting enzyme.[226,227] Angiotensin I converting enzyme plays a role in blood pressure. Inhibiting this enzyme is how the popular class of antihypertensive known as ACE inhibitors works. The *in vivo* significance of these metabolic breakdown products has yet to be established. If you're looking for a foodie high, stick with the Rocky Mountain Colorado brownies for now.

Of the thousands of wheat proteins, gluten is the most abundant and the one with the worst press. For all the negative reporting, it is remarkable how few people actually even understand that gluten is a wheat protein product first described in 1728.[228] It is found in the wheat endosperm where it constitutes about 80 percent of the total protein found in wheat.

Gluten is, however, only one of one thousand one hundred different protein products produced by the expression of over thirty thousand genes within the modern wheat plant.[229,230] The gluten component is produced from a combination of storage proteins known as the prolamins, particularly two proteins known as gliadin and glutenin. These proteins are found only in wheat, rye, barley, and triticale. Triticale is a wheat/rye hybrid.

Gluten is a very heterogeneous and viscoelastic protein. It is what gives dough the ability to rise, bread its chewiness, and a cookie its crumble. All gluten, like all people, are not identical. The glutenin and gliadin subunits that comprise gluten can both vary considerably depending on the particular species of wheat. The end result is that gluten varies considerably depending upon the wheat that it is derived from.

If what you're buying should not contain wheat, barley, or rye then it should be gluten free. Period. End of story. Ham should be pork and salt, maybe a variety of spices, but that is it. Your cheese, meat, and popcorn *should* be gluten free. Labeling and marketing something as *gluten-free* when it is gluten free is like getting charged extra for air. Current analysis suggests that there are about one hundred variations of the specific prolamin proteins that comprise the gluten protein. That means there are a lot of different glutens out there. The gluten found in barley is very different than the gluten found in modern wheat bread, just as a Ferrari is a very different automobile compared to a Ford Pinto. Both are cars, but one is something everyone would love to drive and the other blows up.

Celiac disease, celiac sprue, or gluten sensitive enteropathy is a specifically defined pathologic condition. Like baker's asthma, the condition has been recognized for thousands of years. However, it was not defined until 1887 and the association with wheat not established until the 1940s.[231] It is an immunologically mediated response to the gliadin component of gluten.

Of all the different proteins produced by modern wheat, gliadin is the component believed to be involved in the majority of celiac sprue or gluten enteropathy cases. Once a product containing wheat is consumed, the proteins are digested and broken down. Gluten is further broken down into glutenin and gliadin, which is then further metabolized. If that gliadin molecule fragment contains a certain sequence in a susceptible individual it can become immunogenic. This means that the immune system is activated and a series of events occur. Antibodies are produced, which end up attacking the lining of the person's own intestines. True gluten enteropathy is an autoimmune disease.

This autoimmune response results in chronic inflammation from the ongoing gliadin exposure. This in turn causes ongoing damage to the mucosa or lining of the intestines. This condition has been shown to increase intestinal permeability in susceptible people.[232] A consequence of the inflammation and increased intestinal permeability is maldigestion and malabsorption syndromes.

The gliadin component can also induce a pro-inflammatory state independent of the genetic predisposition to celiac disease.[233,234,235,236] Wheat gluten has been correlated with the development of chronic inflammatory diseases like multiple sclerosis, diabetes, psoriasis, immunoglobulin A (IgA) nephropathy, and rheumatoid arthritis.[237,238,239,240,241,242]

Gastrointestinal symptoms can be part of any of such infirmities caused by chronic inflammation. These symptoms include diarrhea, flatulence, weight loss, fatigue, abdominal pain, weakness, and borborygmus—the medical term for those really loud and embarrassing belly noises.

Other systemic findings associated with these inflammatory diseases can include abnormalities like anemia. This is the most common laboratory abnormality found in patients with CD. This is because iron is absorbed in the proximal small intestine, an area particularly affected by CD. Osteoporosis, osteopenia, and hormonal disorders can also occur. These abnormalities may arise in part from calcium and vitamin D malabsorption as a result of the gut injury. Bleeding disorders may develop due to a deficiency of vitamin K. There may also be deficiencies of folate, vitamin B$_{12}$ or both because of malabsorption. These can cause skin and neurological disorders.

The neurological manifestations include cerebral calcifications, epilepsy, peripheral neuropathy, and a form of postural instability. This is referred to as gluten ataxia. A possible etiology may lay in the fact that the autoantibodies associated with CD also have a strong affinity for the vasculature within the brain. Untreated CD has been associated with the development of strictures, bowel obstruction, and enteropathy-associated T-cell lymphoma. Various other forms of bowel adenocarcinoma are also associated with long-standing CD.[243]

The gliadin particularly correlated with CD is produced by genes on the DD portion of the hexaploid wheat genome. Consumption of the more ancient wheat varieties that lack the DD genome may allow the enjoyment of grain products and benefits of cereal consumption without the risk of inciting celiac disease or gluten intolerance. Some studies have shown that the gluten produced by such cultivars as durum wheat does not initiate the inflammatory cascade of celiac disease in some otherwise susceptible individuals.[244]

This is not surprising. Compared to ancient grains, modern wheat comes in a dizzying array of cultivars, but they are incredibly interbred. Many of these are altered to thrive in specific environments or to meet certain production goals. Although there are an astounding number of different modern wheat varieties, there may actually be less genetic diversity in modern wheat compared to more ancient landraces. Think royal inbreeding: lots of princes, princesses, dukes, duchesses, earls, and innumerable lords and ladies but the same bad teeth and big ears. The family tree of modern wheat is more like a telephone pole than a maple.

The breads made from ancient grains were substantially different than their modern-era counterparts in both their ingredients and their methods of preparation. The method of preparation can also affect the gluten composition of dough. Prior to the Industrial Revolution, lactic acid fermentation was not an uncommon method to make a risen type of bread. A lactose fermentation process, like that used to make sourdough, can actually reduce the gluten content in bread. Less than 20 parts per million (ppm) is consider gluten-free; so something labeled gluten-free has less than 20 ppm, not zero. Bread made by the modern commercial methods has roughly 75,000 ppm of gluten per serving, which is roughly about 4.8 g of gluten per slice. However, when made utilizing lactose fermentation via lacto-bacilli the same wheat yields a sourdough bread with gluten at 12 ppm—gluten-free by the accepted labeling standard.[245]

While gliadin may be unique to wheat, and to a lesser extent rye and barley, there are many other plant proteins that may also induce a somewhat similar immunologic response. The pre–Industrial Revolution diet contained a healthy infusion of fresh fruits and vegetables. However, consumption of plants is not entirely risk-free. Plants don't like to be eaten, and over billions of years have developed mechanisms so they can be left alone.

Lectins are ubiquitous proteins that bind to carbohydrates. They are found in many different kinds of plants and are often resistant to degradation by heat or digestive enzymes. This means that even if you cook your veggies you can still be vulnerable to their untoward effects. When high concentrations are ingested it can lead to diarrhea, nausea, bloating, vomiting, and even death in the case of ricin. A lectin present in soybeans, known as soybean agglutination (SBA), can cause damage to the small intestine when consumed in significant amounts in susceptible individuals. Lectins have been shown to potentially initiate and participate in the inflammatory cascade, yielding a condition not unlike the disease state seen in celiac disease.[246,247]

The pre-Industrial Revolution diet was in many ways similar in composition to that of many contemporary hunter-gatherers; there is very little to no refined carbohydrates routinely consumed. Contemporary hunter-gatherers' carbohydrate consumption is based primarily on fruits and vegetables. Within these societies, carbohydrates generally account for 22 percent to 40 percent and proteins account for approximately 19 percent to 35 percent of the total energy.

Despite consuming protein in excess of the current US governmental guidelines of 15 percent of total energy, there is far less incidence and prevalence of the diseases of modern civilization. Adequate protein intake increases calcium absorption and helps maintain adequate muscle mass and bone health. It also helps reduce the risk for hypertension.[248] Contemporary hunter-gatherers may consume more meat, fish, and seafood compared to what we generally eat. But because their protein is significantly less processed, they are healthier as a result.

Prior to the Industrial Revolution, meat, fish, and seafood were also the major source of fats as well as protein. Modern hunter-gatherer societies derive anywhere from 28 percent to 58 percent of their daily energy needs from dietary fat. The traditional Inuit diet is very low in carbohydrates and very high in animal fat. Yet, despite the high fat content of the traditional Inuit diet, there is a very low mortality rate as a consequence of cardiovascular disease.[249,250]

Another diet high in fat is the traditional diet of Crete, a template for the modern Mediterranean diet. This diet has been shown in many different studies to provide significant cardiovascular and other health benefits. It has been demonstrated to reduce diabetes, heart attacks, and strokes in susceptible populations.[251, 252, 253] This diet is also associated with a decrease in the markers of inflammation.[254,255] Yet this diet generally contains 35 percent to 40 percent of the total energy derived from fat sources. This diet is higher in fat than the modern Western diet, which generally clocks in at around 30 percent of total energy derived from fat. Yet, the incidence of cardiovascular disease and other diseases of modern civilization are one third of that seen in the US.[256] People adhering to a Mediterranean diet eat more fat than their modern Western counterparts, but are significantly healthier.

This highlights the fact that the quality of fat matters. A large percentage of the fats found in the Mediterranean diet are monounsaturated fatty acids from sources like olive oil and polyunsaturated fatty acids rich in omega-3s from sources like fish and from wild plants such as purslane. Where such a diet is the norm, mortality rates from cancer and heart disease are a fraction of what is found where the modern Western diet dominates. Consumption of fats can be beneficial. But the character of the fat matters; personality counts for a lot.

Monounsaturated fatty acids like those found in olive oil can improve blood lipoprotein parameters, reduce LDL cholesterol oxidation, improve insulin sensitivity, and reduce the tendency of the blood to form clots.[257] The qualitative character of the fats, the type of fats you eat, is more important than the absolute amount of fat in the diet.

The balance, or the ratio, of the different types of fats is likewise more important than the absolute quantities consumed.[258] A study looked at people eating a low-fat diet at 22 percent of total energy versus a high-fat diet at 39 percent of total energy. The low-fat regimen is reflective of the contemporary *healthy* approach so often touted through the media. It is promulgated to the masses as the most expedient way to weight loss. This is because cutting the fat is the most prompt and easiest way to reduce calories. The skinny on that approach is that the skinniest may not always be the healthiest.

The high-fat diet in the study was more like the ancient and pre-industrial diets than the modern Western diet. The total energy from fat was similar to the fat composition found in the Cretan diet. The ratio of the different types of fats was kept constant between the two groups: polyunsaturated to saturated; omega-6 to omega-3; and monounsaturated to total fat. The only difference was the amount of fat consumed. After fifty days there was no difference in blood lipoprotein markers traditionally associated with cardiovascular risk—total cholesterol and LDL ("bad") cholesterol.[259] In other words, it didn't matter *how much* fat you ate, it mattered *what type of* fat you ate.

Another study revealed that eating a low-fat, high-carbohydrate diet resulted in higher circulating levels of fatty acids in the form of triacylglycerols and cholesterol esters when compared to a diet low in carbohydrates, but with three times more saturated fatty acids. The typical *healthy low fat diet* mantra resulted in higher blood lipoprotein markers. These higher blood lipoprotein markers are the types of findings that are traditionally associated with an increased cardiovascular risk. It is the kind of finding that results in surgical intervention.

Here a diet with three times more *evil* saturated fat resulted in less risk compared to a high carbohydrate diet. Here it didn't matter *how much* fat you ate, it mattered *what* you ate it with: more fat or more carbs.

What emerges is the reoccurring theme that people are healthy and unhealthy not according to what they absolutely eat, but according to the ratio between what they eat and what their body and their symbiotic gut microbiome has evolved to expect and accept.

There are native populations in the Pacific Islands whose traditional diets may contain up to 45 percent of the total energy derived from saturated fatty acids. This, according to the conventional Western wisdom, would mean they should all be dead men walking. However, these fats are not from flat-line fries and quadruple-bypass burgers. A large proportion of that fat content contains fats like lauric acid. This is because these diets are often rich in coconuts and coconut-derived products; and lauric acid is a principal component of coconut oil. It is also a medium chain saturated fatty acid. That would be the same class, saturated fatty acids, that have been labeled for the last half-century as the great dietary Satan.

Even though their diet is high in fat and particularly saturated fat, their rate of cardiovascular disease is extremely low.[260] Despite the popular notion that continues to paint all saturated fats as the cause of cardiovascular disease and every other diet-related ill, a growing body of evidence argues against it. Many studies show little association between saturated fats like those found in the much-maligned fresh red meat and the risk of cardiovascular disease. [261,262,263]

However, many studies demonstrate a significant correlation between consuming *processed* red meat and the risk of disabilities and diseases of modern civilization such as cardiovascular disease, cancer, and diabetes.[264,265] These relationships correlate with increased mortality as well. How quickly we have forgotten the lessons of the law of unintended consequences, or processing, as the case may be.

In addition to the individual quality of certain fats and their ratios in general, the right mix of specific essential fatty acids (EFAs) also seems to be very important. One of the keys to maintaining proper health and reducing the risk of developing chronic disease may lie in the proper ratio of omega-6 to omega-3 polyunsaturated fatty acids.[266,267,268, 269]

Omega-6 polyunsaturated fatty acids are generally metabolized to produce products that are important in the initiation and maintenance of inflammation. Omega-3 polyunsaturated fatty acids are generally metabolized to produce products that counterbalance the inflammatory state. The delicate balance between the process of inflammation, so necessary to fight infection and repair the body, and the anti-inflammatory processes is a key to homeostasis, health, and freedom from disease and disability.

Diets low in omega-3 polyunsaturated fatty acids have been associated with increased markers of inflammation. But it may not just be that the diets are low in omega-3s, but that they are high in omega-6s. Many foods contain both omega-3 and omega-6 fatty acids, but the amounts of each can vary significantly.

A recent study found that the consumption of organic whole milk may substantially contribute to improved cardiovascular health compared to conventional milk. The researchers reported that the reason appears to be that organic whole milk is 62 percent richer in the omega-3 fatty acids compared to conventional milk. It is also lower in omega-6 fatty acids. This results in an omega-6 to omega-3 fatty acid ratio of about 2.5 for organic milk compared to 6.1 for conventional milk.[270] Prior to the Industrial Revolution, the diets had a much lower omega-6 to omega-3 ratio compared to the modern Western diet.

Fresh grass-fed, naturally raised meat has a story similar to organic milk. It is what would have been consumed prior to the Industrial Revolution. This more organic meat tends to have a much lower omega 6:3 ratio compared to that produced by the modern grain-fed feedlot method.[271,272] The ratio that is found in pre-Industrial Revolution meats resembles the ratio of that obtained from wild game. These ratios are similar to what is found in the diets of contemporary hunter-gatherer societies where the modern diseases of civilization are absent or lacking.[273,274] Although the ideal omega 6:3 ratio is unknown, estimates place it anywhere in the 1:1 to the 2–3:1 range.[275,276]

Prior to the Agricultural Revolution, all meat was originally derived from wild game. Even after the onset of the Agricultural Revolution, animals like cows were allowed to do what animals like cows like to do—wander about and eat grass. Although domesticated, the composition of the meat we consumed remained little changed from the days upon the savanna until the onset of the Industrial Revolution. It is some kind of six-ways-to-crazy that we now have to pay more for food raised in the natural manner it had been produced for thousands upon thousands of years.

Any amount of fat found in any particular animal raised naturally, wild or domestic, will vary by species, age, locale, sex, and season. Under any circumstances in wild game, the predominant areas of fat storage are subcutaneously, under the skin, and within the abdomen. The type of fat found within these areas tends to be composed of saturated fatty acids (SFAs).

The type of fat found in the muscle and other organ tissues of wild game is different. The type of fat found in these areas tends to be composed of polyunsaturated fatty acids (PUFAs) and monounsaturated fatty acids (MUFAs). Taken as a whole, the carcasses of wild game animals tend to yield predominantly PUFAs and MUFAs for consumption.[277] Even when animals such as caribou are slaughtered at the point of peak body fat percentage, PUFAs and MUFAs contribute the greatest percentage of edible fatty acids available for consumption.[278,279,280]

Prior to about 1850 in the US, the vast majority of cattle were raised on pasture and allowed to range freely. The typical age of slaughter was somewhere between four to five years.[281] This had been the norm for many centuries; it was roughly the same rearing method and age at which the Vikings would slaughter their cattle for consumption. That made for a tasty and healthful Thor burger. It keeps an Avenger in fighting form.

The beef produced this way prior to 1850 would more closely resemble in composition that of wild game than its more modernized, megamart-bound descendant. The pre-Industrial Revolution ratios of the different types of fats, as well as the individual fats themselves found in meat was a cow of a different color compared to contemporary offerings.

Prior to the Industrial Revolution, not only was the composition of the meat different with respect to fats, but the preservation methods differed as well. Prior to the latter half of the 19th century, salt was a highly valued and at times extremely expensive commodity. Meat and many other foods were often preserved by salting or salting in combination with other techniques such as smoking. Particularly during seasons when there was a reliance on such preserved foods the dietary sodium intake at this time was actually greater than what is seen today. Compared to some of the ancient diets, we eat *less* salt than they did.

The average twentieth-century European consumed significantly less salt than the average nineteenth-century European, which was well below the 100 g per day seen in sixteenth-century Sweden.[282] By comparison, the average American currently consumes around 8 g of salt, sodium chloride, which translates into about 3.4 g of sodium per day.[283] Most of the world population consumes between 7.5 and 15 g of salt or 3 to 6 g of sodium per day.[284] Although they may have consumed more salt than we currently do, prior to the Industrial Revolution the only other major sources of sodium in such diets, in addition to the preserved foodstuffs, would have come from seasoning and that which occurs naturally in foods.

That is distinctly unlike our modern sources of sodium. Today, there is the addition of compounds such as sodium bicarbonate, sodium citrate, and monosodium glutamate, as well as a slew of other artificial additives and preservatives. The manufacturing method of our modern-day foods significantly increases the sodium content of our processed, prepackaged, and pre-prepared foods. The average American diet consists of about 57 percent processed food. About 77 percent of the daily sodium intake in the modern Western diet comes from the consumption of these processed, prepackaged, and prepared foods. The consumption of all this processed food is the tipping point that skews the sodium-potassium ratio into the unfavorable range. There are also contributions that come from non-dietary sources such as pharmaceuticals. If a person is worth their salt and the ancients consumed more salt of the earth than us, that must make our modern Western diet worth-less.

However, in addition to eating more salt, our forebears also ate a lot more potassium than we do. This means that the sodium to potassium *ratio* remained in balance. In the human body, as in all living creatures, sodium exists in a delicately balanced dance with potassium. Potassium is another essential element necessary for proper bodily functioning and is especially important from a cardiovascular perspective. Among the many important effects of potassium is that it can act to help lower the blood pressure.

The pre-Industrial Revolution diet was rich in sources of potassium such as fresh fruit and vegetables. The importance of these cannot be overemphasized. Vegetables contain four times the concentration of potassium compared to conventional milk, even modern fortified milk. They contain twelve times the amount of potassium compared to whole grains. Fresh fruits and vegetables also contain additional vitamins, minerals, and micronutrients that are simply lacking in the modern Western diet french-fried versions of these. The current recommendations are for about 4,700 mg per day of potassium. The average daily potassium intake for an American is about 3,200 mg for men and only about 2,400 mg for women. The diet of ancient peoples may have had, and contemporary hunter-gatherer societies may have, a potassium intake as high as over 10,000 mg per day.

What passes for fruits and vegetables in the modern Western diet is like what passes for love in Westeros, which is to say the faintest of shades. A potato is a vegetable. When you skin it and drown it in hot vegetable oil like some amusement of King Joffrey, you remove everything of substance and dignity. French fries, freedom fries, Stark House sticks, fast food crispy bits of golden deliciousness, call them what you will; but nutritionally they are fools' gold. Legumes, fish, poultry, even fresh red meat are also great sources of potassium if they are not likewise adulterated by over processing. Thou shall not commit adultery is a clear culinary commandment.

The modern result of the handling of such comestibles is an inversion of the natural sodium-to-potassium ratio. Research has demonstrated an increased cardiovascular risk when the dietary ratio of sodium to potassium is greater than one.[285] The current sodium to potassium ratio in the United States is over 1.3. This is something not experienced in the history of human kind prior to the onset of the Industrial Revolution.

If the key is truly in the ratio, this may explain why so many previous studies have failed to definitively link increased absolute amounts of sodium to cardiovascular morbidity and mortality. As one might expect, while the modern Western diet yields a sodium to potassium ratio greater than 1; the pre-industrial diet had a ratio ≤ 1. A skewed sodium-to-potassium ratio is associated not only with hypertension, but with stroke, kidney stones, osteoporosis, certain cancers, asthma, insomnia, Ménière syndrome, and in some studies a significantly increased risk of death.[286,287,288,289,290,291,292,293,294,295,296,297]

Without an adequate intake of potassium and proper balance, the body cannot build proteins and muscle, metabolize carbohydrates, maintain normal repair mechanisms nor maintain normal cardiac and kidney function. Without potassium and proper renal function it is difficult for the body to properly control its natural acid-base balance.

The very composition of the diet itself can also affect our acid-base balance. As we consume foods and they undergo digestion, absorption and metabolism they tend to release either acidic or basic components into the systemic circulation.[298,299] In general, fish, meat, poultry, eggs, shellfish, cheese, milk, and cereal grains tend to be acid producing. Fresh fruit, vegetables, tubers, roots, and nuts tend to be basic in their effect. Legumes, refined sugars, vegetable, and seed oils tend to be neutral in their effect.

Prior to the Industrial Revolution, the constituents of the diet tended to yield a basic effect. The diet of contemporary hunter-gatherers also tends to be basic in character. A net base producing diet has been shown to help retard the progression of age-related chronic renal insufficiency. This condition is so common in industrialized countries as to be an accepted consequence of the aging process. In what we deem more primitive cultures, it is rare or absent.

Sugar was also infrequent until relatively modern times—infrequent but not unfamiliar. It was well known prior to the Industrial Revolution. Modern sugar, or sucrose in crystalline form, has been in production at least as far back as about 500 BCE, in what is now northern India. By the end of the first millennium BCE, it was well known throughout all of India, Southeast Asia and southern China. From there it spread into the Middle East. The growth of the sugar business followed the medieval spread and expansion of the Arabian Empire and its subsequent trade routes. By the fifteenth century the Europeans had established sugar production from sugar cane in the West Indies in order to meet an ever-increasing demand. However, prior to the Industrial Revolution it remained extremely expensive. This effectively limited consumption. Sucrose was not a significant component of the pre-Industrial Revolution diet.

Neither were vegetable oils. Prior to the Industrial Revolution and the development of mechanically driven steel expellers, most oils made from vegetables or seeds were produced by the rendering and pressing method. These methods date back at least five thousand to six thousand years.[300] However, there is difficulty in extraction utilizing this method. The consequence is limited oil production and increased expense. There were a few exceptions like olive oil, which was widely used and consumed, particularly in the Mediterranean world. There were no hydrogenated vegetable oils in use anywhere prior to the Industrial Revolution.

An underlying commonality among all these varying pre-Industrial Age diets from around the globe is their use of naturally derived, minimally processed foodstuffs. While many of these foods contain some forms of carbohydrates, sugars, salt, and fats, they also contain many important nutrients. This makes them both energy and nutrient dense. These are foods with redeeming value. Arranged in rhythm with natural ratios of consumption these foods feed body, mind, and soul.

A fatal flaw in the modern Western diet is that while its foods may be energy dense, they are often nutrient poor. The onset of the Agricultural Revolution rendered our instinctive survival drivers for sugar, salt, and fat obsolete for the most part. However, it was not until the onset of the Industrial Revolution and the advent of modern agribusiness and the modern food industry that these archaic survival mechanisms were exposed as a potent liability.

These vulnerabilities chain us, our foods displace us and we find ourselves bound to despair; enduring what should be golden years in a blemished existence of infirmity and illness. As a result of intestinal dysfunction and dysbiosis we endure a slow inflammatory simmer. We suffer from chronic disabilities and diseases of civilization: cardiovascular disease, obesity, hypertension, type 2 diabetes, polycystic ovary syndrome, myopia, acne, gout, various forms of malignancy, depression, schizophrenia, autism, Alzheimer-type dementia, Parkinson disease, and autoimmune diseases to name but a few.[301,302,303,304,305]

How did we get here?

In the next chapter we shall see.

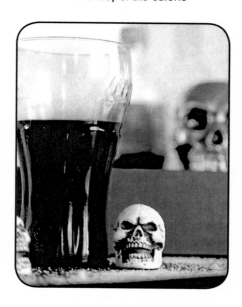

The Modern Western Diet:
A Weakness Exploited and Explained

"Taste me you will see
More is all you need
You're dedicated to
How I'm killing you
Come crawling faster
Obey your master
Your life burns faster
Obey your master..."
~METALLICA, MASTER OF PUPPETS[306]

The Fallacy of the Calorie

Around the world we love numbers. Scientists communicate by numbers. Sports fans obsess about numbers. Health professionals treat by numbers. In a word, Americans and other members of the industrialized world live by the numbers.

We take comfort in the assumption that our numbers cannot lie. After all, the language of math is the language of the Universe. A number, a value, is rigidly defined. There is no room for interpretation. One plus one will never give you five. Numbers, like grains of sand, allow us to draw lines and create boundaries. From there it is a short step to label and categorize. We set minimums to reach and maximums never to exceed. We define the normal from the abnormal and the good from the bad.

But what about the beautiful from the ugly?

Who exactly sets the limits, draws the lines?

The infallibility of numbers is a tall tale we tell ourselves. It is a teddy bear of fuzzy math that gives us comfort in a world of terrifyingly wide-open, foggy gray spaces. The math gives us black and white divisions. But as the timeless bard Jimmanicus Buffettus has sung on more than one occasion, "Math sucks."

Statistics is math based on assumptions. But there is non-numerical wisdom in the adage about what happens when you *ass-u-me*. If the assumption is flawed then it is garbage in, garbage out. Statistics, existing somewhere beyond the pale of damn lies, have long been known to mislead, misdirect, and outright misrepresent the truth. Liars figure and figures lie. This is particularly true if the values they represent are woefully misappropriated and mislabeled.

There are few places of such egregious trespass than within the realm of food and health. It is amazing that when challenged, so many food and health experts, whether food professionals like chefs promoting their *healthy cuisine*, health professionals, self-proclaimed wellness experts or just the generally self-anointed experts, they are all so unfamiliar with the currency of the realm. That currency is, of course, the Calorie.

When confronted with the challenge of defining a Calorie, most people including the majority of the aforementioned experts will simply yammer about like the Mad Hatter on bath salts. Even the government (surprise, surprise) cannot get it correct. This example is part of the US Federal Code regarding food fortification; Title 21, section 104.20, part d:

"(1) a normal serving of the food contains at least 40 kilocalories that is, 2 percent of a daily intake of 2,000 kilocalories … (3) The food contains all of the following nutrients per 100 calories based on 2,000 calorie total intake as a daily standard…."[307]

Which is it, Uncle Senile Sam: kilocalories, calories or, Calories?

The story starts with the Calorie. The Calorie has been around for about two hundred years. It continues to cause confusion on a number of different levels including its very definition. Let us set the record straight now. Exactly when the calorie came into usage is unclear. It was probably sometime during the late 1700s to early 1800s. Among the earliest published was a French definition in 1825.

At that time the Calorie was defined, and continues to be defined, as the quantity of heat needed to raise the temperature of 1 kilogram (kg) of water from 0 to 1° Celsius (C). This was assumed to take place at 1 atmosphere of pressure, or sea level. This is the Calorie with a capital "C". It is critical to note that this measurement reflects the heat produced by a substance. A Calorie originated as, and remains, a thermal unit. To convert it to a measurement of energy, one Calorie is equivalent to 4.186, or roughly 4.2 kilojoules (kJ).

The calorie with a lowercase "c" is defined as the amount of heat required to raise the temperature of 1 g of water 1°C with a temperature change from 14.5 to 15.5°C. According to the current US Dietary Reference Intakes that is equivalent to 4.186 Joules. Therefore, 1,000 calories are equal to 1 kilocalorie, which is also the same as 1 Calorie. All of these contain roughly 4.2 kJ in terms of energy.

How did all this confusion about food and calories begin? The fact that it began with the steam engine is a clue to how little calories have to do with actual food consumption and metabolism. With the invention of the steam engine and the onset of the Industrial Revolution, within the scientific community of the time, there developed a keen interest in trying to determine the amount of work that could be obtained from a machine or system. There is always money to be made in the development of a better mousetrap, or steam engine as the case may be.

In the early 1800s, Nicolas Clément and Charles Dosormes derived a mathematical constant, γ, which is equal to 427 kg-meters/kilocalories. This constant was important because it allowed for the calculation of the amount of energy produced by a system from the amount of heat generated. For a perfectly efficient machine, the amount of energy that could be supplied by different types of fuels, in other words their potential energy, could now be calculated by comparing their different caloric values. It is the way we can determine that burning jet fuel yields more energy than burning a stick of wood.

To determine the caloric value of different fuels, they are placed in a device called a calorimeter. The fuels are then completely burned and the amount of heat given off, as measured by the increase in the temperature of water, is recorded. This is the type of analysis that led to the discovery that using a substance such as coal to power steam engines could yield superior results compared to the same steam engine powered by wood. This is very important when you're buying fuel to power a steam engine, but much less relevant to the health of a human being.

Nonetheless, eventually the inquiry turned toward that most incredible of nature's machines, the human body. During the 1860s an American studying in Germany named Wilbur Olin Atwater became interested in the potential energy of different foods. While the mechanical efficiency of machines at that time was about 8 percent, the mechanical efficiency of humans and animals was estimated at between 20 percent and 30 percent. R2D2 was still a long way off; most physical labor was still done by animals and people. Atwater assumed a human mechanical efficiency of about 20 percent for his calculations.

He looked into supplying the human machine with fuel because of the significant amount of labor still performed by human manual exertion. The purpose of his work was to determine the amount of potential energy available from different types of food. He was looking to help find inexpensive foods that nonetheless potentially provided large sources of energy. The idea was to help provide economical types of food for people who had to perform strenuous physical labor. He was Moses at the granaries because dead slaves make no bricks. It was the search for fuel to get the job done, not food for health and wellness that Atwater was researching.

From Atwater's perspective, if a 70 kg person consumed 1 pound of fat at 20 percent mechanical efficiency, it would provide the energy to move 4,270 m. This is roughly the equivalent to traversing Pike's Peak (4,302 m or 14,114 ft.). His only concern was that of adequately powering the human machine to perform work. His purpose was to help identify economical yet energy-dense foods so that people could execute the necessary labor. It had almost nothing to do with health, and most certainly nothing to do with nutrition as we now understand it. Atwater was looking for cheap fuel. While both the meaning and intent of his pursuit were clear to Atwater and his contemporaries, it is something that has become confabulated with a more salubrious meaning over the ensuing decades.

There is a very simple reason as to why Atwater chose to label the potential energy of food with a thermal heat unit, the Calorie.

When he began writing the first of his five articles in 1887, the Calorie was the only applicable unit available in the English dictionaries of the time.[308] From this time and for almost one hundred years until the late 1960s and early 1970s foods were then defined in terms of the Calorie.

The relationship between the Calorie with a capital *C* and a calorie with a lowercase *c* was first defined in 1879 by Marcellin Berthelot, a French chemist. He noted that the Calorie with a capital *C* was the equivalent of 1,000 calories. The actual term kilocalorie was not introduced until 1907, and not readily adopted until the widespread implementation of the metric system in the 1950s. Since the major purpose of adopting the metric system in the US seems to have been to assure you need two sets of socket wrenches, it is of little surprise the description of food energy remained a muddled affair.

The confusion regarding the different terms remained rampant until about 1970, when professional organizations recommended that all nutrition texts change from Calories to kilocalories. However, after more than one hundred years in the public vernacular the term Calorie remains firmly embedded in the communal psyche. No one recognizes Frederick Austerlitz or Marion Morrison but everyone knows Fred Astaire and John Wayne. The public's caloric confusion continues.

Over a hundred and twenty-five years after its introduction the Atwater system is still the standard that is used. Some of the caloric value of food is determined today as it was in Atwater's time. That method is by the use of a bomb calorimeter. The caloric value of foods is determined by the heat that is generated when the food is completely burned.

Within this device, the food to be studied is completely incinerated and reduced to carbon powder. The bomb calorimeter measures the heat, in calories, that is given off when the food is completely burned. This is how the caloric value of food was originally determined. This value represents simply the absolute potential energy of certain foodstuffs; in other words the amount of heat that might be released if your body processed it by incineration. There are not many absolutes when it comes to human physiology. However, you absolutely do not process food by turning all to ash and naught, unless you are Sauron, The Great Eye.

The other, more commonly utilized modern approach still uses the Atwater system. In applying this alternative method the calories are not determined by directly burning the foodstuffs. Instead, the total caloric value is calculated by adding up the calories provided by the percentages of protein, carbohydrate, fat, and alcohol. The fiber component is usually subtracted from the total carbohydrate before calculating the calories. This approach uses the average values of 4 kcal/g for protein, 4 kcal/g for carbohydrate, 9 kcal/g for fat, and 7 kcal/g for alcohol.[309] However, these average values were originally determined by the bomb calorimeter method and then averaged. They are, in a sense, even more deceptive, inaccurate, and misleading than the values determined by complete combustion of the actual food.

If we examine foodstuffs with an eye toward their substantive values—the vitamins, the minerals, the types of fats, the types of carbohydrates, the different protein and fiber compositions, and the like—it is obvious that the caloric value of food speaks nothing toward these. When it comes to identifying the true value of food, the value depends on both quality and quantity.

Calories are only about quantity. Calories provide for a simple numerical quantification in comparison of foods. It makes it easy. But the more important question is, does it make for an accurate assessment? Evaluating foods based solely on caloric comparisons is like calculating the value of different automobiles based exclusively upon their fuel mileage. Such an analysis does not take into account the different features, jobs, terrain, and needs that are met and filled by the different classes of vehicles and the different choices and specializations within each class. You don't feed the cows out of the back of your Bentley.

If anyone has ever compared the published estimated fuel mileage of any vehicle against the actual fuel mileage of said vehicle once it is in their possession, they know there can be quite substantial variation. In fact, the variation is the norm. The same holds true for the caloric value of any naturally obtained food. The actual caloric value of food yields can vary from person to person, just as a gallon of gas can yield different fuel mileage for cars of the same make and model year.

The caloric value can also vary from apple to apple, even though there is a single value for an average apple. Given the differences that arise from production location, size, and a host of other innumerable variables, the caloric value of any particular food may vary from 10 percent to 20 percent. Therefore a 100-Calorie apple may actually range anywhere from 80 Calories to 120 Calories. That makes comparing apples to apples extremely problematic before one ever gets to compare apples to oranges.

Yet people tend to operate on the assumption that the numbers are set in stone, are absolute in value, and that less is healthier. Such faulty logic can be dangerous. Operating from the premise that fewer calories translates into a more healthful food choice can lead to conclusions that defy common sense. Extrapolating that logic to its ultimate end point would result in the conclusion that a completely artificial, zero calorie beverage is a more healthful choice than an apple containing roughly one hundred Calories. It is a conclusion that we know to be pure folly.

Such extrapolation of the caloric approach yields a simple query; are calories useful?

As a relative, comparative guideline the answer is, *Yes*.

With understanding, they can supply some incremental, comparative information regarding the quantitative value of various comestibles. They are a rough guideline. They are not a codex; they are not the law. They are not a substitute for reading the label and knowing the qualitative components of the food we eat.

Even detailing the caloric value on the label should be approached with a bit of trepidation. The amount of calories listed on the label can be deceptive. By manipulating the size of the serving portions into unrealistic amounts, the advertised caloric content can belie a false sense of assurance. A lazy overreliance on simply comparing calories can transform these numbers from a potentially helpful adjunct into a modern weapon of mass confusion. And when it comes to food, mass confusion can easily become mass consumption.

If you really need a calorie guide to determine whether the apple consisting of 100 Calories is a more healthful choice than the Heart Attack Grill quadruple bypass burger clocking in at 9,982 Calories you need to reassess your method of food valuation. You need to use some bloody common sense. Food choices *still* have Darwinian implications.

The problem with the modern Western diet is not only in its composition and its resultant effects. It is in the way we evaluate it. It is in the way we attempt to gauge, assess, and solve the problems it creates. We tend to calculate the worth of the food by simply looking at the number of calories it contains. We quantify it, assign it a number, and that number is its value.

That value is based on an assumption. If we consume fewer calories, we will lose weight. If we lose weight we can achieve the ideal body mass index (BMI) as indicated on some governmental chart. Attaining the ideal BMI confers supposed health and wellness. QED, we consume fewer calories and we live happily and healthfully ever after.

But the pot of gold at the end of the ideal BMI rainbow is as much a farce as the caloric road to Oz. The body mass index (BMI) is categorized as follows (measurements in kg/m²):

Underweight BMI < 18.5

Normal or Ideal BMI 18.5 – < 25

Overweight BMI 25 – < 30

Obese – Grade 1 (or mild) BMI 30 – < 35

Obese – Grade 2 BMI 35 – < 40

Obese – Grade 3 (or morbid) BMI > 40.

According to both the Centers for Disease Control and the World Health Organization: "A crude population measure of obesity is the body mass index (BMI), a person's weight (in kilograms) divided by the square of his or her height (in meters). A person with a BMI of 30 or more is generally considered obese. A person with a BMI equal to or more than 25 is considered overweight."[310,311]

The BMI is what is currently used to define normal, overweight, and obese individuals. It is based on the assumption that the BMI is a great (read: unfailing) measure of fitness and fatness.

But is it?

The BMI is in essence a guideline developed in the nineteenth century. Lambert Adolphe Quetelet was a Belgian polymath. He became interested in the social sciences and in the study of what was considered normal. Being a mathematician and a statistician, he defined normal as a certain percentage of a population that fell under a Gaussian, or normally distributed, bell-shaped curve. The population from which he derived what would later become the BMI consisted of several hundred European Caucasian male army conscripts in 1832. From this he developed the Quetelet Index of Obesity.

In 1972 Ancel Keys compared the Quetelet Index of Obesity against several other easily obtainable clinical measures of obesity. These down-and-dirty measures were compared to the more rigorous assessments of body fat and obesity available at the time. It was found that amongst the quick and easy, the Quetelet Index of Obesity exhibited the best correlation when looking at large populations. Ancel Keys coined the term "body mass index" and both the label and the definition were later adopted by the World Health Organization and the Centers for Disease Control. Both Adolphe Quetelet and Ancel Keys cautioned that while an adequate population measure, the results of the BMI should never be applied to individuals. In the definition above the WHO and CDC acknowledge that the BMI is a crude population measure of obesity. Despite the acknowledged caveats, using it as an individual measure of obesity is, of course, exactly how we use it today. In fact, an individual's BMI is a mandatory collectible data field on every approved electronic health record according to the Affordable Care Act.

Despite governmental acceptance of the BMI as a gold standard, there is an ongoing debate about the accuracy and ultimately the utility of such a measure. On the opposite side of the scales, physicians, statisticians, researchers, and other scientists are asking whether a measure that defines about two-thirds of the population as overweight or obese is a harbinger of doom or simply an inaccurate or outmoded measure.

One of the major problems of BMI is that it does not measure fat; it measures your total body mass, which includes not only fat but lean body mass such as muscle. While the BMI does correlate with percentage of body fat, it correlates more generally with bone density and mass.[312] A study examined the contradictory findings when defining overweight and obesity by a more time-consuming but more accurate measure such as triceps skinfold thickness versus the quick and easy BMI calculation. The study found that the BMI findings were consistently about 10 percent higher than a more rigorous measure.[313] Some world-class athletes like rugby player Jonah Lomu have a high BMI. According to BMI measurements Arnold Schwarzenegger and Sylvester Stallone are or were all obese or overweight during their buff Terminator and Rocky heydays.

Quetelet and Keys cautioned against the use of the BMI to make an individual diagnosis. There is an inherent danger in trying to apply a singular population characteristic to any individual. The difference between normal and overweight, or overweight and obese, can be as little as 0.1 kg. Yet the difference between members of the same category can be as great as almost 5 kg. This fact translates into potentially huge differences in the outcomes between people placed in the same category, while there are minimal, if any, differences at different groups separated at the borders.

The reduction of the definition of overweight from 27 kg/m^2 to 25 kg/m^2 in 1998 suddenly made thirty million Americans overweight who were not overweight the day before.[314] In Australia, the United Kingdom, and most recently the US, governmental and other organizations have adopted obesity definitions against the recommendations of their own scientific advisory panels.[315] The vote of the American Medical Association's House of Delegates in favor of labeling obesity as a disease went against the conclusions of the association's own Council on Scientific and Public Health. The Council had reached the conclusion "that obesity should not be considered a disease mainly because the measure usually used to define obesity, the body mass index, is simplistic and flawed."[316]

According to the World Health Organization and in the definition accepted by the Centers for Disease Control, "Overweight and obesity are defined as abnormal or excessive fat accumulation that presents a risk to health."[317] This places both overweight and obese categories as different stops on the same disease train. A disease is defined as "a disordered or incorrectly functioning organ, part, structure, or system of the body resulting from the effect of genetic or developmental errors, infection, poisons, nutritional deficiency or imbalance, toxicity, or unfavorable environmental factors; illness; sickness; ailment."[318]

Since the BMI does not directly measure fat, accepting the BMI as the gold standard for the definition of overweight and obese, which are diseases caused by fat, is beset with peril. It is like getting a speeding ticket because your car looks like it can go fast. This is the *ecological fallacy*, where relationships found in aggregate level data are wrongly assumed to apply at the individual level.

People driving a certain sports car are more likely to exceed the speed limit. But just because you drive that model sports car does not mean you are guilty of speeding. Take a group of people who drive Lamborghinis and a group of people who drive Priuses. For every person driving a Prius who gets a speeding ticket two people in the Lamborghini group will get a speeding ticket, on average. However, just because *you* drive a Lamborghini doesn't make *you* automatically twice as likely to get a speeding ticket as the yuppie driving a Prius. The averages that hold true for large populations completely fall apart at the individual level.

This is one of the great challenges of the practice of medicine. Studies are done on treatments that are applied to large numbers of very narrowly defined patients. When these results are then attempted to be applied to a broader population and individuals in particular, the results may no longer be applicable. Medicine may study populations, but *healing* is still an individual art. These same difficulties arise when trying to apply the results from any particular BMI group to an individual in that group. Interpreting this data becomes even more troublesome when the relationship is not a straight line.

And of course, the relationship between BMI and mortality is not a simple straight line. It is what is referred to as a *J*-shaped curve; it more resembles a Nike swoosh than anything else. At a BMI less than 18, the underweight category, mortality increases. This increase in mortality is not simply the result of wasting conditions like those associated with cancer or other severe, systemic illness. Likewise, at some point increasing weight is *always* associated with an increasing risk of morbidity and mortality. Somewhere, at the bottom of that swoosh is a sweet spot of healthy weight with the lowest risk of disability and disease.

What is not clear is where that spot is located. Conventional wisdom would place it in the healthy weight category; a BMI between 18 and 25. Yet it may come as a surprise that the conventional wisdom may be neither conventional nor wise. Many studies have shown the healthiest group may be those in the overweight category. In some studies the maximum benefit actually includes the mildly obese category.

A meta-analysis of almost one hundred previous, smaller studies was published in 2013 in the *Journal of the American Medical Association*.[319] The study comprised almost three million people around the world and is one of the most comprehensive analyses to examine the relationship between mortality and BMI to date. The researchers found that the lowest mortality rates were not in the ideal BMI group. It was the overweight group that had the lowest mortality rate, with a statistically significant six percent reduction over the ideal group.

In fact, the mortality rate of the ideal or normal BMI group was actually the same as the Grade one, or mildly obese, group. Grades two and three, obese and morbidly obese, did show a significantly increased risk. However, in terms of total numbers the individuals in those groups represent a small fraction of the 67 percent of all Americans who are classified as either overweight or obese. It should also be noted that, unfortunately, grades two and three are among the faster growing classifications. At some level of increasing weight, there is *always* going to be an increased risk of mortality, but where that boundary lies is far from clear. Where the bottom of that J curve sits, no one really knows.

To add to the confusion many studies show that for people with certain disease states, like congestive heart failure, it is the overweight and mildly obese groups that have a superior survival rate, not the ideal body weight group.[320] This holds true even though obesity is listed as a risk factor for the development of such conditions.[321]

Cardiologists are still grappling to understand this phenomenon, known as the *obesity paradox*. The number of studies confirming the reality of this paradox grows. And this obesity paradox isn't just Dr. Phil looking in a mirror. The obesity paradox refers to a number of well-done studies showing that among patients with established heart disease, other medical conditions, and even the general population at large, those who are overweight or even mildly obese by BMI standards fare better and survive longer than those of *normal* or *ideal* weight. In short, obesity is generally recognized as a risk factor for the development of cardiovascular disease. But many studies of patients with the disease have shown that the best survival rates occur not in the ideal body weight group but in those groups that are either overweight or mildly obese.[322]

A study pooled the data from five previous studies examining over twenty-five hundred patients, both men and women over age forty with newly diagnosed diabetes (DM).[323] Participants were classified as normal weight if their BMI was 18.5 to 24.99 or overweight/obese if the BMI was 25 or greater. Although only about 12 percent of the study group was normal weight, they had the highest rates of total, cardiovascular, and non-cardiovascular mortality. After adjusting for other variables, the *ideal* weight group still had higher mortality levels in every category. The study concluded that adults "who were normal weight at the time of incident diabetes had higher mortality than adults who are overweight or obese."

Another study done at The University of California found that adults with heart failure who were overweight or obese had lower risk of death. In addition to BMI, the study also included waist circumference as a measure of risk. In men, a waist circumference of forty inches or more indicates a high-risk group. For women, it is thirty-seven inches or more that is considered high risk.

Heart failure is a condition for which previous studies have suggested obesity to be a risk factor. Heart failure has many causes, but the end result is a condition in which the heart muscle is weakened and unable to pump efficiently enough to meet the demands of the body. A condition, by which all conventional wisdom should suggest, is exacerbated by increased weight.

That's not what the data showed.

The survival of the overweight and obese groups was superior to both underweight (a known higher risk group) and those with a "normal" BMI. Not only was the risk of death lower, but also the higher weight groups were less likely to require a heart transplant or suffer other related morbidities. The study examined approximately 2,700 heart failure patients. The participants were followed for two years. The study found men with a high waist circumference and a high BMI were more likely to survive and were less likely to need a heart transplant.

Overweight and obese women also fared better than normal-weight women. The cardioprotective effect was significant: men with a normal BMI and smaller waist circumference had a 34 percent higher risk for adverse outcomes and normal weight women had a 38 percent higher risk for adverse outcomes. An interesting hypothesis suggested by the study's authors involves increased serum lipoproteins. These molecules are made of proteins and fats and often act to transport fats throughout the body. The authors suggest these molecules may have potent anti-inflammatory properties.[324]

Heart failure patients are not the only very sick cardiovascular patients to show increased survival at the overweight and mildly obese BMI range. Patients suffering from critical aortic stenosis who underwent a relatively new cardiac procedure are among the latest to exhibit the paradox. Critical aortic stenosis, which commonly affects the more elderly patients, involves a narrowing of the aortic valve. The aortic valve is out the outflow of the left ventricle and helps regulate the flow of oxygenated blood to the brain, organs, muscles, and throughout the body.

When this valve becomes narrowed, or stenotic, it can severely limit the outflow of needed oxygenated blood and result in passing out spells known as syncope, heart attacks, congestive heart failure, cardiomyopathy, and ultimately death. Until recently, the only effective way to have a satisfactory long-term outcome was to have open-heart cardiopulmonary bypass surgery with implantation of a mechanical or a bio-prosthetic valve.

Recently techniques have been developed to perform this procedure in a much less traumatic fashion. A catheter is inserted, much as is done in a routine cardiac catheterization, and a balloon containing a metal stent and a valve is passed across the aortic valve expanded. A new artificial valve is implanted with the old native valve pushed out of the way up against the arterial walls.

Whenever a relatively new technique like this is developed, investigators are always sorting through the data to help identify predictors that indicate whether a patient will do well with the procedure or identify a patient at potentially higher risk with a particular approach. A French study looked at such predictors in patients undergoing the aforementioned aortic valve replacement technique known as transcatheter aortic valve implantation (TAVI).[325]

What they found confirms previous data regarding the obesity paradox. After other variables were adjusted, those patients who were overweight had a 26 percent reduction in their likelihood of mortality compared to normal weight individuals. In other words, if your BMI placed you in the overweight category you were 26 percent less likely to die within the year following the procedure compared to someone who had a BMI that placed them in the *ideal* category.

If you were in the obese category, your likelihood of dying was reduced by 29 percent. Of note, the vast majority of the obese patients were in what is considered mild or grade 1 obesity, with a BMI from 30.0 to 34.9. Those who were underweight, with a BMI less than 18.5, formed the highest risk category in terms of major vascular complications and the lowest survival. One-year survival was 67.9 percent for underweight; 73.6 percent for *ideal* weight; 77.4 percent for overweight; and 80.3 percent for obese patients.

An important caveat is that this study was observational and not randomized in any fashion. Additionally, all the patients were considered such high risk that traditional surgery was not an option, so this procedure was utilized. The study examined over three thousand patients with a mean age of eighty-two from January 2010 to October 2011. In general, survival and mortality curves for those who are underweight continually have a higher risk and mortality than the normal or overweight category. What is interesting in this study is that like other studies examining the obesity paradox, the overweight and mildly obese patients had improved survival compared to what is identified currently as an *ideal* or *normal* BMI measurement.

The true ideal BMI may even turn out to be different based on ethnicity and gender. Because the BMI does not take into account lean body mass such as muscle, it can overestimate obesity in certain ethnic groups while underestimating it in others. Many physically fit people, including actors and athletes with very low percentages of body fat, register as obese when judged solely by their BMI. Other groups that tend to have larger bone and muscle mass, such as African-Americans, may be labeled obese when they are in fact quite fit. Conversely, ethnic groups with slight frames like Asians may appear to be healthy by BMI measurements when that in fact is not the case.

Are there more accurate measures we should use? Should we be looking at fat distribution and body polymorphisms?

Other less commonly used measures such as waist circumference and the waist-to-hip ratio seem to correlate better with the risk of morbidity and mortality. This is because evidence continues to accumulate that it is not just weight—which includes lean muscle mass and fat—but where the adipose tissue deposits that correlates with risk. Studies suggest that it is the dreaded *belly fat* that has the connection to death and disease.

A study from the University of Minnesota found that the waist-to-hip ratio strongly correlated with the risk of sudden cardiac death. The research evaluated data on about fifteen thousand people who had participated in the Atherosclerosis Risk in Communities (ARIC) study, which enrolled individuals ages forty-five to sixty-four at baseline in 1987 to 1989. Over a mean follow-up of about twelve years, there were three hundred cases of sudden cardiac death, defined as a death that occurred within one hour of symptom onset when witnessed or within twenty-four hours of being seen alive when unwitnessed.

A waist-to-hip ratio greater than 0.85 for women, and greater than 1.0 for men, is considered high risk. In this particular study, for those in the top quintile of waist-to-hip ratio (0.97 and higher for women and 1.01 and higher for men), the risk of sudden cardiac death was a relative 40 percent greater compared with those in the lowest quintile (less than 0.82 for women and less than 0.92 for men). BMI, waist circumference, and waist-to-hip ratio measures of obesity were all evaluated for an association with sudden cardiac death.

After adjustment for age, sex, race, education level, smoking status, family history of coronary heart disease, diabetes, LDL cholesterol, hypertension, prevalent coronary heart disease, heart failure, and left ventricular hypertrophy which are all known risk factors for sudden death, only the waist-to-hip ratio emerged as a significant predictor of sudden cardiac death. The BMI did not correlate with risk. Selcuk Adabag MD, the lead author of the study, remarked that it is unclear why the waist-to-hip ratio appears to be more informative than waist circumference or BMI. He hypothesized that it may have to do with the correlation between abdominal fat deposition and increased inflammation.[326]

Among the shortcomings attributed to the BMI measurement is that where the weight is located may be as critical, if not more so, than the total volume.[327] A study presented at the European Society of Cardiology meeting in August 2012 demonstrated that normal-weight individuals with belly fat have the highest cardiovascular risk.[328] Francisco Lopez-Jimenez, senior author on the study and a cardiologist at the Mayo Clinic in Rochester, Minnesota, commented that those with normal overall weight but with significant belly fat or visceral adipose tissue (VAT) have "the highest death rate, even higher than those who are considered obese based on BMI." Compared to normal individuals, risk of cardiovascular death was 2.75 times higher, and the risk of death from all causes was 2.08 times higher for those with the jelly belly. This may explain why these people in fact, never seem very jolly.

The key seems not to be in the amount of fat, *per se*, but in determining the connection between fat and increased inflammation. That may depend on the type of fat and its deposition. It may depend ultimately on where that bottom of the *J* lies. What is ideal today may be more deadly tomorrow. This is counter-intuitive to the conventional wisdom, but in agreement with studies like the previously mentioned BMI meta-analysis. Researchers have suggested that the survival benefit may be related to an absolute greater percentage of body fat, not just due to a misleading BMI.

A study into this obesity paradox demonstrated that body fat was an independent predictor of mortality. Higher body fat meant improved survival in those with stable coronary heart disease. This is even though a higher body fat has previously been suggested to be associated with conferring an increased risk of developing coronary heart disease. Even eliminating the small percentage of underweight patients (6 of 570) who demonstrated a 50 percent mortality rate did not change the overall significance of the findings. Using more direct measures of body fat and lean body mass, the investigators followed this population of patients for more than three years.

They found the group with the highest survival rate and thus the lowest mortality were those with the highest body fat and lean mass index. The highest mortality was in those with a low body fat and low lean mass index. This skinny group had almost a threefold increased risk of death.[329] Those with both fat and lean body mass, such as muscle, lived longer than those without fat or muscle. *Skinny Girl* be dead girl.

Another much larger study examined more than fifty thousand patients with ST-segment elevation myocardial infarction, or a big heart attack. After adjustment for all other variables, there was higher in-hospital mortality in the *healthy* BMI group compared to the overweight or mildly obese. The *ideal* BMI group had identical in-hospital mortality to the obese group. The only group with a higher in-hospital mortality for heart attack than the *ideal* group was the morbidly obese.[330] In other words, if you have a heart attack, your best chance for survival is to be in the overweight or mildly obese category.

So the paradox emerges and hangs awkwardly in the air like an ill-timed dog fart. Obesity is considered a risk factor for many diseases, including coronary artery disease (CAD), diabetes, heart failure, and certain types of cancer. However, many studies of patients with cardiovascular disease, including heart failure, hypertension, atrial fibrillation, CAD, and other diseases have demonstrated an inverse relationship between obesity and increased morbidity or mortality.

Many of the measurements used to determine obesity in these studies utilized the BMI methodology. Often, the seemingly contradictory results of these studies were explained as a failure of the BMI. Yet, emerging data suggests that there is a fat threshold below which there is increased risk of disability and disease. Just as there is a maximum above which the same risks exist.[331]

The bottom of that curve, the place to be, may not be where we currently define *normal, ideal* or *healthy*. It may be with the group we currently define as *overweight*. This, of course, begs the question—with respect to the target and goals—do we have it wrong?

It is a question with interesting implications. Millions of dollars have been invested and continue to be invested at all levels and in innumerable programs to help those falling outside the parameters of an ideal body mass index. The impetuses for such interventions are more statistics showing roughly two-thirds of the US population overweight or obese.

According to these classifications approximately 40 percent of adult US men and about 30 percent of adult US women are overweight. This category, if the data is to be believed, is actually the healthiest group with the lowest mortality. If we also consider the fact that those in the obesity grade one, or mildly obese category, have the same mortality as those in the normal BMI category, then the magnitude, if certainly not the mass of the problem, seems somewhat less daunting.

Such analysis provides curious insight. It would suggest that for the vast majority of the population, the rise in the incidence and prevalence of the disabilities and diseases of modern civilization is not attributable to simply being fat. If it is not simply the *quantity* of what we consume that is the problem, then perhaps the problem is simply the *quality* of what we choose to consume.

The importance of the quantity of consumption appears to manifest at the extremes of the BMI *J* curve. Those less than a certain BMI are consistently at increased risk. The percentage of those obese (grade two) and morbidly obese (grade three) continue to rise inexorably like a gently baking Cinnabon. This group also seems to truly be a population at risk.

The non-profit RAND Corporation completed a study published in the *International Journal of Obesity* in which they found that "the percentage of American adults who are one hundred or more pounds over a healthy weight has skyrocketed since 2000."[332] In 2000 the rate of severe obesity was 3.9 percent; in 2010 it had increased nearly 60 percent to a rate of 6.6 percent. This applies to the small but massive group that would be considered severely or morbidly obese. It is defined as those with a BMI equal to or greater than forty (obesity grade 3).

In spite of defining the boundaries, the healthiest of the BMI defined groups is still under debate; the "normal" or "ideal" is likely neither. But what does it say about policy implementation, on a national and international level, that literally may have been slightly off the scales? The obesity paradox brings into question the very risk of obesity, as it is currently defined, itself. Many studies have demonstrated that those who are obese but physically fit have no increased health risk compared to their non-obese counterparts. The caveat was that the fit-but-obese population also did not suffer from any of the diseases of modern civilization like metabolic syndrome or diabetes, conditions associated with underlying inflammation. Such an approach should give us pause.

Much like the French Paradox of the late 1990s, the current obesity paradox remains an enduring mystery, a Bermuda Triangle of medicine. Caloric restriction was once touted as a path to the fountain of youth. It was held by some that reducing consumption could lead to longevity. This has been debunked. Some earlier data using worms and mice had suggested that reducing daily caloric intake might add years of life.

A study which examined caloric restriction in monkeys over several decades was published in the journal *Nature*. It exposed some of these previously held myths. "One thing that's becoming clear is that calorie restriction is not a Holy Grail for extending the lifespan of everything that walks on earth," said Rafael de Cabo, an experimental gerontologist at the US National Institute on Aging in Baltimore and lead author of the paper.[333]

What is no mystery is that the BMI provides a crude population-level measure and is utilized for its convenience and simplicity, not necessarily for its precision and accuracy. Yet, despite these limitations, the BMI continues to be increasingly used in clinical practice to diagnose obesity and has found its way into clinical, bureaucratic, and regulatory guidelines for which it was never intended.[334]

Taken by itself BMI is simply irrelevant for clinical decision making and will necessarily result in the over-treatment or under-treatment of millions of individuals deemed to be in one category or another simply because their body weight divided by the square of their height happens to fall below or above a rather arbitrary cut-off.[335]

Perhaps the discussion about the foods we eat needs to be less about calories and our BMI and more about the content of what we eat. We must strive for individual wellness, not government-mandated numbers. Wellness, which includes good physical health, should be each individual's goal. It must be individually nurtured, not uniformly impressed.

Wellness requires choice and participation by election. To try to achieve some ideal without any respect for the individual situation, while perhaps expedient, is ultimately poorly conceived. It is of the utmost importance to strive for metabolic health as opposed to simply targeting a BMI number through blind caloric restriction. And then assuming that magic number somehow universally confers health and wellness upon an individual. Health and wellness cannot be measured by just stepping on a scale.[336] You cannot simply quantify your way to good health.

Neither can it be achieved through imbalance. Most dietary programs tend to focus on exclusion. There is a single bad guy to blame. Eliminate the offender, and weight loss and good health return like Forrest Gump reruns on TBS. There are low-fat, low-carb, high-protein and all manner of approaches based on some form of restriction. Despite any initial weight loss success, such programs based on constraint of certain food groups ultimately fail. Only 17 percent of people maintain 10 percent of the weight loss for greater than one year. That number is optimistic; it is likely considerably less. Regardless, it is estimated that over five years over 95 percent of such diets fail to maintain the initial weight loss. Many of these folks end up weighing more than when they started.

More importantly, such limiting approaches have metabolic consequences. A remarkable study examined three popular tactics.[337] There was a low fat–high glycemic approach. This is the typical low-fat diet scenario. There was a low fat–low glycemic approach. This is the typical low-glycemic, reduced-carbohydrate diet. Finally, they examined a very low carbohydrate approach. This reflects an Atkins type diet.

The participants consumed the same number of calories on each diet. They also rotated between the various diets with a washout or stabilization period between each of the differing methods. The only variable was the composition of the diet. But the dietary composition of the macro and micronutrients affects a myriad of metabolic and hormonal pathways.

The researchers measured the resting energy expenditure (REE). This is the equivalent of your basal metabolic rate. It is the baseline energy you require to function. They examined the total energy expenditure (TEE). This is how much energy you burn in a day including what you use for various physical activities.

They measured serum leptin, the hormone released from adipose tissue that burns fat and suppresses hunger. They measured cortisol levels, a stress steroid hormone and elevated levels correlate with the deposition of belly fat. They also measured thyroid hormone levels, which correlate with the metabolic state of the body.

They examined markers of metabolic syndrome, a pre-diabetic inflammatory condition and associated with the diseases of modern civilization. Finally they measured C-reactive protein (CRP), a marker of the body's inflammatory state. The higher the CRP, the more generalized inflammation is occurring.

The results would mind-freak Criss Angel.

The drop in resting energy expenditure and total energy expenditure was greatest in the low-fat group. The drop in thyroid hormone was also greatest in this group. This suggests that a low-fat diet acts to shut the body's metabolism down. Without adequate fat intake the body goes into starvation mode slowing down the entire body's functioning. Not what you are looking for if you want to burn calories and lose weight. People suffer through workouts to kick up their metabolism; no one wants their diet to shut it down.

The least effect on the REE, TEE, and thyroid was observed with the Atkins diet. Awesome! That must be the answer. Except the Atkins diet resulted in the greatest increase in cortisol. Since that stress hormone is associated with increased deposition of the dangerous belly fat we would want to stay away from that. We want to stay away from the Atkins approach because it was particularly associated with the greatest increase in CRP. That indicates that this dietary method caused the greatest overall inflammation. The low-fat diet recorded the lowest CRP levels. That sounds enticing until you realize that the low-fat diet also had the greatest increase in markers of metabolic syndrome. No one wants to diet and sacrifice only to suffer from the diseases of modern civilization. We need to strive for more than leaving a good-looking and fit-appearing corpse.

The strictly low glycemic index approach remained mediocre, consistently intermediate in effect. It was neither best by any measure nor worst. But every approach had some effect of the body's state of inflammation and metabolism.

The authors conclude that this type of information should "challenge the notion that a calorie is a calorie from a metabolic perspective" (p. 2632).[338]

That is when it comes to food; a calorie is not a calorie is not a calorie. The calorie is a fallacy. The BMI is misdirection. There is no salvation in deprivation.

Fats: Displaced and Dissed

Over half of the caloric energy in the typical modern Western diet comes from refined grains, refined sugars, and refined vegetable oils.[339] If you're smirking with self-satisfaction that you don't eat any of that stuff as you wipe the mayo from your whole wheat sandwich off the page: just hold on there, Jared. Many of these grains, sugars, and oils are further processed and combined into various baked goods, breads, cereals, snack foods, soft drinks, desserts, condiments, and salad dressings. These are the Trojan horses at the gate, and in your mouth.

A greed for fats and the ability to procure them enabled the success of the human species. Since the onset of the Industrial Revolution the consumption of added fats and oils has increased. The increase has been particularly substantial over the last sixty-five years or so. But these ain't your great, great grandmother's fats and oils. Despite the conventional wisdom that the increase in fats and oils is primarily due to more butter and burgers, the fats plead to disagree.

Paula Deen notwithstanding, this increase reflects mostly refined vegetable oils. Although the category of fats does contain butter and meat, the average per capita consumption of butter in the US has remained fairly stable since the 1970s at about four and a half pounds per person. That is about a 50 percent reduction since 1950. Likewise, the use of lard and beef tallow has decreased 57 percent since 1950. It represents only about six pounds per capita in the US. Over the last half-century Americans have consumed less butter, lard, and tallow during the same time period the diseases of modern civilization have continued to plague us with an ever-increasing intensity.

The increase in added fats and oils has been primarily driven by the increase in refined plant-based oils. Prior to the Industrial Revolution, meat, poultry, and seafood served as the primary dietary source of fats and oils. However, in just over the last fifty years starting in roughly 1950, there has been about a 60 percent increase in the consumption of salad and cooking oils. This is a reflection of an increase in the consumption of fried foods, snack foods, salad dressings, mayonnaise, and sweet baked goods.[340] This category now accounts for a greater percentage of per capita fat consumption than meat and poultry.

The main source of fat in the average American's diet doesn't come from eating a steak. It can be found in the deep-fried croutons that swim in the artificially flavored salad dressing that covers up a limp offering of vegetables. It is found in the sweet baked rolls that sit in the basket next to the salad. The presumption of a meal like this as a healthy choice is wrong on more levels than Ben Affleck as Batman. Unfortunately, this US dietary trend mirrors those seen in other industrialized countries around the world.

Prior to the Industrial Revolution and the development of mechanically driven steel expellers, most oils made from vegetables or seeds were produced by the rendering and pressing methods. These are the same labor-intensive methods humankind has been using for at least the last six thousand years.[341] Such factors made the widespread use of vegetable oils prior to the Industrial Revolution, with a few exceptions like olive oil, less commercially viable. The modern industrial methods utilizing steel expellers or the more recent hexane extraction process allow the production of vegetable and seed oils on an industrial scale. Vegetable and plant oils, like HFCS, are now about as hard to come by as a Gordon Ramsay expletive.

Prior to the Industrial Revolution there were no hydrogenated vegetable oils. It was just over one hundred years ago, in 1897, that vegetable oils were first solidified utilizing the process of hydrogenation.[342] This process introduced trans-fatty acids (TFAs), particularly trans-elaidic acid, into the food chain in significant quantities.[343] Trans-fatty acids are rarely found in unmodified natural foodstuffs. Vaccenyl acid and conjugated linoleyl acid are the two naturally occurring trans-fatty acids found in extremely small concentrations in food products derived from ruminants. They occur at levels less than 0.1 percent. A natural diet does not contain any significant amounts of TFAs. The modern Western diet produces TFAs like the Kardashians produce late night video fodder, which is to say way too much, way too often, and way too personally in your face.

Although it was appreciated at the time by some that the creation of such items was wholly unnatural, the science of the time could find no fault. These concerns over the effects of consuming hydrogenated oils were voiced as early as the first part of the twentieth century. However, it was not until the 1990s that enough scientific evidence accumulated to support the discontinuation of their use. Even then, it was 2006 before the FDA required any labeling regarding trans-fatty acids.

Trans-fatty acids, virtually unknown in the human natural food pathways before the Industrial Age, have now been recognized as a significant dietary source contributing to disease and disability. It is increasingly recognized that consumption of significant amounts of these types of compounds lead to the creation of a chronic low-grade pro-inflammatory state within the human body.

It took over a century from their creation for science and government to figure out eating lots of stuff not found in natural food wasn't such a good idea. Leaving containers of trans fat–rich margarines out on a hot summer's day will result in a puddle reminiscent of hamster urine. But where natural food such as butter would attract insects and other animals eager to consume it, nothing will touch this stuff. For all our superior intellect and technological achievement it took more than a hundred years to ascertain it might not end well if you fancy the completely unnatural.

Yet, people still may be unwittingly consuming trans-fatty acids despite current regulations and their best intentions. The present labeling requirements may be misleading with respect to consumption. Think you can eat all you want because the label reads "No Trans-Fats"? Think again.

Based on current recommendations, if a serving of food contains less than 0.5 g of trans-fatty acids the label is legally allowed to read no trans-fats. *Any* food containing hydrogenated vegetable oils is likely to contain *some* amount of trans-fatty acids. The key here is the serving size, which is whatever the manufacture decides it should be.[344] A serving size may be five snack chips. If each serving size contains 0.49 g of trans-fatty acids, the label can read no trans-fatty acids. Eat ten chips and you consumed 0.98 g of trans-fatty acids. Current guidelines recommend no more than 1.11 g of trans-fatty acids per day. Eat another five chips you've blown your trans-fatty wad.

The second-largest contributor to fats and oils in the modern Western diet comes from the consumption of meat, poultry, fish, and seafood. Like many of the other foodstuffs discussed, meat has undergone a significant qualitative change over the last two hundred and fifty years.

Prior to about 1850, the vast majority of US cattle were raised on pasture, allowed to range freely, and brought to slaughter somewhere between four to five years of age.[345] This is how the majority of meat and poultry had been produced since the Agricultural Revolution. The aftereffect was to have meat that in composition resembled that of wild game.

Like many other things, both our food and our food pathways were forever changed by the Industrial Revolution. One of the great impacts of the Industrial Revolution was not only its direct effect on foods and food production with technological innovations such as mechanical rollers and steel expellers, but also its incredible effect on transportation. The effect of transportation forever altered the food pathways of the modern world.

The Industrial Revolution brought with it the steam engine and the mechanical reaper. The mechanical reaper changed the face of grain harvesting and utilization by substantially increasing yields. The steam engine became the railroads that revolutionized transportation during the nineteenth and twentieth centuries. The combination of improvements in the grain harvest and the ability to ship both grain and cattle forever reshaped commercial meat production. The modern practice of feedlots and fattening, of slaughterhouses, warehouses, and distribution had been born. By 1885 in the US, the average age of slaughter for beef cattle was reduced to about two years.[346] The meat of younger animals produced by this method exhibits the familiar marbling pattern found in contemporary mega-market beef. The marbling is the result of excessive fat between the muscles. This beef tends to have a higher concentration of SFAs and a higher ratio of omega-6 fatty acids to omega-3 fatty acids compared to wild game, pasture, grass-fed, or free-range beef.[347,348] By the 1950s, the familiar modern feedlot factory had become the norm. Today, a twelve hundred pound steer with 30 percent body fat can be brought to slaughter in just fourteen months.[349,350] Although unheard of just two hundred years ago, 99 percent of the beef consumed in the US is now produced utilizing this factory grain-fed feedlot method.[351] Choice is an illusory stage show to distract the masses into believing it truly exists.

In the 1970s there was an aggressive campaign to reduce the percentage of fat, and particularly saturated fat, in the American diet. By all accounts, this campaign has been successful. However, this has had no impact on reducing the disabilities and diseases of modern civilization. In fact, it may have had quite an unintended effect.

Taken as a class there is significant evidence that saturated fatty acids do not increase the risk of cardiovascular disease, including the risk of stroke or heart attack.[352,353,354,355,356,357, 358,359] Much of the study of fats, and particularly saturated fats, has focused solely on their impact on blood lipoprotein levels. This is then extrapolated to increased rates of disease. It has not examined the results of manipulations and substitutions in the complex web of interactions and processes that occur within our body and in which fats play such a pivotal role.

It seems not so much the class or even amount of fat *per se* that is consumed, but the ratios and specific types of fats; the quality is the vital variable. Combine the character of the fat with the total energy intake; add in the reduced energy expenditure associated with a modern, more sedentary existence, and your equation begins to yield obesity, disease, and disability. When you sit all day and pop enough chocolate-covered yodels to fill a Slim Whitman album the problem isn't just the saturated fat—or your glands.

After over fifty years of research, there is no strong evidence that consuming a diet low in saturated fat helps anyone live any longer or any better.[360] Both Julia Child and her husband Paul lived a healthy life until they passed at ninety-two years of age. Both consumed a typical French diet, rich in fresh and wholesome natural foods as well as saturated fat. The traditional French diet has anywhere from 37 percent to 42 percent of the dietary energy derived from fats and about 16 percent derived from saturated fat. It is higher in both total fat and saturated fat than the modern Western diet. However, the traditional French diet demonstrates cardiovascular morbidity and mortality at a fraction of what is seen in those consuming the standard American fare.[361,362]

A study funded by the National Institutes of Health (NIH) re-examined the data from the Sydney Diet Heart Study, which was conducted from 1966 to 1973.[363] This new analysis was published in the *British Medical Journal* in 2013. The original study examined 458 men who had experienced a heart attack or other coronary event. The study group had the saturated animal fats in their diet replaced with polyunsaturated fats from corn, sunflower, and safflower oils. All of these are potent dietary sources of linoleic acid, the dietary source for omega-6 PUFAs.

The group consuming more polyunsaturated fatty acids from vegetables had a 16 percent rate of death from heart disease. The group eating saturated fats from animal sources had a 10 percent death rate. These differences were statistically significant.[364] A possible explanation is that because omega-3 and omega-6 fatty acids interact, high ratios of 6:3 can result in a pro-inflammatory state and lead to worse health outcomes. Yet the conventional wisdom remains to replace all saturated fats, particularly animal fats, with vegetable-derived oils. Substituting the unnatural for the natural in our diet is playing with a nutritive Ouija board; you just may regret who you invite to the party.

The AHA's current guidelines recommend that most people consume at least 5 percent of their total daily calories from omega-6 fatty acids. However, the clinical benefits of the omega-6 poly-unsaturated fatty acids like linoleic acid have yet to be established. There is also increasing evidence that high ratios of omega-6:3 can result in a pro-inflammatory state. Current blanket recommenda-tions that most people consume at least five percent of their total daily calories from omega-6 fatty acids and replace saturated fats with oils high in PUFAs, in the words of Philip Calder, professor of nutritional immunology at the University of Southampton, "may be misguided."[365] The answer lies in proper ratios and balance, not exclusion and excess.

The type of fats, or the quality, in the diet makes a critical dif-ference. Replacement of just 1 percent of the dietary energy derived from refined carbohydrates with *saturated* fatty acids such as lauric, myristic, and palmitic acid increases both LDL and HDL cholesterol and therefore has no significant impact on the LDL to HDL ratio; a potent measure of cardiovascular risk.[366] However, the reduction of the refined carbohydrates can have dramatic and positive health benefits. This is in keeping with other studies that have shown that the types and ratios of fats consumed are more important than rela-tive and absolute amounts.

Lauric acid, a medium chain fatty acid commonly found in coconut oil, actually decreases the total cholesterol to HDL ratio compared to a similar diet where carbohydrates are eaten instead of the fat.[367] Eating this saturated fat produces a blood lipoprotein level associated with less cardiovascular risk compared with a similar diet with less fat. Eat more fat, even more *saturated* fat, and reduce your cardiovascular risk. It's a fat, fat world.

Stearic acid, commonly found in animal fat, does not have any appreciable effect on LDL or HDL cholesterol levels. Second verse, same as the first; please repeat: stearic acid, commonly found in *animal fat*, does not have *any appreciable effect* on LDL or HDL cholesterol levels. In theory, replacing just 10 percent of the dietary energy derived from refined high-glycemic index type carbohydrates with energy derived from omega-3 and monounsaturated rich fats such as grapeseed, olive, or soybean oil would significantly improve the total cholesterol to HDL cholesterol ratio.[368] This, in theory, would significantly reduce the risk of cardiovascular disease. This, in plain English, means less heart disease by eating more fat.

This may be due in part to the fact within the groups of saturated fatty acids, monounsaturated fatty acids, and polyunsaturated fatty acids it appears that further specificity is required. It is not just the class of fat, but the specific type of fat that may be most important. Mounting scientific evidence suggests that the specific type of fat consumed is of much greater import than the absolute amount.[369]

Since the Industrial Revolution there has been a continuing displacement of saturated fat for increasing amounts of polyunsaturated fats. With respect to the polyunsaturated fatty acids there is accumulating evidence that the proper ratio of n-6 omega to n-3 omega PUFAs may be one of the keys to maintaining health and decreasing the risk of developing chronic disease.[370,371,372]

Diets associated with a low intake of n-3 omega PUFAs have been associated with an increase in markers of inflammation.[373] It is interesting to note the observational correlation between low levels of EPA and DHA and the high incidence of depression associated with the adherence to a modern Western diet. Patients with depression tend to have low EPA and DHA levels and an elevated omega-6 to omega-3 ratio.[374] In rats, low levels of omega-3 PUFAs are associated with increased turnover of serotonin[375]—the natural happy juice that drugs such as Paxil, Lexapro, Zoloft, Celexa, and other selective serotonin reuptake inhibitors (SSRIs) keep floating around in your noggin.

Consuming a diet that is excessively rich in omega-6 PUFAs can displace other fatty acids and tilt the omega-6 to omega-3 ratio into the unfavorable range. Conversely consuming fats, which are rich in the omega-3 fatty acids such as EPA and DHA, can have positive effects on endothelial function, blood pressure, and triglyceride levels, and have anti-thrombotic, anti-atherosclerotic, and anti-inflammatory effects.[376,377,378] Fats such as these may reduce the development of abdominal obesity, type 2 diabetes, and other inflammatory conditions including the neurodegenerative disorders such as Alzheimer-type dementia, Parkinson disease, ALS, multiple sclerosis, and depression.[379,380]

With the onset of the Industrial Revolution it became feasible to commercially produce plant-derived oils from seeds and vegetables. Most plant-based oils have an inherently high n-6 to n-3 omega PUFA ratio. This is because a majority of the plants that are used to supply vegetable oils are rich in linoleic acid (LA), the primary dietary source of omega-6 PUFA.

The majority, and an ever increasing percentage, of the fats and oils in the modern Western diet are derived from LA-rich vegetable and seed sources, which displace the saturated fats and the n-3 omega PUFAs in favor of the n-6 omega PUFAs.[381] This can result in chronic inflammation and lead to disability and disease.

The situation is only exacerbated by the consumption of modern meats with their altered fat profile. Modern industrial meats tend to have a significantly elevated n-6 to n-3 ratio. Fresh grass-fed, naturally raised meat similar to what would have been consumed prior to the Industrial Revolution tends to have a lower omega-6 to omega-3 ratio, resembling more the ratio found in meat from wild game.[382,383]

It is not just the meats that are out of kilter. There's been an entire dietary shift in the omega-6 to omega-3 ratio. At the same time there has been increased consumption of omega-6 linoleic acid (LA) there has been decreased consumption of omega-3 PUFAs such as eicosapentaenoic acid (EPA) from fresh vegetable sources and docosahexaenoic acid (DHA) from marine sources. The overall result is a much greater consumption of omega-6 compared to omega-3 PUFAs.

The typical Western diet as a whole tends to have a ratio of omega-6 to omega-3 exceeding 15-16:1 or higher.[384] This high ratio is consistently found in countries with a high incidence of cardiovascular disease.[385, 386] While the ideal ratio is unknown, estimates place it in the 1:1 or 2-3:1 range.

This is comparable to the ratio found in the diets of contemporary hunter-gatherer and pre-Industrial Revolution societies, where it is estimated to be between 2:1 and 3:1.[387,388] Within these groups the diseases of civilization, so prevalent among those consuming the modern Western diet, are absent or lacking. Among the Japanese, who have one of the longest average life expectancies on Earth, the range is typically 4-8:1.

From the 1970s to the present, Americans heeded the warnings and advice of government and health care experts to reduce the percentage of fat, especially saturated fat in the diet. Over roughly the same time period, Americans also heeded similar advice that is likewise still widely disseminated; they decreased their daily cholesterol intake from around 700 mg to less than 300 mg per day.[389] Despite this, there's been minimal, if any, appreciable impact on the risk of developing of heart disease. Other disabilities and diseases of modern civilization such as diabetes continue to increase at a terrifying pace.

Cholesterol, necessary for proper health, is a critical component of every cell in your body. It is essential for the proper integrity and function of cell membranes. It is required for the production of many different hormones such as estrogen, testosterone, and vitamin D.[390] Cholesterol is necessary for proper digestion of dietary fats. Cholesterol plays a major role in our nervous system by ensuring proper nerve transmission. Without cholesterol, we don't live.

How does *dietary* cholesterol enter the fray? Dietary cholesterol is like a third string backup to Peyton Manning—it just doesn't get much playing time. Although it is somewhat dependent on genetics, in general dietary cholesterol does not play a major role in determining cholesterol levels.[391] People end up not eating butter or eggs because they fear the saturated fat and cholesterol. But losing the butter does not result in a reduction in blood cholesterol levels.[392] Neither does avoiding or replacing the eggs.[393] That is why professional organizations such as the American Heart Association ultimately had to retract its egg ban. Eggs are now considered part of a healthful diet. The lack of a significant dietary effect on cholesterol levels is why statins are such a big business, although many attribute their beneficial effect not to a direct effect on cholesterol reduction but on their anti-inflammatory effect.

Despite all the hoopla and expert marketing, the fact remains that our cholesterol levels are not primarily determined by the amount of cholesterol we ingest. Of greater impact on blood cholesterol levels are the consumption of certain saturated fats and the consumption of trans-fats.[394] The consumption of trans-fats has been shown to unequivocally contribute to higher blood levels of LDL cholesterol and to accelerate and facilitate the initiation of the atherosclerotic process.[395]

Any manipulation of a system, whether by addition or subtraction, invokes to some extent the Law of Unintended Consequences—with possibly negative outcomes. Hormone replacement therapy (HRT) for post-menopausal women was based on the extrapolation of the desirable effects these hormones had on blood pressure and cholesterol levels (sound familiar?). It is no longer routinely prescribed today due to the serious increased risks of heart attacks, breast cancer. and strokes associated with this therapy.

The conventional wisdom and approaches to weight loss and the purported healthy practice of replacing saturated fat in the diet with carbohydrates, particularly high glycemic carbohydrates, is wrong. The equally fallacious extrapolation that all vegetable oils or mono and polyunsaturated fats are good and that all animal or saturated fat is bad likewise needs to be purged from the public psyche.

Think about that next time you want to pass up the grass-fed steak, fresh veg, and potato with real butter for some industrially processed deli meat held together with guts and gluten piled high on a refined white flour sub roll drowning in some artificially flavored sauce resembling more a bloody bowel movement than a superior salutary choice. "Eat fresh," hardly.

Sugars and Carbohydrates: Lies, Lies, Sweet Little Lies

Following the Agricultural Revolution, absolute sugar consumption changed little. People still consumed large amounts of vegetables, although a portion of the carbohydrates now came from cereals and grains. Sugar consumption would have continued to wax and wane with the seasons. Most sweet treats would have come in the form of cyclically available fruits and additional sweeteners such as honey.

With the dawning of the Industrial Revolution, there was little initial change with respect to sugar consumption. The granulated crystalline form of sucrose, which had been around since about 500 BCE, [396] would have been somewhat more accessible with the colonial spread of successful sugar cane plantations into the West Indies, India, and other places. Despite this increased production, sugar remained expensive even after the onset of the Industrial Revolution. It was white gold for the pirates of the Caribbean, not because they had a sweet tooth but because it was valuable, and because rum is made from the sugar cane leftovers.

In 1815 the average per capita refined sucrose consumption was only about 6.8 kg per person in Great Britain. By 1970, that had risen to 54.5 kg.[397] In the US refined sugar consumption was a similar 55.2 kg per person in 1970. In the ensuing thirty years it rose to 68 kg per person—almost a 20 percent increase.[398] This drastic increase in sugar consumption has occurred over only about the last one hundred years, with the biggest spike in the last fifty. Today sugar seems to be the principal hidden ingredient within the modern Western diet. It is the *sweet* in the *sweet meat* that describes typical American fare. Sugar borders on its own food group.

In addition to devouring more sugar, during this time period there has been a significant qualitative change in the type of sugar consumed as well. Sugar remained a relatively expensive commodity up until the 1970s, when high fructose corn syrup (HFCS) was introduced as an extremely cheap alternative to pure crystalline sucrose. It has become the crack ingredient of processed foods.

High fructose corn syrup is a deadly cheap and ubiquitous mixture of the two simple sugars, fructose and glucose. It is utilized in mainly two liquid forms. HFCS 42 (42 percent fructose) is the form most often found as an additive to foods and baked goods. HFCS 55 (55 percent fructose) is the form most often used to sweeten beverages.

Since its introduction into the food supply, HFCS has contributed an ever-larger portion of the sugar consumed. The availability of such an inexpensive sweetener has facilitated its dissemination in a number of products as well as eased any quantitative restrictions. Corn-derived sweeteners now account for an almost 10 percent greater per capita consumption than sucrose in the US, and similar trends exist in other industrialized nations.[399] In other words, not only has the overall consumption of sugar exploded, but also corn-derived sweeteners are the predominant type of sugar consumed.

The why is in the dollar. HFCS made using sugar cheap. It costs next to nothing to supersize your sugary soft drink using HFCS. It costs nothing to add a little subliminal sweetness to your hamburger bun. It costs zilch to make those condiments and salad dressings turbocharge your taste buds and dial up your sweet zone pleasure.

Because of the massive quantities consumed, HFCS has introduced a volume of fructose into the modern Western diet that has never before been encountered. A diet high in fructose is associated with potential ill health effects such as hyperlipidemia, obesity, and insulin resistance that may lead to the development of diabetes and cardiovascular disease.[400]

There are also differences in the way sucrose and HFCS are metabolized. When human beings ingest sucrose, insulin is released along with the hormone leptin, which is released from fat cells.[401] The net result of this is to induce satiety and make you feel pleasantly full. It is why dawdling over small dessert can help you leave the table completely fed up, but in a good way— at least until the check arrives.

The consumption of foods sweetened with HFCS produces the opposite effect. It acts to reduce insulin and leptin levels.[402] By potentially not shutting down the hunger drive, the consumption of HFCS-rich foods leaves the door open for rampant overconsumption. A diet high in fructose can facilitate the development of insulin resistance, a hallmark of type 2 diabetes.

This is because not all carbohydrates, sugars, or even simple sugars are created equal. Fructose is metabolized via a different sugar pathway from glucose. As previously noted, unlike glucose, when you consume fructose it does not stimulate insulin secretion. Because of its unique metabolism, it has a number of distinctive physiologic effects.

Chief among them, fructose has an ability to affect the composition of fats. It does this by causing a shift in the balance from oxidation to esterification of non-esterified free fatty acids in the serum.[403,404] It stops you from burning fat.

When you decrease your fat metabolism, you increase your fat storage. Also unlike glucose, fructose metabolism occurs primarily in the liver. These differences may contribute to the observation that meals high in fructose attenuate the normal postprandial suppression of ghrelin.[405]

Ghrelin is a hormone that acts to increase hunger and drives us to eat. Ghrelin is the hunger gremlin. Fructose hurts us two ways. First, fructose does not shut off the normal hunger response that got us eating something in the first place. Secondly, it hits the mute button on the satiety response. You pop all the energy-dense, nutrient-poor calories you can into your cakehole to the tune of "I can't get no satisfaction." Fructose turns us into a modern day tubby Tantalus.

There is none of the natural packaging that occurs in fruits and other natural sources of fructose when HFCS is added to processed, pre-prepared, and prepackaged foods as a cheap sweetener. This has more than weighty implications. Those who consume fructose from sources like fresh fruit versus consumption from added sugar sources like HFCS in soft drinks suffer less hypertension. Consuming just over two 20-oz. HFCS-sweetened colas[406] per day increases the risk for blood pressure greater than or equal to 160/100 mmHg by 77 percent.[407] That blood pressure can turn into a real stroke of bad luck.

When fructose or HFCS supplies at least 25 percent of daily calories, risk factors for coronary heart disease such as triglycerides, LDL ("bad") cholesterol, and apolipoprotein B will rise significantly.[408] Reducing intake can reduce cardiovascular risk factors. In people with hypertension who also consumed a significant amount of sugar-sweetened beverages, reducing their intake by just one 12-oz. sugar-sweetened beverage per day yielded great benefit. They lost weight and reduced their blood pressure in excess of that expected from weight loss alone.[409]

Just because the current HHS/USDA recommendations allow an opportunity for up to 25 percent of daily calories to come from such sources as HFCS-sweetened beverages doesn't make it a good idea. The FDA also allows thirty fly-eggs per 100 g of pizza sauce.[410] The pizza and soda deliveryman might as well be Freddy Krueger in a chef's jacket.

The increasing consumption of sugars over the last fifty years mirrors the increase in such diseases of modern civilization as type 2 diabetes.[411] Other diseases of modern civilization such as hypertension and metabolic syndrome have been associated with the corresponding consumption of sugar-laden drinks. The incidence of these conditions can be reduced by simply reducing the amount of sugar-sweetened beverages consumed.[412]

Paralleling the increased use of HFCS and the rise in type 2 diabetes is the overall replacement of carbohydrate sources like dietary fiber with refined carbohydrate products.[413] Starting around 1980, there was an increase in the total energy intake of Americans by over 500 kcal per day. In other words, starting around 1980 Americans started to consume significantly more calories per day in addition to consuming a diet qualitatively different from anything mankind had consumed prior to two hundred years ago. About 80 percent of this increase was in the form of carbohydrates, particularly refined carbohydrates.

In 1909 Americans consumed approximately 500 g per day of dietary carbohydrate. Almost 6 percent of that was in the form of dietary fiber. Almost a century later, in 1997, Americans still consumed about 500 g per day of dietary carbohydrate. The amount of carbohydrate that the average American consumes per day has not changed over the last one hundred years. However, almost 40 percent of fiber consumption had been replaced by highly refined carbohydrates such as refined flours, sweets, and food items containing high fructose corn syrup. What has changed in the last one hundred years is the *type* of carbohydrates that are eaten.[414]

The glycemic index (GI) was introduced in 1981. Using glucose as the standard at 100, the GI provides a measure of how quickly a certain food raises the blood sugar, or blood glucose, level. The glycemic load (GL) measures the same effect, but also takes into account the amount of carbohydrate per serving size. The GL attempts to account for both the quality and the quantity of the food consumed, with respect to its impact on rapidly raising blood sugar levels.

While often touted as the ultimate standard by which to craft various diet programs utilizing the proven science of the glycemic index, both the GI and GL are subject to a number of important limitations. Foods within the same category will vary by variety, ripeness, cooking methods, processing, and even the length of time they have been stored.

While both the GI and GL assess the effects in isolation, foods are rarely consumed that way. The combination of foods can have a dramatic impact on blood sugar. Protein and fat in conjunction with carbohydrates as part of a meal tend to effectively lower the GI of the carbohydrate components. This response is also different from person to person, and even in the same person the response can vary daily.

Accepting the limitations of the measure, the GI and GL nonetheless provide a comparative basis by which to examine contemporary foodstuffs. A GI value less than 55 is generally considered low while a value over 70 is considered high. Unprocessed vegetables and fruits generally exhibit low glycemic indices. This state was the primary form in which fruits and vegetables were consumed prior to the Industrial Age.

Conversely, refined sugars and grains tend to be in the high category. This includes foods commonly marketed at the health conscious such as whole wheat bread (GI 71), Cheerios (GI 74), shredded wheat cereal (GI 75), and corn flakes (GI 81). Frosted Corn Flakes? They're Gr-r-reat at inducing a diabetic coma!

Almost 40 percent of the total energy found in the modern

Western diet comes from refined sugars and grains. This is a diet that predisposes us to a chronically elevated hyperglycemic and hyperinsulinemic state.[415] A diet consistently high in such high GI foods results in higher sustained blood glucose and insulin levels compared to a lower GI diet.[416,417] Such a sustained spike in the blood glucose level triggers not only the insulin response, but initiates a sequence of events throughout the entire gastrointestinal tract. This affects us indirectly through our gut microbiome as well as affecting us directly.

The high circulating insulin levels have a direct effect on a key enzyme involved in cholesterol production: hepatic 3-hydroxy-3-methylglutaryl-coenzyme A reductase or, as it is more commonly known, HMG-Co-A reductase.[418] Insulin acts to stimulate this enzyme and causes the liver to make more cholesterol.[419] This is the same enzyme blocked by the popular and profitable class of cholesterol-lowering drugs known as statins.

The effects of such a diet can also increase triglycerides and result in an increase in circulating levels of small dense LDL ("bad") cholesterol. It can have unfavorable effects on the HDL (good) cholesterol.[420,421] These high glycemic diets are associated with hypertension, elevated plasma uric acid[422] and increased markers of inflammation.[423]

Such inflammatory effects include increased oxidative stress, pro-inflammatory cytokine production, protein glycation and disposition towards a pro-coagulant milieu.[424,425,426,427] Such an inflammatory response triggers atherosclerosis.

High glycemic index diets are also associated with insulin resistance, obesity, metabolic syndrome, and the unfavorable lipid profile. If you'll take the high-glycemic road, you will be in the hospital before those who take the low road. And you and your true love will never meet again, on the bonnie, bonnie banks o' Loch Lipitor. A diet that replaces the high-glycemic carbohydrates with high-quality proteins has been shown to mitigate the high glycemic diet effects.[428]

A study prospectively evaluated over fifty-three thousand men and women. The researchers replaced the dietary saturated fatty acid with carbohydrates that had a high glycemic index. What they found was that those folks eating high GI carbs instead of *saturated fats* significantly increased their risk of heart attack.[429] By way of explanation, remove the evil saturated fat from the diet and replace it with processed high glycemic carbohydrates, say like one slice of white bread at a GI of 70,[430] and you are *more* likely to have a heart attack.

The take away message is that the long-standing weight loss and purported healthy practice of replacing saturated fat in the diet with carbohydrates, particularly high-glycemic carbohydrates, is misguided. Your tuna-drowning-in-mayo sandwich on an entire loaf of bread, supersized bag of chips, and a cooler of HFCS sweet tea isn't a healthy choice. It is a down payment on a coronary stent.

The average American now derives around half of their total energy from carbohydrates. Of the remaining half about a third comes from fats, and about 16 percent from protein.[431] Highly processed and refined carbohydrate products, often packing in HFCS sweetness and omega-6 pro-inflammatory vegetable oils, are nutritionally-lacking IEDs: Inflammatory Energy Densities.

The chronically elevated glucose and insulin levels that accompany consumption of these foods lead to insulin resistance and metabolic syndrome—the precursors of diabetes and other diseases of modern civilization.[432,433,434,435] High levels of glucose may likewise initiate an immune response, which may result in conditions like Alzheimer disease and in association with high levels of cortisol it has been shown to directly impair memory. [436] Avoidance when it comes to ingesting highly refined white powdery substances is a pretty good rule of thumb.

Avoiding the carbohydrates by switching to non-caloric alternatives like artificial sweeteners may not lead to any better health benefits. Artificial sweeteners have only existed since the advent of the Industrial Revolution with the development of saccharine in 1879. It was not commonly used until 1917 during World War I when sucrose was in short supply.

Like fructose, artificial sweeteners may confound the normal pathways for fat storage and utilization.

But chronic consumption can have longer lasting and deeper ramifications. Chronic consumption of such artificial constructs can alter normal physiologic responses. They can depress your metabolism and interfere with the regulation of normal sweet-tasting foods.[437] When you eat something sweet, your body is expecting carbohydrates, sugars. A physiologic chain reaction is put in motion to ready the troops for arrival of said comestibles. Defaulting on delivery, time after time, has consequences. Over time, the actual brain response patterns can be altered.[438]

Another important consequence of the way modern foods are

processed, packaged, and pre-prepared is their effect on vitamins, minerals, and other micronutrients. Refined and highly processed sugars contain essentially no vitamins or minerals. Refined seed and vegetable oils are likewise energy sources in the modern Western diet that provide little to no micronutrients. A consequence of consuming diets high in these types of foods is displacement. By consuming foods with little to no nutritional value, nutrient-dense foods, those with significant nutritional value, are displaced from the diet. In searching for the Holy Grail of a scrumdillyicious and nutritious, healthful diet, we are not … choosing wisely.

Comprising over 36 percent of the total energy in typical American diet, refined sugars and vegetable/seed oils cause significant displacement.[439] This creates the opportunity for potential vitamin, mineral, and micronutrient deficiencies. This in turn, of course, opens the door for disability and disease. Such deficiencies can mimic the damage to DNA caused by radiation and may instigate or play a causal role in the development of various cancers.[440] Within the US it is estimated that between 2 percent and 20 percent of the population may not even consume half of the recommended daily allowance of a number of these micronutrients. Despite the promise of easy redemption from supplement manufacturers, there are no such indulgences for purchase. It is easier for a camel to pass through the eye of a needle than for you to replace what you miss in the diet with supplementation.[441,442]

Access to all forms of carbohydrates and sugars is no longer subject to seasonal availabilities, regional access, or economic constraints. These refined carbohydrates and all their synthetic brethren are cheaper and more ubiquitous than at any other point in history. The devil's kiss is sweet to taste.

Salt: Blood, Sweat, and Tears

Without salt there is no life. We can give no blood, there is no sweat, and we can shed no tears. In the early days of prehistory, ancient humans sought out sources of sodium like modern-day herbivores and chimps. When our diet is primarily plant-based sodium becomes an essential supplement. Later, as hunter-gatherers, there was little need for exogenous sodium with the diet rich in animal flesh. If you eat enough meat, you can get all the sodium you need. In some contemporary hunter-gatherer societies where they consume a significant amount of meat, there is very little, if any, additional salt required in the diet.[443]

With the development of the Agricultural Revolution, salt became an intensely valuable commodity. The bulk of the diet was plant-based, with vegetables, cereals, and grains constituting the majority portion. Salt was necessary not only for human health, but also for the health of all the domesticated livestock. Salt was recognized for its health-giving properties. The Roman word for salt, *sal*, is where our word for salt originates. The Roman word derives from *Salus*, the Goddess of Health.

Salt was not only necessary for health, it was necessary for life. Prior to the Industrial Revolution salt was the major method of food preservation. If salt consumption is examined on an expanded timescale, we currently consume less salt compared to historical intakes. The Industrial Revolution with the changes to food pathways by transforming transportation have all but eliminated the dependency on salt for the preservation of foods. The average American currently consumes around 8 g of salt, sodium chloride, or about 3.4 g of sodium per day.[444] This is over 50 percent less than just two centuries ago; and less than 10 percent of what sixteenth-century Swedes likely consumed.[445]

From a broad perspective, we are consuming less salt than we ever have. And the amount has stabilized over the last half-century. However, over the same fifty years there has been a dramatic increase in the incidence and prevalence of hypertension and heart disease.[446] During the same time period the incidence and prevalence of the other disabilities and diseases of modern civilization have likewise reached dire proportions.

If we are currently consuming less salt than at any other time since the Agricultural Revolution and suffering more disease, where have we spilled the salt? What are the sinister demons? What has changed?

One of the major changes to the way we ingest our daily sodium has only occurred in the last fifty to seventy-five years. Our sodium no longer comes solely in the form of sodium chloride, or common table salt. It now comes in the form of a number of preservatives, stabilizers, enhancers, and additives: sodium bicarbonate, sodium ferrocyanide, monosodium glutamate, sodium nitrate, sodium stearoyl lactylate, sodium acetate, sodium acetate, sodium acid pyrophosphate, sodium adipate, sodium alginate, sodium aluminosilicate,

sodium aluminum phosphate, sodium ascorbate, sodium benzo-
ate, sodium bisulfate, sodium bisulfite, sodium carbonate, sodium
carboxymethylcellulose, sodium caseinate, sodium citrate, sodium
cyclamate, sodium dehydroacetate, sodium diacetate, sodium dihydrogen citrate, sodium dihydrogen phosphate, sodium DL-malate,
sodium erythorbate, sodium ferric pyrophosphate, sodium fumarate, sodium gluconate, sodium hydrogen carbonate, sodium hydrogen DL-malate, sodium hydrogen sulfite, sodium hydroxide, sodium
hypophosphite, sodium L(+)-tartrate, sodium lactate, sodium lauryl
sulfate, sodium metabisulfite, sodium metaphosphate, sodium ni-
trite, sodium O-phenylphenol, sodium phosphate, sodium potassium tartrate, sodium propionate, sodium pyrophosphate, sodium
saccharin, sodium sesquicarbonate, sodium stearoyl lactylate,
sodium stearyl fumarate, sodium sulfate ... you get the idea. Sodium
comes in more forms than Bubba Gump shrimp.

The average American diet consists of about 57 percent processed foods.[447] This source contributes approximately 75 percent
to the daily sodium intake.

More than 40 percent of the daily sodium ingested by the average American comes from just ten prepackaged, processed food
sources: breads, cold cuts, pizza, poultry, soups, sandwiches, cheese,
pasta, prepared meat dishes like meatloaf, and snacks.[448] With some
agencies and experts calling for 1,500 mg of sodium as the recommended daily allowance, ordering a healthy turkey sandwich with
two slices of bread and four slices of deli turkey would exceed your
daily allotment coming in at over 1,500 mg for that item alone. That
is without any condiments.

The average American also spends about fifty cents of every
food dollar dining out. Many restaurants, particularly fast food establishments, use prepackaged and highly processed foods. In such
establishments food is not prepared under the auspices of a chef,
with an eye toward taste and quality ingredients. It is assembled by
minimum wage workers for maximum profit. Therefore, a significant
amount of sodium is derived from these pre-prepared sources.[449]
Only about 5 percent of daily sodium intake comes from salt added
to properly season fresh food, as a chef may do. Even if you add
more salt at the table, this would only add about 6 percent to the
daily intake. Another roughly 10 percent is inherent in food itself.
The remaining sodium consumed comes from other sources such
as pharmaceuticals.

In the modern Western diet, non-dietary compounds like pharmaceuticals can be significant contributors to the daily sodium load for certain individuals. There is a bit of irony to taking pills for hypertension, many of which contain sodium in the form of sodium starch glycolate or other forms, when we are told that it is the consumption of sodium that causes hypertension in the first place. A recent study performed in the United Kingdom examined more than a million patients over seven years. Those taking sodium-containing drugs of any type had a death rate 28 percent higher than those who did not.[450]

What is more important than the absolute amount of sodium consumed is the ratio of sodium to potassium. One of the major problems with all the processed, pre-prepared, prepackaged, and preserved foods is not just the added sodium. It is the processing of natural foods that corrupts the sodium-to-potassium ratio found in such natural foodstuffs. The risk of morbidity and mortality increases when the dietary ratio of sodium to potassium is greater than one.[451]

A meta-analysis comprising over a million participants worldwide was performed at Harvard University. They found an increased cardiovascular risk and an increased risk of developing diabetes when highly processed meat products were regularly consumed.[452] Consuming four ounces of fresh red meat (beef, pork, or lamb) each day did not increase cardiovascular risk or the risk of developing diabetes. However, consumption of just two ounces each day of *processed* meats (bacon, sausage, deli meats) increased the risk of a cardiovascular event over 40 percent and the risk of developing diabetes by 19 percent. A study examining almost a half million people worldwide found no increased risk of death, cardiovascular disease, or cancer with the consumption of fresh red meat at any level.[453] But there was a clear relationship between *processed* red meat and cardiovascular disease, cancer, and death.

One of the largest studies to date examining red-meat consumption and stroke risk was performed in Scandinavia. The researchers studied more than forty thousand Swedish men ages forty-five to seventy-nine over ten years.[454] The researchers found that consumption "of processed meat, but not of fresh red meat, was positively associated with risk of stroke."

That increased risk of stroke from processed food was over twenty percent. Dr. Robert Eckel, a professor of medicine at the

University of Colorado and a past president of the American Heart Association (AHA), also noted that the group with the highest intake of processed meat in the Swedish study also had a healthier diet overall, including more fruit, vegetables, and whole grains. Stop and note that: a supposed healthier diet with more vegetables and whole grains and a worse outcome. Dr. Eckel commented that this "suggests that the effects of processed meat may confound the benefit of a heart-healthy diet."[455] Then why award the fast food places that serve it your seal of approval, AHA?

Another study out of Sweden examined ten previous trials looking at data from almost 270,000, examining those who suffered strokes. They found that the higher the potassium intake, the less the risk of stroke.[456] A multi-country study demonstrated decreased all-cause mortality with increasing potassium consumption.[457] A study in the United States examined over 12,000 people for all-cause mortality and cardiovascular risk as part of the Third National Health and Nutritional Examination Survey (NHANES III). What they found was that in over fifteen years the group with the highest risk for heart attacks and death had the highest ratio of sodium to potassium in their diet.[458]

Such findings are a result of the disruption of the natural sodium-to-potassium ratio. But the modern Western diet disrupts this natural ratio not only through the addition of sodium-containing compounds to all the processed, prepackaged, pre-prepared, and preserved foodstuffs. It is not just the loss of potassium when processing meats and seafood. It is displacement. Because refined carbohydrates and added fats continue to constitute an increasing percentage of the US diet, they tend to displace foods such as fruits and vegetables, which are the primary sources of dietary potassium. Even with the fortification of flours, milk, breads, and other similar foodstuffs, you simply cannot match the power of nature's fruits and veggies. Vegetables contain four times the concentration of potassium compared to milk and twelve times the concentration compared to whole grains.

The current fear being mongered about is that prolonged consumption of the high sodium diet could result in hypertension and an increased risk of cardiovascular disease. This is the basis of the current recommendations; although the evidence for positive health outcomes following interventions utilizing strictly a reduction of dietary sodium is lacking.[459,460,461] It seems clear that the focus should be on the restoration of the proper balance. Chasing such meaningless absolutes is like waiting for Godot to come bring you a fruit basket.

This unnatural perversion of the sodium-to-potassium ratio was not present before the modern methods of food production, processing, and packaging. In addition to hypertension and stroke this alteration of the natural sodium-to-potassium ratio has also been associated with kidney stones, osteoporosis, certain cancers, asthma, insomnia, Meniere syndrome, and even a significant increase in the risk of death.[462,463,464,465,466,467,468,469,470,471,472,473]

There is evidence that the modern Western diet with its skewed ratios and displacement of natural foods causes all the ill effects we wish to lay at the feet of a char-grilled scapegoat seasoned with salt and replete with saturated fat and cholesterol. But the disabilities and diseases of modern civilization are not the result of the absolute amounts of salt, cholesterol, or saturated fat we eat—especially when we're consuming less sodium, saturated fat, and cholesterol than ever before. The substantiation that our displacing diet with its emphasis on items like refined carbohydrates and processed meats causes our ills dates back well over a century.[474] Now it is time to seek out the veracious grains amongst the chaff.

Modern Wheat: Separating the Chaff and the Chuff

Although cereal grains have been consumed since Neanderthals were our neighbors, it was not until the Agricultural Revolution that they assumed a staple role in the diet.[475] Even today, within isolated groups of hunter-gatherers, cereals and grains are rarely consumed as a year-round source of sustenance.[476]

The rise of grains to dietary prominence, and particularly wheat, began in the Levant at least ten thousand to thirteen thousand years ago. From that time until the Industrial Revolution, wheat changed little in form and function. That has all changed within the last fifty years. The ancient wheat and the foodstuffs prepared from them are as far removed from what is on the mega-market shelf as Miley is from Mozart.

These ancient grains were substantially different than their modern era counterparts in both their innate attributes and their methods of preparation. From the beginning of their consumption over forty-five thousand years ago until the Industrial Revolution, all grains were stone ground. The ancient stones worked slowly, and unlike modern commercial roller-milling methods, produced very little heat.

With the onset of the Industrial Revolution the method of stone grinding was replaced with modern roller milling methods. These modern commercial methods allow for vast increases in production capacity—which comes at a price. The modern commercial rollers also produce heat, which can oxidize and destroy valuable phytonutrients.

The result of stone grinding is very little oxidation or destruction of the nutrients and other important phytochemicals. The flours also contain bits of the bran and germ as well as the endosperm. These pre–Industrial Age stone ground flours were particularly rich in dietary fiber, essential fatty acids, protein, vitamins and minerals, as well as starch.

Because modern refined flours are devoid of both the germ and bran they are basically just endosperm-derived starches. The highly refined flours of the modern Western diet consist of uniform, particulate endosperm, bereft of any contributions from the germ or bran. They are nothing but refined carbohydrates. Such flours have only existed for the last 250 years or so.[477]

Like hydrogenated vegetable oils, the increased use of refined white flour for bread production at the time of its introduction was resisted. In 1880, May Yates founded the Bread Reform League in London promoting increased consumption of whole-meal bread for nutritional reasons. In 1909 she proposed a minimum standard of 80 percent flour extraction rate. This composition was known as *standard bread*, and is where the modern term standard white bread is derived from.

However, data from the scientific community at this point in history was lacking and experts and critics countered that there was no validity for her claims. Ostracized and ridiculed, she nonetheless persevered. Over thirty years from the founding of the Bread Reform League, May Yates finally received some scientific support. In 1911, Gowland Hopkins's research suggested that standard bread contained "unrecognized food substances" that were essential for health. These substances were later determined to be vitamins.[478]

At this time flour also began to be bleached, a process that makes the flour the familiar white powder we are used to seeing today. Prior to actively whitening the flour with bleaching and oxidizing agents, flour was left to sit for several months. Slow exposure to oxygen would naturally condition the flour.

Dr. Harvey W. Wiley crusaded against bleached flour and other food additives and adulterants of the time. The case against bleaching flour was heard before the US Supreme Court. In 1914 the justices ruled that flour could not be bleached or "adulterated" in any way.[479] However, it was never actually enforced.

Many of the common bleaching agents used in the US are currently banned elsewhere. These whitening agents affect the carotenoid content, or the colored portion, of flour. This in turn affects the nutritional composition of the entire flour. These modern refining processes end up increasing the caloric density by over 10 percent, reducing the dietary fiber by 80 percent and dietary protein by almost 39 percent.[480] Bleached white flour, so omnipresent today, has been commercially produced for less than one hundred years.

The rise in consumption of such refined grains has followed a similar trajectory as that of refined sugars. Refined-grain consumption represents approximately 85 percent of the total cereal-grain consumption in the US.[481] Refined grains contain 400 percent less fiber (by energy) versus whole grains. When people try to compensate by consuming more whole grains, it can be difficult to know exactly what you are getting. The labeling can be deceiving. Many of the modern foodstuffs labeled as whole grain or containing whole grains are actually made from significant amounts, if not a majority, of refined white flour. This is partially because many totally whole grain foods cost more to produce.

It is also because whole-grain foods that contain the bran or germ will contain essential fatty acids. Fatty acids are oils, and oils can oxidize and become rancid. This results in a decreased shelf-life. Flour that is labeled *whole wheat* commonly has over 70 percent of the germ removed in order to increase the shelf life.

Fortified white wheat flour may have some of the micronutrients lost to modern processing added back, but it often contains none of the macronutrients, including the fiber and protein, that are found in the bran and germ. The voluminous consumption of refined carbohydrates, which lack dietary fiber, along with the displacement of fresh fruits and vegetables by refined carbohydrates and added fats and oils, render the modern Western diet a sugary glazed black donut hole of nutrition and dietary fiber.

Fresh fruit contains twice, and fresh vegetables contain almost eight times, the amount of fiber found in whole grains. Fruit and vegetables supply not only the insoluble fiber found in cereals and grains but significant amounts of soluble fiber as well.[482] Fiber is nature's little colon sweeper and keeps our symbiotic gut bacteria healthy and happy.[483,484]

Since the Industrial Revolution these qualitative and quantitative changes to the diet have resulted in an unprecedented dearth of dietary fiber. A deficiency of dietary fiber has been associated with a number of gastrointestinal and circulatory maladies.[485] Diets high in fiber have been shown to alleviate these conditions as well as reduce total cholesterol and LDL ("bad") cholesterol, and to help control caloric intake by facilitating satiety.[486]

The ability to bulk you up notwithstanding, fiber is important for intestinal health by keeping your little bacterial residents in good spirits. Bacteria, like residents of Napa Valley and all of France, love to ferment. When dietary fiber undergoes fermentation by bacteria within the human intestine it produces short chain fatty acids, like butyric acid. Butyric acid, which is also a component of butter, has been shown to be anti-inflammatory and antibacterial, and to help prevent intestinal permeability and potentially the development of colon carcinoma.[487,488,489]

Diets such as those of the ancients or modern hunter-gatherers do not in general contain significant amounts of refined carbohydrates, added fats and oils, refined sugars, or processed foods. They do contain high levels of dietary fiber and they also lack the association with the disabilities and diseases of modern civilization.[490] The standard American diet does not even meet its own recommendations for daily dietary fiber intake.

While the processing methods for cereal grains have substantially changed the character of this comestible over the last two hundred to two hundred fifty years, both the refining and bleaching practices actually predate the arrival of the most commonly grown and consumed wheat species today: dwarf and semi-dwarf bread wheat.

The modern cultivars of dwarf and semi-dwarf wheat were derived in the 1950s from an experimental Japanese semi-dwarf variety known as Norin 10. The new semi-dwarf and dwarf varieties derived from Norin 10 provided significantly increased yields, both by virtue of increased fruit production and increased hardiness.

Wheat naturally grows tall upon a rather slender stalk. The

business end, the fruit that contains the cereal grain sits atop the stalk. If you try to increase the yield, the plant is vulnerable to collapsing under its own weight. These plants are also vulnerable to natural environmental occurrences such as high winds, hail, rainstorms, and the like that can also result in stalk breakage. All of these events can result in significant crop losses.

However, dwarf and semi-dwarf varieties are shorter and sturdier. This platform provides an opportunity for significantly increased yields, both by virtue of increase through production of fruit and increased hardiness. Following their development in the 1950s, they were cultivated worldwide as part of the Green Revolution led by Norman Borlaug from the United States throughout the 1960s. The introduction of these higher-yield cultivars during this time period is credited with saving millions of people around the globe from starvation.

In no small part because of this initial success, by 1999 dwarf and semi-dwarf bread wheat varieties comprised over 93 percent of the global wheat grown.[491] The small remaining percentage of wheat cultivated that is not modern bread wheat is a combination of durum wheat and lesser amounts of emmer, einkorn, and spelt varietals.

The majority of the dwarf and semi-dwarf bread wheat varieties grown today can trace their lineage back to Norin 10.[492] The consequence of this is that the majority of the wheat consumed today, in all its various forms, is from a cultivar that has been in existence for less than seventy years. The dramatic rise in the last fifty years of health issues associated with wheat make much more sense when we realize that it is not we who have changed, but the wheat that is different. Pay no attention to the straw man behind the gluten-free shopping zone; if we only had a brain.

The practice of manipulating wheat is nothing new. The wheat plant has been genetically manipulated for millennia. The ancestors of Norin 10 have been unable to survive in the wild since the Industrial Revolution. During the early 1880s, John Bennett Lawes performed the famous Broadbalk experiments in Rothamsted, England. In 1882, he left part of his wheat crop unharvested. He then monitored its growth year after year as it competed against native vegetation. By 1885 there were only a few spindly, pathetic wheat plants left.

This highlights one of the repercussions of such manipulations. Modern wheat cannot grow without modern agricultural techniques and intensive supplementation. That means massive amounts of nitrogen fertilizers and other chemicals must be added to the soil. The protein content of modern wheat, even when grown under the same conditions, can vary as much as twofold simply as a result of the amount of nitrogen fertilizer applied. There is evidence that the amount and type of fertilizer used with modern wheats not only affects the amount of proteins, but also their expression and types. Genetic manipulation can triple the protein expression as well.[493] But as the saying goes, there is no free lunch, or in this case free sandwich bread.

Modern wheat, along with rice and corn, is one of the "big three" cereal crops. In 2007, six hundred million tons were harvested worldwide.[494] Cereal grains and particularly wheat have become an integral part of modern agriculture's attempts to feed an ever-burgeoning worldwide population. The carbohydrates and proteins derived from wheat and wheat products are a staple for many populations throughout the globe; it is an important protein source for both humans and livestock.

Today there are over twenty-five thousand types of bread wheat propagated to grow across a wide range of environmental conditions.[495] There are varieties that have been selected to grow in drought-prone areas; others to grow in areas of heavy rainfall, while still others are adapted to colder regions or other unique conditions and climes. Still others have been transformed for increased yields.

Recently, in 2013 genetically modified (GMO) wheat was found growing in an Oregon field.[496] As a consequence of such alterations, modern varieties may be more immunogenic and potentially less healthful than more ancient types of wheat.[497,498,499] Most of the starch found in wheat products is digested in the small intestine. Significant amounts of modern wheat's easily digested carbohydrates may rapidly increase the blood levels of glucose. This can cause elevated and persistent levels of insulin to circulate and thus perhaps in this way contribute to the current rise in type 2 diabetes and obesity.[500]

A diet like the modern Western diet, which is very high in the consumption of refined grains, has other potentially serious health consequences. Modern wheat varieties also appear to contain significantly lower amounts of various minerals compared to more ancient varieties.

Modern semi-dwarf cultivars introduced in 1968, when compared to archived grain samples, show significantly less of the essential elements zinc, iron, copper and magnesium. These reductions are significant, ranging from 18 percent to 29 percent.[501] These more ancient varieties may not only contain higher levels of important nutrients and minerals, but they may have higher levels of plant sterols and antioxidants than their more modern progeny.[502]

It has been shown that diets high in refined cereal grains can induce vitamin-D deficiency[503]—itself increasingly being recognized as a significant contemporary health issue of such magnitude that it is referred to as a silent epidemic.

Low vitamin-D levels have been associated with various types of cancer, autoimmune diseases, susceptibility to infection, muscle diseases, osteoporosis, hypertension, insulin resistance, cardiovascular disease, and an increase in all-cause mortality.[504,505,506,507] Diets based on refined cereal grains can also affect the levels of such nutrients and minerals as biotin (vitamin B_7), vitamin B_6, magnesium, calcium, iron, and zinc.[508,509]

Wheat gluten has been correlated with the development of multiple sclerosis, diabetes, psoriasis, immunoglobulin A (IgA) nephropathy, and rheumatoid arthritis.[510,511,512,513,514,515] Gluten is a protein found in wheat and to a lesser extent barley and rye. It is composed of glutenin and gliadin, both of which can vary considerably depending on the particular species of wheat. The gluten from modern wheat is different in composition than the gluten from more ancient species such as durum wheat, although there is obviously some overlap.

Gliadin is the component of gluten believed involved in the majority of celiac sprue, also known as celiac disease (CD) or gluten enteropathy, cases. It has been shown to increase intestinal permeability in susceptible people.[516] Gliadin can also induce a pro-inflammatory state independent of the genetic predisposition to celiac disease.[517,518,519,520]

In persons with CD, the T cells of the immune system end up responding to a specific spot on the gliadin portion of the gluten molecule. A majority of the persons with CD share the human leukocyte antigens (HLAs) DQ2 and/or DQ8, indicating a specific genetic predisposition. Having this genetic weakness is like having an operating system on your computer that is susceptible to hacking. If the computer virus finds the right sequence—weakness—all hell breaks loose. If the gliadin molecule has the right key, it finds the T-cells and causes inflammatory havoc.

More than 95 percent of people with true CD have the HLA DQ2 antigen.[521] If you have a first degree relative with CD, your likelihood of having the disease increases by 10 percent to 20 percent. Having CD nearly doubles your risk of cardiovascular disease.[522] It also increases your risk of abnormal heart rhythms and heart failure. A specific portion or epitope between the glutamine and proline residues of a particular α-gliadin subtype seems to be the primary instigator. This area on the α-gliadin subtype holds the key to the hack.

There are specific epitopes of the alpha gliadin protein that are particularly associated with the development of celiac disease in susceptible individuals. These are known as the glia-α9 and the glia-α20 epitopes. An immunogenic response to glia-α9 is found in a majority of the patients who suffer from celiac disease. Most cases of true gluten enteropathy, CD, are due to a genetic weakness to a part of the gluten molecule that expresses a protein sequence known as glia-α9.

Compared to more ancient varieties the glia-α9 epitope is expressed to a much higher degree in modern semi-dwarf and dwarf wheat varieties.[523] This suggests that the increased utilization and consumption of modern wheat varieties may contribute to the development of increased incidence and prevalence of wheat-related diseases and associated conditions.

The affected individuals' tissue transglutaminase (TTG), a digestive enzyme, reacts with this α-gliadin fraction. The result is a deamidation product yielding peptide byproducts. This occurs as a result of converting the glutamine residue in the α-gliadin subunit of the gluten molecule to a glutamate. In other words, when you eat some wheat products your digestive enzymes break off the chunk of the protein that causes the problem and modify it. It is like activating a computer virus by opening the email.

The CD4+ T cells then release inflammatory cytokines in response to the products of this reaction and the chain of events resulting in true celiac disease are unleashed. However, much like automobiles, gliadins come in a variety of shapes, sizes, and models. Naturally occurring gluten with gliadin components that do not initiate this T-cell mediated reaction (and thus do not exacerbate CD) have been demonstrated.[524,525] Not all wheat gluten is created equally.

The majority of the allergenic epitopes seem to be related to the DD (of the AABBDD hexaploid wheat) genome. The introduction of the DD genome improved the overall bread-making properties of the modern bread wheat varieties of *Triticum aestivum*. None-theless, the cost may have been the introduction of a potentially allergenic protein: an antigen that may be more highly expressed in modern semi-dwarf and dwarf wheat. The immunologic response is a result of the amount of exposure measured both by the quantity and duration.

Paralleling the concern over celiac disease and gluten intoler-ance, there has been an increase in the expression of celiac disease–related T-cell stimulatory epitopes by dwarf and semi-dwarf varieties of modern wheat.[526] In other words, the more modern varieties of bread wheat being grown and harvested may be delivering increased allergens in addition to increased yields compared to their predeces-sors. Not only is the lunch not free, the sandwich bread may kill you.

The prevalence of celiac disease may have increased slightly during approximately the last fifty years.[527,528] This increase corre-lates with the implementation of the Green Revolution in the 1960s and the widespread planting and subsequent domination of wheat production by modern derivatives of the Norin-10 dwarf and semi-dwarf wheats.

Consumption of more ancient wheat varieties that lack the DD genome may allow the enjoyment of grain products and benefits with a decreased risk of inciting celiac disease or gluten intoler-ance.[529] Some studies have shown that the gluten produced by such cultivars as durum wheat does not initiate the inflammatory cascade of celiac disease in some otherwise susceptible individuals.

Although there are an astounding number of different modern wheat varieties, there appears to be a high degree of expression of the celiac disease initiating, T-cell stimulatory epitopes glia-α9 and glia-α20. This may be because genetic study reveals *less* diversity in the modern varieties as compared to the more ancient landraces. In one study that examined thirty-six modern varieties only one ex-hibited low levels of expression of the glia-α9 protein. Data such as this suggests that toxicity of modern wheat has increased. This type of data also suggests that the use of ancient grains such as einkorn, emmer, durum, and related species could yield less toxic side-effects and potentially even superior nutritional value.

It may not be necessary to abandon the consumption of wheat, but simply to vary or change the type of wheat and wheat prod-ucts we consume. Diseases such as CD do not manifest unless you have the genetics and these genetics are exposed in a susceptible environment. You only get a computer virus if your operating system has a weakness *and* it is exposed and acted upon. The diseases of modern civilization depend upon our genetic predisposition and the environment unto which we expose it. The environment where all that happens is the gut microbiome.

The Intestinal Microbiota: Time for a Gut Check

It is critical to understand the importance of the evolutionary perspective in order to comprehend the origin, nature, and ongoing challenges when dealing with modern human health issues. Since our nuclear DNA changes at a rate of about 0.5 percent per million years we remain essentially unchanged from the very first *Homo sapiens* that appeared over two hundred thousand years ago on the East African plains.

Yet our genetic predisposition does not act in isolation; it interacts with our environment. That interface can produce several potential outcomes. The outcomes range from having no appreciable effect whatsoever to resulting in death. In between those two extremes are intermediate changes that may result in disability and disease. Some of these may affect us at a younger age and prevent us from successfully procreating. This is bad from a species-survival perspective, not to mention individual disappointment.

Other outcomes may not impact our ability to reach the reproductive age and reproduce. They may not even affect the overall life expectancy. However, they may significantly impact the quality of health in those post-reproductive years. This potentially negative form of adaption was recorded by Darwin as far back as 1859.[530]

An example of an adaption that may have at one time helped us survive but now has been turned against us is what is called the "thrifty genotype."[531] Until the most recent times, the ability to survive periods of famine conferred a significant survival advantage. In essence, the ability to be metabolically "thrifty", and be extremely efficient in terms of both energy usage and the ability to store energy as fat, endowed a benefit to the individual that could be passed on to their offspring. If you were metabolically efficient, you would store extra energy as fat. With lots of fat in the bank you could weather the lean times, in a very literal way. From a survival standpoint, fat was where it's at.

This genotype that was previously a boon is a curse for obesity in our modern world. We live in a society in which there is little need for physical activity to survive. All around us are endless offerings of energy-dense foodstuffs available 24/7/365. The result is you can plump up faster than the Pillsbury doughboy doing yeast hits.

But it is not the gene *per se* that causes the obesity. If you have those genes in one environment, you survive and reproduce. If you have those genes in another environment, they remove you from your apartment with a forklift. It is not the genes that express the disease; it is the environment.

There is also a similar phenomenon called the "thrifty phenotype."[532] In this instance, malnutrition at particular times during the prenatal period could cause both physical and metabolic changes within the fetus. These adaptions as a response to stressors can predispose it to diseases at a later period in life. Such effects can be seen in the babies that struggle to develop in hostile environments, such as when the mother is a heavy smoker. These babies are often underweight when they are born.

A low birth-weight is associated with the development of coronary artery disease, obesity, type 2 diabetes, stroke, osteoporosis, polycystic ovary syndrome, abnormal vascular compliance, endothelial dysfunction, insulin resistance, compromised hypothermic-pituitary-adrenal (HPA) axis, and schizophrenia in adulthood.[533] Disabilities and diseases such as an increased percentage of body fat, and even areas of fat storage, may not manifest until these children reach adulthood. They may suffer from abnormalities of fat storage, such as preferentially storing fat in the abdominal cavity, abnormalities that are associated with significant health risks much later in life.[534,535] The bill comes home to be paid with interest much later in life, even though the original tab was rung up *in utero*.

From a Darwinian perspective, the intrauterine adaptions allow an organism's individual survival. The adaptions allow the organism to survive and to reach reproductive age. The price that is paid is the development of disease and disability after the reproductive years. This is of little consequence from a species-survival viewpoint. Clearly, as studies with monozygous twins have shown, as we age our environment has a greater and greater impact in the expression of our phenotypes.[536]

Our diet is arguably our most important environmental interaction. One important consequence of the way modern foods are processed, packaged, and pre-prepared is their effect on vitamins, minerals, and other micronutrients. This can have tremendous ramifications with regard to our own internal environment by affecting the composition of our gut microbiome.

Refined and highly processed sugars and oils contain essentially no vitamins, minerals, or micronutrients. However, refined sugars and vegetable/seed oils contribute almost 40 percent of the total energy in the typical American diet and by sheer volume they have significant potential to deracinate more nutrient-dense foods.[537]

This can culminate in disability and disease directly or indirectly resulting from deficiencies of folic acid, vitamin B_{12}, vitamin B_6, niacin, vitamin C, vitamin E, iron, or zinc, to name a few. Many of these deficits can cause pathologies that mimic damage to DNA. These deficiencies also impact the gut microbiome, which depends upon us to deliver the micronutrients needed for bacterial health.

Too often, we only view bacteria in light of infection and disease and seek their eradication with antibiotics. The truth is that is only half the equation. The correct bacteria are necessary for life; they are the *pro-biotics*. Disrupting and decimating them with poor dietary choices does not leave a vacuum. Nature abhors a vacuum. If we create an undesirable internal neighborhood, the less desirable characters will move into it; you will create your own gut ghetto. And like any dangerous neighborhood, you enter at your own peril; the consequences of such intestinal inequity may result in the development of such diseases as cancer.[538]

The acid-base environment also affects the composition of the gut microbiome. As we consume foods and they undergo digestion, absorption, and metabolism they tend to release either acidic or basic components into the systemic circulation.[539,540] The replacement of fresh fruit, vegetables, and other basic foodstuffs has culminated in a diet producing a net acid load of 50mEq per day.[541] An acidic diet can compromise renal function as we age and create a vicious cycle of increasing acidosis. This can also affect which types of bacteria co-habitate within us.

This increasing acidity compounds the problem in the elderly. Such a diet is in contradistinction to the pre-Industrial Revolution diet, which was basic in nature. Such a diet has been demonstrated to aid in the prevention and treatment of conditions that plague our twilight years such as osteoporosis, muscle wasting, kidney stones, hypertension, and asthma. It has also been shown to retard the progression of age-related chronic renal insufficiency.[542,543,544,545,546,547,548,549,550,551]

It is also not just the corruption of naturally occurring compounds that may cause issue. There is a potential for interactions that occur secondary to changes modern foodstuffs may undergo as a result of extreme heating, irradiation, ionization, pasteurization, sterilization, or other forms of food packaging and processing. A number of different compounds, known as advanced glycation end products (AGEs) and advanced lipid oxidation end products (ALEs), have been identified as a result of these types of processes.[552] These compounds have been associated and implicated in the complications related to diabetes.

Although the exact contribution from these compounds is currently an area of intense investigation, it is not thought that these compounds exert a significant effect by ingestion. Oral bioavailability is thought to be extremely low, secondary to poor absorption within the gastrointestinal tract and the fact that these products tend to be resistant to enzymatic or chemical hydrolysis. [553] However, we know little of how they are metabolized or interact with our gut microbiome.

A recent study portended the potentially significant role these compounds may play in manifesting the disabilities and diseases of modern civilization. The Trial to Assess Chelation Therapy (TACT) randomized diabetic patients age fifty and older who had experienced at least one prior heart attack to a regimen involving up to forty separate three-hour infusions of a chelation-therapy solution, disodium ethylenediaminetetraacetic acid (EDTA), ascorbic acid, magnesium chloride, potassium chloride, sodium bicarbonate, B vitamins, procainamide and a small amount of standard heparin (a blood thinner).

Chelation is a process where molecules or compounds bind metal ions. It has been in use since World War I as an effective way to remove potential fatal heavy metals. Certain molecules capture a heavy metal ion and escort it out of the body, reducing or eliminating its toxic effect. Think of it as sending your pup to fetch a ball (that is a metal ion) and Fido grabs it and brings it back, removing it from the field of play

The diabetics who received the treatment experienced an 18 percent drop in the trial's primary end point. The patients receiving the infusion were 18 percent less likely to die, suffer another heart attack or stroke, undergo coronary artery bypass grafting, get a stent placed, or be admitted to the hospital for angina. Despite the remarkable benefit seen in diabetic patients, for patients without diabetes there was no difference in outcomes whether participants received the chelation therapy or not.

"When we broke composite down to look at our secondary end points, we found that we had about a 40 percent reduction in total mortality, a 40 percent reduction in recurrent MI, and about a 50 percent reduction in mortality (in patients with diabetes)," said Gervasio A. Lamas, MD, one of the lead researchers of the study.

Dr. Lamas remarked that many diabetic complications appear to be the result of the accumulation of advanced-glycation end products. AGEs involve metal-catalyzed oxygen chemistry for their formation. As such, chelation of metal ions may prevent manifestations such as cardiovascular disease in diabetic patients.

"The reason this is exciting is—if this is borne out by additional experimentation—it is a way of treating the complications of diabetes that we have simply missed the boat on for decades, not knowing that metal chemistry was needed to form the advanced-glycation end products," Dr. Lamas concluded. [554,555]

The etiology of such chronic diseases involves an exceedingly multifaceted interplay of environmental factors, genetic factors, and complex nutritional factors. Perhaps there is no greater example of this intricate interaction than where it all happens: the human gut microbiotica. The human gastrointestinal tract is the ultimate interface between our genetics and our environment. It is here that the ultimate outcome of what we ingest is tempered by the razor thin microscopic margin of our symbiotic bacterial charge.

It is a population of well over a thousand different species. It is estimated that the number of bacteria in the human gut is over one hundred trillion while we consist of around ten trillion or so cells. Up to 90 percent of the cells within your body are actually intestinal bacteria. Altering upwards of 90 percent of anything can fatally disrupt homeostasis. But fluctuating in between the normal, healthful bowel and acute severe systemic illness lays the slow grind of chronic low-grade inflammation.

One of the potential consequences of being in a state of continuous low-grade inflammation is that a stimulus that might ordinarily elicit only a mild immune response becomes exaggerated. This hyper-inflammatory response is known as the systemic inflammatory response syndrome (SIRS). This is associated with cellular or tissue damage, scarring and fibrosis and can lead to the formation of a type of immune paralysis known as compensatory anti-inflammatory response syndrome (CARS). The characteristic of CARS is badly weakened immune defense system and a susceptibility to infection.[556] Keeping the immune system burning all the time ultimately weakens its ability to respond. Chronic continuous low-level inflammation from an unhealthy gut microbiome may manifest as secondary infections.

Triggered from within the gastrointestinal tract this pro-inflammatory background produces increased oxidative stress, pro-inflammatory cytokine production, protein glycation, and a disposition toward a pro-coagulant milieu throughout the entire body. Inflammation is the mechanism by which atherosclerosis, diabetes, metabolic syndrome, rheumatoid arthritis, inflammatory bowel disease, and other metabolic diseases and injuries are believed to develop.[557,558]

The ongoing inflammation directly affects the gut as well. Gut inflammation leads to detrimental changes resulting in increased intestinal permeability and a repetitive cycle of ongoing, low-grade chronic inflammation.[559,560] Increased intestinal permeability is a condition in which the gut becomes leaky. The normally tight seals between the cells that line the gut no longer seal well. All sorts of compounds including bacteria and toxins then can potentially enter the bloodstream and circulation. It's like opening the Wal-Mart doors on Black Friday with the barbarians at the gate.

Recent evidence suggests that people who suffer with inflammatory bowel disease are more likely to have significant complications from heart attack and stay in the hospital significantly longer. Indeed, just having inflammatory bowel disease is now recognized as a risk factor for having a heart attack.[561] Several different types of gastrointestinal cancers as well as lymphomas have also been associated with this type of injury.[562] These damaging alterations to the normal gut flora reduce the normal bacterial diversity and have also been implicated in the development of obesity by modulating human lipid metabolism.[563,564] These types of distortions have far-reaching implications.

Does our gut microbiome play the key role in the disposition of abdominal fat and the risk of developing the diseases of modern civilization?

Our health status depends not only on the quantity and quality of the food we ingest, but also the time course over which we consume it. The immediate effects are amplified and modified by the time course of cumulative exposure. The Grand Canyon was not made in a day or even a year. It appeared because of the persistent and relentless application of varying forces over time.

Atherosclerosis does not occur in a day; it is the result of years, even decades, of ongoing inflammation. If you eat garbage for twenty-nine days out of the month, eating a salad on one day is not going to buy you much absolution. At any time, an individual can be expressed by his or her metabolic phenotype. This metabolic phenotype is a snapshot in time of where you are and what processes, for good or for bad, are affecting you. Even among people who eat the same exact food, because of baseline genetic differences, their metabolic phenotypes can be quite different. The inter-individual variation to different foodstuffs is extremely high.

There are persons who have a variant lipo-oxygenase genotype. If these people consume high amounts of omega-6 fatty acids they are susceptible to an inflammatory reaction resulting in atherosclerosis of the carotid artery. In contrast, those without the variant do not exhibit significant atherosclerosis independent of the fatty acid intake.[565,566] Two people can live in the same house and eat the same exact diet. If the diet is rich in omega-6 fatty acids and one person has the variant and the other doesn't, one may have a massive stroke and the other no disease. If both eat a diet high in omega-3 fatty acids and low in omega-6, neither has any disease. It is the environment, the diet, which bring the potential for illness to full manifestation.

Everyone has that annoying friend who eats whatever he or she wants and never gains an ounce. It has been found that certain individuals are genetically immune to the effects of a high-fat diet. What this implies is that the consumption of a high-fat diet does not universally lead to weight gain, despite what circulates for dietary law in the media. These individuals habitually consume a high-fat diet and remain lean and are therefore labeled as having high-fat phenotypes. Then there are others who seem to gain weight by breathing and are labeled as having low-fat phenotypes.[567]

We all know this to be true. We see that incredibly annoying friend eat whatever he or she wants. They chow down on insane amounts of food and never seem to gain a pound. Across the table from them, watching them intently while gnawing on nothing more than a carrot stick, wallowing in a pool of his own drool sits our other friend. He seems to gain weight just by thinking about food.

A study examining mice yielded some insight into why findings like this may be.[568] The gut microbiome from four sets of human twins, with one obese and one lean twin, were implanted into certain strains of mice. Half the mice had their guts colonized with the gut flora from a fat twin. The other mice received the gut flora from the genetically identical, but lean twin.

All the mice ate the same food and the same amount. However, the mice implanted with the gut microbiome of obese individuals gained weight. The mice implanted with the gut microbiome of lean individuals remained thin. It was not the calories or even the food that made the mice fat or lean. It was what bacteria grew in their gut. But the food choices ultimately have a large impact on what grows in your garden.

But this is where the tale with the mice gets even more intriguing. Some mice implanted with the obese microbiome were then placed in a cage with the mice implanted with the lean microbiome. All the mice moved into the same apartment and ate the same food. Because mice like to eat each other's feces, every mouse in the house now had a mixed gut microbiome. All the mice stayed lean. That is one golden colon.

Fortunately, for human beings there are other methods short of a poo-poo platter to improve our gut microbiome; although, the concept of a therapeutic turd transplant has actually been going on for many years. Surgeons have long transplanted the gut flora of healthy individuals to treat patients with symptoms of chronic diarrhea. It works. A metabolically healthy gut reduces disability and death.

A less invasive method was recently shown to be quite effective in treating infants with cyanotic congenital heart disease. These are children born with life-threatening heart-defects. They require complex and immediate surgery and often suffer a high mortality from any number of complications.

A group of these high-risk babies were given a specified probiotic cocktail. Those who received the beneficial gut bacteria had an over 35 percent reduction in death.[569] Having a healthy gut and being metabolically healthy kept more of these critically ill infants alive. This held true even when the cause of their high mortality was critical heart disease and the stress of high-risk operations.

A diet that promotes a beneficial gut microbiome and results in low levels of inflammation predicts long-term cardiometabolic health—regardless of your weight or body mass index (BMI) status.

It does not matter if you are overweight or ideal weight; what matters is that you are healthy. And our health starts at the intersection of our environment and our genetics: our gut.

The products of certain gut microbiota have been shown to predict the risk of cardiovascular disease in humans.[570] The atherosclerotic plaques associated with cardiovascular disease have been shown to contain the bacterial DNA of gut microbiota; and the amount of inflammation correlates with the amount of bacterial DNA in the plaque.[571]

Patients with symptomatic atherosclerosis and atherosclerotic plaques were found to have an increased intestinal concentration of bacteria from the *Collinsella* species. Patients without disease were found to have higher levels of the bacteria from *Roseburia* and *Eubacterium* species.[572] All three of these bacterial species are gram-positive types of bacteria. It is possible that certain species like *Collinsella* produce products that initiate an inflammatory reaction.

An initial bacterial product known as a tri-methylamine (TMA) is released into the bloodstream and metabolized in the liver to form a product known as tri-methylamine-N-oxide (TMAO).[573] This compound is believed to cause macrophages, normal infection fighting white blood cells, to form foam cells—one of the earliest markers and initiators of atherosclerotic disease. It is the macrophages that ingest the oxidized the LDL ("bad") cholesterol in the walls of the arteries. They then become known as foam cells and are believed to instigate the inflammatory reaction that ultimately leads to cardiovascular atherosclerotic disease. The way to a person's heart may indeed be quite literally through their stomach.

A study looking at more than four thousand people over three years who underwent elective coronary angiography were followed for the development of a major cardiovascular event like death, heart attack, or stroke. Those with the highest levels of TMAO had over two-and-a-half times the likelihood of having one of those events versus those with the lowest levels.[574] Another byproduct of this same compound can form a cancer-producing nitrosamine under weakly acidic conditions. [575]

Other species like *Roseburia* and *Eubacterium* may produce cardioprotective compounds like beta-carotene and lycopenes.[576,577] The fact that some of the health benefits associated with such compounds may depend on their bacterial production in the large intestine might explain the failure of so many approaches based on simple dietary supplementation. When ingested, many of these compounds may never reach the large intestine intact. Our diet is the single most important determinant in the composition of our intestinal microbiota. And it appears that they may be the single most important determinant in how our genetics are ultimately expressed within the environment we live in.

The short time period over which our diet has been altered from the Industrial Revolution to the present does not allow for genomic adaption. Many of the polymorphisms that are now associated with certain disease states have likely been part of the original human genome. In other words, for the most part the genes that are associated with the diseases of Western civilization do not manifest as such unless they're exposed to the proper environment. It is perhaps more useful to view this genetic and environmental interplay as genes that will manifest in a negative environment. The more conventional approach labels these as disease-causing genes.

As previously discussed, the major interventions that have resulted in an overall increase in average life expectancy have been improvements in engineering and sanitation; reductions in childbirth mortality, childhood diseases, and infections; and success in mitigating the effects of disasters like droughts and famines.[578] It has not been interventions that directly improve us. Human potential longevity remains unchanged from the time of our most distant forebears.

The diseases of Western civilization tend to occur after the reproductive years, and dietary and environmental efforts to address them may not contribute substantially to change the average life expectancy. However they could significantly contribute to a reduction in the last three decades of life that the average American spends with such chronic disabilities and diseases. Such an approach also may potentially significantly decrease overall health-care expenditures.

We no longer have agriculture, a pursuit designed to produce the best possible food product. It has been increasingly replaced since the Industrial Revolution by agro-industry's pursuit to produce the most product and maximize profit. We have been on the short end of the agribusiness and modern food industry stick. It is time for us to reclaim our right to metabolic health. It is time to reverse the curse with our own Intestinal Revolution.

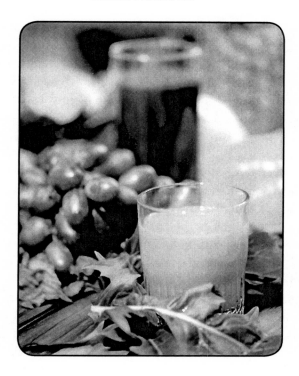

The Program

"My God, What have I done ... How did I get here?"[579]
~"Once In A Lifetime," The Talking Heads

As we waste away in our nutritional desert, we emerge double-dipped and deep-fried with the disabilities and diseases of modern civilization. Unnatural accumulations of visceral adipose tissue, belly fat, are the hallmark of the modern Western diet phenotype. We have become androgynous because male or female, everyone at every age looks a wee bit preggers. We are *Homo sapiens body habitus horribilus*.

On the surface the chronic excess caloric intake and decreased caloric expenditure that results in morbid obesity and subsequent health issues appears a simple fix—just eat fewer calories. Yet, it is anything but simple. Beyond calories-in-versus-calories-out there is underlying metabolic regulation, energy expenditure, physiologic processing by both our bodies and by our individual and symbiotic gut microbiome, sleep cycles, genetics, behavior, and food intake, all affected by both quantity and quality of what we choose to consume.

Among groups there is great inter-individual variation. It is not just that the French eat an entirely different diet than the Eskimos; but within France there is a gamut of cuisines. There is also gamut of opinions about those cuisines. Get a group of your friends together and ask who wants what to eat. You will get a number of different answers, and potentially violent disagreement. Food can be right up there with politics, religion, and sports as topics to avoid in large group conversation.

Within any given environment there can be great intra-individual variation as well. We change what foods we desire on a regular basis. This forms some of the basis as to why restrictive diets tend to fail; they are in opposition to our very nature to seek varied foods and to seek out certain food characteristics. If you want to get people to eat something, just tell them they can't have it.

All this serves to challenge the notion as to what actually constitutes a normal response to food and diet. Many studies have found that the healthiest groups as measured by survival are not those at an *ideal* or *normal* body weight as defined by the BMI, but overweight or in some cases even mildly obese. This questions even the basic premise of what size we should or shouldn't be, let alone what regimen we should or should not follow: a Mediterranean, Japanese, Inuit, low-fat, glycemic index, no-carb, high-fat, liquid-meal-replacement, or screw-it-all-give-me-a-G&T diet?

Given the evolutionary predilections for what constitutes a healthful diet and the incredible variation seen worldwide it begs the question of who should actually set the definition for what is a healthy weight and what is the standard diet.

Who is to say?

Such conclusions, or lack thereof, highlight the fact that ultimately our goal must not be a predefined number achieved at any cost, but improved health and wellness. We must become metabolically healthy. It is imperative to understand that over time genes become adapted to the environment; the environment does not adapt to our genes. We must positively maximize the interaction point of our genes and our environment. That point is our gut microbiota. We need an *intestinal revolution.*

And to achieve that we must start with our food, for a number of reasons and on a number of levels. What you eat is in your wheelhouse and directly wired into your funhouse. That is why eating food is an experience, not just an exercise in subsistence. It is why food comforts us and makes us feel good. Only the soulless consume simply for existence; the tasteless among us are truly the walking dead.

Yet food is also the basis for our very health. You cannot gorge with reckless abandon. You need proper nutrition, although it may not be what conventional wisdom would have you believe. Master this domain, become the captain of your own cuisine and it opens the door for incredible opportunity. And the first port of call for this voyage must be to restore quality into our food making decisions. We must assess food value in terms of quality, as well as quantity.

We routinely assess the value of many things as a function of both quantity and quality. Offered a hundred old five-inch, black-and-white televisions from 1960; or one ninety-inch, internet-ready, super high definition, three-dimensional television; most everyone will choose the one. We understand that the one has more value than the many because the quality component so dramatically outweighs the quantity component in the calculation of value. Yet, when it comes to assessing food value we so often base it solely upon quantity.

While at some unconscious level the extra-large portions are favorably received, it causes us to *consciously* confuse the value—particularly with respect to the quality component—of what we eat with the sheer quantity of how much is stuffed into a take-away bag. During the Stone Age, the more grass-fed, organically raised mastodon you could chow down on, the greater the value; no one was using money and pretty much all the mastodon were the same. Quality was not a variable; meat was meat.

The same principle simply does not apply in today's world where we first have to sort out choices between real food and pseudo-phood. By neglecting quality and equating quantity with value our hardwired individual survival instincts betray us. Customers return again and again innately satisfied with the consumption of mass quantities of industrially manufactured substances. At some point we lose the ability to discern between real food and the food-like products. Eventually, we even lose the ability to taste anything real at all. It all becomes an addiction to satisfy a craving for supersized quantities of sugar, salt, and fat. It is the food equivalent of slurping antifreeze to feed an alcohol addiction.

Properly seasoning the food, vibrant flavors and judicious

spicing also leave an impression of how we perceive a meal. That can ultimately impact how much we eat. The ability to combine smell, taste, and taste sensations increases our dining satisfaction, and we become satisfied with less compared to a bland version of the same meal.[580] Within the brain the areas that control taste, satiety and emotion all overlap. The same areas that respond to the mouth feel, viscosity, odor, texture, and the pleasantness of fat are also associated with satiety and other important physiologic signals.[581,582] It is why sex and food are conjoined twins.

We also respond positively to the taste and textures found in a varied diet; we respond positively to natural variety. The diet upon which *Homo sapiens* evolved and thrived was one rich in vegetables, which provided a much-needed source of the omega-3 essential fatty acid ALA. It was consumed in a natural balance with the omega-6 essential fatty acid LA. The environment yielded terrain rich in dietary sources of other fatty acids such as arachidonic acid (AA), EPA, and DHA. Certain types of saturated fatty acids were consumed in harmony with these mainstays of the diet. There were none of the skewed ratios seen after the onset of the Industrial Revolution and no such things as trans-fatty acids.

It is not rocket science. It is basic biology, literally. Real world evidence continues to accumulate. Within those atherosclerotic plaques—which ultimately manifest as heart attack, stroke, peripheral vascular disease, or other forms of cardiovascular disease—can be found bits of DNA from gut bacteria. This indicates that there is a powerful connection between what we eat, our gut microbiome, our genetics, and the presence or absence of certain disabilities and diseases.

A workable definition of the modern Western diet is a diet that consists of an overabundance of modern wheats, sweets, processed meats, and deep-fried treats. It is not just a quantitative issue; the carbohydrates are refined, the meats are adulterated, and the fats altered. There is oft nary a vegetable or fruit to be seen, unless it is a French-fried potato.

The result is a diet that is energy dense and nutrient poor. It is high in sodium and low in potassium and other valuable minerals, vitamins, and micronutrients. It is a monster. And worse, it is a monster that has become our master. This puppet master can be recognized by the 4 P's of the modern Western diet: (over) processed, (artificially) preserved, prepackaged, and pre-prepared foods. These are the Four Horsemen of our dietary apocalypse.

Today, we picnic upon the plains of Mc Megiddo. And now that we are here, where do we go and how do we get there? We need to find a position of balance. We need to restore ourselves to a point of homeostasis. That point is a locus of Nature. Here, in harmony with ourselves and our environment, we can prevent and reverse the disabilities and diseases of modern civilization.

How we get there is in two steps. The first is an intensive thirty-day program to reboot our gut microbiome. The second is to expand and adapt the thirty-day program so that it becomes our daily operating system. We replace our modern Western–diet death-style with a positive lifestyle for health and wellness.

Step One: Juice Detox, Days 1–3

The program starts with a juice and detoxification regimen. Depending upon your individual response and the specific regimen you choose, you may vary the length of the juice detoxification regimen from a minimum of forty-eight hours to longer than the recommended three days.

An approximately forty-eight hour to seventy-two hour regimen is probably the easiest to practically execute for those who work, travel, or otherwise have hectic and busy schedules. You can start it on a Friday and finish it by the time you have to return to the fray on Monday. The length of time to remain on a juice fast can vary from two to sixty days, depending on the program.

However, particularly for those who have not had much experience with this practice and have not previously undergone a prolonged juice-detox, it is best to start with a two to three day regimen. It is worse to completely break a longer planned fast than to successfully transition from a smaller time frame detox directly into a new dietary regimen. For anyone but those experienced or extremely motivated, going beyond a week can be extremely difficult. Depending upon the approach, particular juice fasting plans can result in certain deficiencies when engaged in for prolonged amounts of time.

Subsisting on juices for an extended period is not meant to become a permanent diet. However, once you start you will likely notice a difference. If you enjoy the taste, textures, and the way the juicing makes you feel, incorporate it into part of your regular diet after the juice-detox period is complete. You can expand the juicing concept by mixing it with active culture yogurt and using it as a breakfast replacement, and if not every day then perhaps several days a week. You can use it as a meal replacement, a snack replacement, or just a mid-day pick me up.

This is Nature's energy drink.

During the first forty-eight to seventy-two hours of the program, juicing serves to help us rest and reset our gastrointestinal systems. Juicing allows us to fire up the body with the equivalent of nutritional jet fuel. By undergoing the juicing process, the phytonutrients, vitamins, and minerals are provided in a form that requires minimal digestive effort.

Three days of juicing is not a quick fix for all your health care woes. It is not a quick weight-loss solution. Approach the first seventy-two hours as if you are crossing a bridge. Let this period serve as a gateway to a more healthful you.

There are many juicing programs and juicers available on the market today. Simply find one that works well for you. You do not want to buy the juice that is sold at the mega-market. Most of those choices consist primarily of fruit juices. They are often loaded with preservatives, additives, and flavors enhancers. The processing that many of these juices undergo eliminates or alters the very phytochemicals and vitality found in fresh vegetables and fruits that we are trying to capture.

The juicing program that is recommended is made with a juicer that compresses fresh fruits and vegetables. It will also extract and remove the pulp. This is what we will consume for the first seventy-two hours. While it may seem that investing in a juicer for a three-day juice fast is an expensive proposition, it will serve you in the long term.

As previously mentioned, you may wish to repeat the cleansing, reset, and reboot effect associated with such practices. More likely, you'll want to incorporate some form of daily juicing into your permanent regimen. High-end juicers often offer more options, easier cleaning and are often built to hold up to the rigors of a daily juicing program.

The shopping list for the first part of our journey to becoming Grassroots Gourmets™ is very simple. Buy produce. If you have a farmers market or other source of seasonal, fresh, organic fruits and vegetables this should be where you source them. During the juicing detot period go heavy on the vegetables, and light on the fruits.

Too much fruit can result in high levels of ingested glucose and fructose. Without the pulp and fiber that is found in the naturally occurring packaging there can be some concern over the effects of the rapid absorption of such sugars.

Some of the best fruits and vegetables to juice are those that are firm with high water content. These include but are not limited to: carrots, apples, celery, beets, cabbage, ginger, oranges, limes, lemons, berries, and all varieties of leafy greens. You can also add a variety of herbs for different flavors.

Also, make sure that with respect to vegetables, during this period as well as throughout the thirty-day program, you chase the rainbow. Using vegetables and fruits of all different colors assures a wide variety of phytonutrients and antioxidants. Some vegetables and fruits that you may think would work well like bananas and avocados don't produce good juice. However, feel free to experiment with what is seasonally available and don't be afraid to try combinations and readily use substitutions when necessary.

Many people are concerned about some discomforts they may feel during the detoxification process. Over the long haul, there is no doubt that juicing will make you feel better and healthier and infuse you with more vigor and vitality.

During the short run, everyone's responses can be slightly different. Much of this depends on your starting point. You may respond very positively with near instantaneous feelings of increased energy and alertness. Others may feel slight discomfort from hunger pains. Still others may feel very sluggish, grumpy, and tired. If you are one of the latter, that is another reason to limit the length of time to forty-eight to seventy-two hours.

There are a few general guidelines that can help minimize any distress. Although you will be drinking a lot of juice, also remember to drink lots of water as well. Even with the juice, one should strive for roughly eight ounces of water eight times a day. Water consumption is important to maintain proper hydration levels, for the functioning of all body systems and to aid the body in eliminating toxins.

The goal of our program is to restore ourselves to a point of homeostasis, a point of health and wellness. This is not a diet of caloric restriction. So, during the juicing and detox process, do not worry about limiting your calories. In fact, most good juicing programs would recommend a minimum of four to five hearty juices and up to ten to twelve glasses throughout the day to keep your energy levels up.

It is important to remain active during this phase as well. However, don't go overboard with physical activity or exercise. You don't want to pick the weekend you start the juice detox as the time you begin training for a marathon. Continue your usual level of physical activity and engage in a moderate exercise but avoid intense, prolonged physical stress.

Also, since juicing can take some time, don't be afraid to prepare ahead. If you have some time in the morning, you can prepare your vegetables and fruits for the entire day so you can simply run them through the juicer when you need them. Alternatively, you are not going to lose much benefit if you make all your juice ahead of time and then just store it in the pitcher to use throughout the rest of the day. Either of these approaches can eliminate some of the fuss.

If you decide to utilize the juice detoxification for more than three days, it is recommended to add some condensed greens powder or similar supplement to the juice. You may also add this from the very beginning if you like. These supplements can help avoid the nutritional gaps and deficiencies that can occur with prolonged juicing.

Step One B: Chase the Rainbow, Days 1–30

When selecting vegetables, start with a base of green. This applies to the juicing and detox phase as well as your menu planning from now until forever. Since the beginning of *Homo sapiens* our dietary palate has always been composed of mostly green stuff.

It was not until the onset of the Industrial Revolution with the changes to food and food pathways that vegetables and fruits started their moribund slide off our culinary table. It has reached a crescendo over the last fifty to seventy-five years with the ever-increasing displacement of fruits and vegetables from the diet in favor of refined carbohydrates and plant-based oils.

Dark green, leafy vegetables are a keystone in our intestinal revolution. Salad greens, kale, spinach, broccoli, bok choy, watercress, mustard, and other greens are rich in vitamins A, C, E, and K. They provide a tremendous source of many of the B-complex vitamins. They contain essential minerals like iron, magnesium, and calcium as well as many trace elements.

But we want to build our program, our diet and ourselves on the principles of diversity and inclusion. We don't want a monotone existence and we shouldn't have a monochromatic diet. We want to add all the fruits and vegetables of the rainbow: whites, oranges, yellows, reds, blues, indigos, and purples. Each of the different colors that differing fruits and vegetables bring to the party highlights a variety of phytochemicals, antioxidants, and important compounds like carotenoids, flavonoids, melanins, and porphyrins.

Just make sure your richly colored choices are unadulterated. Just two parts per million of citrus red dye No. 2 can make those oranges on the shelf pop and look extra nutritious and delicious. One of the advantages of buying organically is that such artificial dyes cannot legally be used on fruits and vegetables that are labeled organic.[583]

Be extremely wary of fruits and vegetables that are heavily processed. These food-like items generally lose their natural color during the processing. To compensate, and make you think they are fresh, nutritious, and delicious, manufacturers usually add artificial colors. Just because the Skittles are bright does not make them more nutritionally redeeming than a plain old white onion. An onion, by the way, that contains vitamin C, vitamin B$_6$, folate, chromium, manganese, molybdenum, phosphorus, copper, and a number of sulfur-containing phytonutrients. None of which are found in Skittles.

With organic vegetables and fruit the more intense the hue, the greater the likelihood that the increased vibrancy represents an increased density of nutrients. These vitamins, minerals, and phytonutrients run the gamut of actions. Folate promotes heart health and helps prevent certain birth defects. It is necessary for proper DNA duplication and repair. The vitamins are necessary for proper bodily functions and for preventing disability from conditions like osteoporosis. Without trace elements like selenium there is no proper heart functioning. The powerful antioxidants have a broad range of anti-inflammatory effects protecting the brain and helping to reduce age-related diseases like Alzheimer-type dementia.

Organic fruits and vegetables have several distinct advantages over their conventionally produced brethren.[584,585] They are nutritionally superior and contain less toxic heavy metals, nitrogen, and significantly less pesticides. By consuming organics, it is estimated that you receive the equivalent of eating an additional one to two fruit and vegetable servings per day.[586]

That is extremely important as fruits and vegetables play such an important role in supplying us with potassium. It is a combination of the increased sodium from highly processed and adulterated foods combined with the displacement of fresh fruits and vegetables that have altered our natural sodium-to-potassium ratio. The restoration of a sodium-to-potassium ratio of less than one is critical in our prevention and treatment of the disabilities and diseases of modern civilization.

By including a rainbow of different colored fruits and vegetables we also restore to our diet its innate high levels of fiber. Unlike cereals and grains, which when unadulterated can supply significant levels of insoluble fiber, fruits and vegetables are our primary source for soluble fiber. This dietary component is critical for the maintenance of a healthy gut microbiome. It is the soluble fiber that provides a substrate for gut bacteria fermentation. Happy gut bacteria are fermenting bacteria.

Unlike refined carbohydrates to which insoluble fiber may be added back, fruits and vegetables are generally quite low in their respective glycemic indices. This can help prevent and reverse such conditions as type 2 diabetes. Because of nature's packaging the consumption results in sugar and carbohydrate metabolism that does not enhance visceral adipose deposition and other unnatural fat accumulation. It results in a metabolically healthy body with a healthy body weight.[587] The Dietary Guidelines for Americans recommends increasing average intakes of fruits and vegetables.

Eating a variety of fruits and vegetables protects against the development of other diseases of modern civilization such as cancer. Several large studies have shown that high vegetable intake may lower the risk of precancerous colon polyps by 30 percent to 40 percent. Such consumption may also lower the risk of breast, stomach, skin, cervix, and lung cancers.

With a base of green add all the colors of the rainbow. Do not think of fruits and vegetables in terms of "better" or "worse" with respect to their color, any more than you should judge a person by his or her skin color. Each colorful offering is nutritionally unique with its own nutritional benefits. The consumption of a wide variety of fresh, unadulterated fruits and vegetables provides a number of health benefits including preventing the inflammation that is the root cause of the disabilities and diseases of modern civilization.

Step Two: Probiotics, Days 1–30

Probiotics are a hot topic these days. There are many different brands being introduced almost daily and hundreds are sold across all forms of media. Celebrities and wellness enthusiasts offer up all sorts of suspect salutatory reasons for you to buy their particular brands.

Hence, here are the caveats. The FDA has not approved any health claims for probiotics. However, just because the FDA has not put their seal of approval on it, does not mean that this cornerstone of our metabolic health is unimportant. The scientific research on the importance of the gut microbiome is beyond reproach.

The regulation of probiotics depends upon the products' intended use. It may be regulated as a dietary supplement, a food ingredient, or a drug. Most probiotics are sold as dietary supplements. These do not require FDA approval prior to marketing.

Dietary supplement labels may make claims about how the product affects the structure or function of the body without prior FDA approval, but they cannot make health claims. Health claims state that the product reduces the risk of a certain disease or diseases. Such claims require the FDA's approval.

A product that is marketed as a drug must meet the highest standards. It must demonstrate both safety and efficacy and be verified in clinical trials. This data must then be submitted to the FDA for review and approval before it can be sold.

The FDA and other organizations like the European Food Safety Authority have rejected hundreds of health claims made by the makers of probiotics. This is not a rejection or denial of the fact that such a strategy may provide health benefits. What it highlights is that a clearly reproducible cause-and-effect relationship that bears out under scientific scrutiny is lacking.

In attempting to isolate and quantify responses in such complex systems, it is paramount to remember that scientific axiom: absence of evidence is not evidence of absence. There is any number of potential reasons for the shortcomings of such submissions. Many trials examined only one or a few of the many bacterial species that coexist within us on a daily basis. Even within the same species, there are many different types or strains. *E. coli* is a normal member of our intestinal horde. However, the specific strain *Escherichia coli 0157:H7* causes a hemorrhagic colitis that can result in death.

It is likely that there is a complex interplay between the different probiotics, just as there is a complex interaction between animals and plants in any given environment. The beneficial effect of some bacteria may not be some vitamin or nutrient they directly produce. They may produce products that suppress the development of more pathogenic bacterial species. They may also occupy a niche that prevents a more undesirable bacterium from moving in.

Many of the earlier studies also did not take into account the importance of prebiotics or their environment. Planting acorns in the Antarctic will not yield oak trees. Add to this the fact that there is likely an exact combination of probiotics and a certain ratio of these probiotics that works best with an individual's unique genotype or genetics. Also add in the following facts that each individual's genetics affect to some degree the nature of his or her intestinal inhabitants, the number of microbial guests, the various species and strains, the impact of all the varieties of food we eat, the impact on our emotional state which can affect our gastrointestinal metabolism and the equation quickly reaches Big Bang proportions.

Despite the complexities that make it challenging to tease out any sort of probiotic benefits, the initial research is quite encouraging. Currently a large number of probiotics are marketed as adjuncts for specific gastrointestinal conditions such as infectious diarrhea, antibiotic-associated diarrhea, irritable bowel syndrome, and inflammatory bowel disease. Probiotics have also been aimed at preventing specific conditions such as tooth decay, gingivitis, and periodontitis. A number of studies support their adjunctive use in these situations.[588]

Although the study of probiotics is a relatively new area of investigation, their use in fact is not new at all. Throughout most of the history of humankind from the Agricultural Revolution up until the Industrial Revolution, fermentation was an important method of preservation. Ancient peoples consumed lots of probiotics in many different forms every day. They just didn't know it. Fermented products containing such probiotics are still popular today in northern Europe, the Middle East, and throughout Asia and Africa.

The modern study of probiotics is generally recognized as beginning in the early twentieth century. It was during this time that Nobel laureate Elie Metchnikoff first hypothesized in *The Prolongation of Life: Optimistic Studies* that ingesting microorganisms could have substantial health benefits for humans. For this, he is remembered as the *father of probiotics.*

The term probiotic refers to living microorganisms. The term was first introduced in 1953. Today, the World Health Organization's 2001 definition is the generally accepted definition: "live microorganisms which, when administered in adequate amounts, confer a health benefit on the host." The term itself derives from the Latin *pro* meaning "for" and the Greek βιωτικός (biotic), meaning "life." This stands in contradistinction to the more familiar "antibiotic."

In most cases, probiotic refers to certain bacterial species and some yeast. Part of the problem is that we only know a small bit of information on a few of over the potentially one thousand different bacterial species that inhabit our gastrointestinal tract. We know nothing about potential yeasts, fungi, and viruses that also likely play a role.

The bacteria that are packaged in probiotic preparations are species that are similar or identical to the beneficial microorganisms naturally found in the human gut. These bacteria may have been studied in certain disease states and found to yield some sort of healthful benefit when taken on a regular basis.

Much like a nuclear reactor uses fuel to produce energy and waste products, what you eat combines with your gut microbiota to fuel your personal bioreactor. This bioreactor aids your digestion, provides nutrients, and not only helps form the basis of the immune system, but helps regulate it. The largest collection of lymphoid tissue in the body is in the intestine. Just a few of the essential nutrients produced here include members of the B vitamin complex, vitamin K, and some short-chain fatty acids. And that is only what we know to date.

It is also unappreciated that just like a nuclear reactor, your personal bioreactor delivers usable fuel. Up to 10 percent of your daily energy needs can be derived from the byproducts of these good bacteria in your gut. As the previously discussed rodent study suggests, the difference between a healthy weight and morbid obesity may be in the composition of the gut bacteria, not so much in the calories you consume.

The key here is to help repopulate our gut microbiome with the right balance, the right ratio, of the probiotics that are beneficial for us. If you decide to use a supplement, look for one that contains some *Lactobacillus* and *Bifidobacterium.*

There are many specific types of bacteria within each of these two broad groups, and health benefits associated with one type may not hold true for others. It is unclear at this time what are the best number and combination for maximum benefit. As the human gut may contain several hundred microbial species, brands with more than one type of probiotic would seem to be the most desirable choice. However, this currently remains scientifically unconfirmed.

Be sure the ingredients and strains are identified on the label. There is no way to adjudicate the safety of unidentified mixtures. Make sure the supplier is reputable. There have been many instances where samples have been tested only to find all of the probiotics are dead.[589]

Lactobacillus species such as *Lactobacillus bulgaricus, casei,* and *acidophilus* are found naturally occurring in many yogurts and soft, fresh cheeses. Make sure the yogurts have live active cultures. This particular bacteria acts to convert lactose and other sugars into lactic acid. For the many people who may be somewhat lactose intolerant, consumption of such foods with this species of bacteria may be particularly helpful.

There is some research that indicates *L. acidophilus* may also be helpful at reducing cholesterol levels.[590] Other controlled trials have shown that *Lactobacillus GG* can shorten the course of infectious diarrhea in infants and children. Limited data does suggest that probiotics reduce antibiotic-associated diarrhea by as much as 60 percent when compared with a placebo.

Streptococcus thermophilus has nothing to do with disease. These bacteria are also found in yogurts and cheeses. They appear to produce some nutrients that are important for normal growth and metabolism.

Bifidobacteria species appears to be extremely important in the maintenance of normal gastrointestinal health. A gut microbiome rich in *Bifidobacteria* species may be less susceptible to gastrointestinal infections, inflammatory conditions like irritable bowel syndrome, and constipation. This species of bacteria produces not only lactic acid but also some very important short chain fatty acids. The short chain fatty acids are absorbed and metabolized by our bodies. Such products may help prevent certain types of gastrointestinal cancers.[591]

Some studies suggest that certain probiotics may help in the treatment of inflammatory bowel disease. They may extend the periods of remission among those who suffer from ulcerative colitis. There is a specific complication of surgery used to treat ulcerative colitis, known as pouchitis. Here too, probiotics may be of benefit. They may also aid to decrease the rate of relapse among those who suffer from Crohn's disease. Probiotics may also be of use in maintaining urogenital health, particularly female urogenital health.

In an article in the issue on probiotics published in a 2008 edition of the medical journal *Clinical Infectious Diseases,* the authors listed several conditions in which probiotics may be of benefit. They concluded that strong evidence exists for utilizing probiotics in the treatment of acute diarrhea and antibiotic-associated diarrhea. It may also be useful for atopic eczema (a skin condition most commonly seen in infants). Promising applications include: childhood respiratory infections; tooth decay; gastroenteritis relapses caused by *Clostridium difficile* bacteria after antibiotic therapy; and inflammatory bowel disease. Studies also indicate that probiotics may reduce side effects associated with treatment for *Helicobacter pylori* infection, the cause of most stomach ulcers.

A systematic review suggests that there is strong evidence that probiotics may reduce the risk of necrotizing enterocolitis, a severe intestinal condition of premature newborns. Other studies have found evidence that a strain of *Lactobacillus reuteri* might slow the growth of certain tumors, and that *Lactobacillus acidophilus* may play a role in helping prevent rotavirus infection. The rotavirus is the most common cause of infectious diarrhea in infants and children worldwide. Other potential future applications include use in reducing cholesterol levels, treating obesity, and managing irritable bowel syndrome.[592]

There are two ways to get our probiotics. One is in a supplemental pill or other packaged form. The second is through the consumption of certain types of food. Certain yogurts and cheeses can contain active cultures. Just remember that the live bacteria are very sensitive to oxygen, light, and extreme temperature changes. Therefore make sure that the yogurt you purchase has a label that reads *live and active cultures.* Many brands that play to the health benefits of live active culture yogurt are actually heat-treated or pasteurized. This kills the probiotics.

There are also many other foods that contain live probiotic cultures. Look for foods that are naturally fermented. Foods that contain fermented soy like miso or fermented cabbage like sauerkraut contain healthy doses of probiotics as long as the label reads *live and active cultures.* Other sources of probiotics include other forms of pickled vegetables like kimchi, fermented bean pastes such as *tempeh* or *doenjang,* or other dairy products such as kefir and buttermilk.

In some situations the initiation of probiotics may be contraindicated. Probiotics are sold under the premise of GRAS, generally recognized as safe. This is because they already exist in a person with a normal digestive system. During a time of acute gastrointestinal illness or any illness that results in a lowered immune system, all programs such as this should be placed on hold. If you have any significant underlying gastrointestinal problems or medical condition, always consult a physician before the initiation of such a program as this.

The most common side effects from probiotics, when they are experienced at all, are mild gastrointestinal side effects such as gas. However, the long-term, cumulative effects of probiotics use, especially in children, are unknown. Probiotics should not be used in critically ill patients.

Our understanding of probiotics is a work in progress. There are a plethora of probiotic products that are marketed for many different uses. There can be large variation between the different probiotic preparations; cheaper isn't always better and greater expense does not assure quality. The scientific understanding of how these complex and symbiotic pathways and relationships work in health and illness is still accumulating.

The use of probiotics is but one adjunctive strategy in a program to help reset, reboot, and restore metabolic health to our gut microbiome. A 2011 Agency for Healthcare Research and Quality assessment of the safety of probiotics concluded that the current evidence does not suggest a widespread risk of negative side effects associated with probiotics. However, the data on safety, particularly long-term safety, are limited, and the risk of serious side effects may be greater in people who have underlying health conditions.[593] Remember the following points in utilizing probiotics.

Probiotic products may contain different types of probiotic bacteria and have different effects in the human body. The effects will vary from person to person.

Do not replace medically proven treatments with unproven products and practices. Do not use probiotics as a reason to postpone seeing your health care provider about any health-related problem.

If you are pregnant or nursing a child, consult your or your child's health care provider.

The long-term effects of any probiotic administration in children are unknown. This program is specifically for adults.

Anyone with a serious underlying health problem should consult with their health professional prior to taking probiotics.

Step Three: Feed the Need, Days 4–30

It does no good to keep taking probiotics if you don't feed them. Like a goldfish, a kitten, a puppy, or sea monkeys these are living organisms and need to be fed. What they live on are the bits we cannot digest. Soluble fiber and other dietary components that we don't utilize as a source of nutrition become food for our probiotic organisms. These gastric flotsam and jetsam are better known as prebiotics: the naturally occurring, non-digestible substances that promote the growth and/or activity of potentially beneficial micro-organisms. The fiber that passes through undigested by us or our bacterial minions is the insoluble fiber component.

Because the modern Western diet is so low in fruit, vegetable, and fiber consumption, it supplies much less of these prebiotics.[594] The consumption of specific prebiotics has been shown to enhance a healthy gut microbiome and prevent the growth of pathogenic bacteria.[595] The consumption of prebiotics improves the absorption and utilization of important minerals.[596] Interestingly, the increased absorption of such minerals as calcium only occurs when levels are low or need is high. This suggests some sort of modulating physiologic effect as opposed to simply an increased binding and delivery of large amounts of calcium.[597] Somehow, feeding our bacteria helps them help us when we need it. It is intestinal insurance of sorts.

Naturally occurring prebiotics are foods that are rich in fructo-oligosaccharides (FOS), such as inulin, oligofructose, and galacto-oligosaccharides (GOS).[598] Prebiotics come in several flavors. These flavors are based on the degree of polymerization of the molecules. There is the long chain version, which contains from nine to sixty-four units per molecule. Inulin is a long chain prebiotic fiber. Being longer in length, these prebiotics are digested more slowly.

Short chain prebiotics contain two-to-eight units per molecule. Oligofructose is a short chain prebiotic and undergoes digestion much more rapidly than the long chain versions. Full spectrum prebiotics contain two to sixty-four units per molecule. Oligofructose-enriched inulin (OEI) is an example of a full spectrum prebiotic.

You can purchase prebiotic supplements, just as you can purchase probiotic supplements. When the two are packaged together they are often labeled as symbiotic supplements or simply *synbiotics*.

However, prebiotics occur quite naturally in fruits and vegetables that contain soluble fiber. Although they may contain a majority insoluble fiber, other whole cereals and grains can also supply significant amounts of soluble fiber and function as prebiotics. Prebiotics are found in many foods, including bananas, honey, garlic, onions, leeks, asparagus, artichokes, soybeans, chicory, Jerusalem artichoke, raw dandelion greens, and burdock. Naturally occurring synbiotic combinations, such as bananas with live-culture yogurt, or vegetables stir-fried with miso, cost less than supplements and have the added benefit of being delicious. Even with cooking, these foods retain the bulk of their prebiotic benefit. It is a way to feed your own beneficial bacterial buddies at a fraction of the price of supplementation.

When prebiotics were combined with probiotics they exhibited a synergistic inhibitory effect on pre-cancerous gastrointestinal lesions.[599] The combination also reduced fasting glucose, hemoglobin A1c, total cholesterol, LDL cholesterol, oxidized LDL cholesterol and apolipoprotein B levels (a lipoprotein associated with increased cardiovascular risk) in type 2 diabetes patients.[600] In patients with irritable bowel syndrome the addition of prebiotics improved symptoms.[601] The consumption of prebiotics increased the production of beneficial short chain fatty acids like butyric acid in the human colon by the gut microbiome.

Remember, fruits and veggies and other cereals and grains that are good sources of soluble fiber are good sources of prebiotics. Try to get at least two to four servings of prebiotic-rich foods a day.

Step Four: The Baking Dead, No Modern Wheat, Days 4–30

Modern wheat will kill you, just not for the reasons you think. The success of such programs that eliminate all wheat and wheat products for all time, and programs like the paleo approach, which eliminate all cereals and grains, are successful because they eliminate modern wheat. But that approach is a bit like throwing the baby out with the bathwater.

You don't have to go gluten-free, just be free of modern wheat. Avoid all products, even so-called whole-wheat and whole-grain products, that are made from modern bread wheat. Unfortunately, since most of the wheat gluten that is used as an additive is derived from modern bread wheat, just about any modern processed food that contains gluten is tainted by the use of modern bread wheat.

This does make shopping more difficult.

However, there are some easy options. Obviously, avoid the pre-packaged breads, cookies, cakes and other modern wheat-containing foods and snacks. If you're shopping like a Grassroots Gourmet™, which we will discuss in the following sections, you are already minimizing your purchase of processed, refined, and adulterated foods. You are also avoiding the junk foods and fast food products.

Even with the elimination of modern wheat, there are a wonderful and enchanting variety of other cereals and grains to explore. Don't feel like your only choice is highly processed, polished, microwave white-rice. There are many varieties and heritage types of rice. There are varieties of red rice, green rice, and black rice just to name a few. These add unique flavors and textures to many dishes. Wild rice is a great addition to any meal and need not just be used once a year as a stuffing. Wild rice is not actually an Asian-type rice at all, although as the seeds of a type of grass they are somewhat related. These are great sources of vitamins, antioxidants, many phytonutrients, and fiber, both insoluble and soluble.

Taking a page from other cuisines around the world, beans and lentils also provide a wonderful alternative source of flavorful starches. These are also great sources of protein, vitamins such as folate (vitamin B_9) and thiamine (vitamin B_1), other phytonutrients, and insoluble fiber, and they can function as prebiotic material. These legumes lower cholesterol, aid in the control of blood glucose levels, and are rich sources of such minerals as molybdenum, manganese, iron, phosphorus, copper, and potassium.

Corn, oats, and barley also offer an expansive list of non-wheat options. Just make sure to shop for and purchase the less adulterated and processed forms. Stone-ground oats and corn offer a superior nutritional profile when compared to those from mass-produced modern roller methods. Some of the heritage and more ancient varieties offer unique tastes, textures, and nutritional characteristics compared to varieties that have been bred predominantly for the purpose of mass production.

There are also options like quinoa, buckwheat, and kaniwa. Kaniwa hails from South America and was a staple food of the Incas. It was able to grow where other staples including quinoa could not. Therefore, it provided a dependable source of food for this ancient empire. Although it looks like a cereal grain, it is actually the seed of a broad-leaved goosefoot plant related to quinoa. The approximately

1 mm, dark seeds are a great source of protein, fiber, calcium, zinc, and iron. The seeds are also about 16 percent protein, equivalent to the highest protein-containing wheat. Kaniwa is also rich in antioxidants and certain types of amino acids.

You also don't have to give up the breads, rolls, crackers, and pizza crusts. Just make them the way they have been made for most of civilization's history. Make them with ancient grains. In addition to bread, biscuits, and rolls made from barley, rye, and oats you can use ancient wheat grains. The gluten proteins and many other proteins found in these ancient grains are different from that found in modern bread wheat. The predominant ancient grains that are readily available today include spelt, kamut, durum, emmer, and einkorn.

These ancient grains are increasingly popular among foodies and cutting-edge chefs. There is increasing availability in terms of getting the ancient grains and buying ancient-grain products. There is now an abundance of recipes and information for cooking and baking with them. Although the flours made from them can yield foods that are a bit denser than those made from bleached modern bread wheat, they do deliver a more intense flavor and unique texture.

These ancient grains are also rich in essential fatty acids, protein, minerals, and both soluble and insoluble fiber. They are rich sources of phytonutrients and antioxidants, often displaying a superior all-around nutritional profile when compared to modern bread wheat.

Do execute a little caution when confronted with the label "farro wheat." Technically, the term refers to emmer wheat. If the wheat product carries an IGP designation, *Indicazione Geografica Protetta*, from the Tuscany region of Italy then you can be sure that it is emmer. What is labeled as "farro wheat" from other countries may be barley, spelt, or even modern wheat in its more raw form.

Likewise, if you purchase dried pasta from Italy you can be sure that it is made from the ancient grain, semolina durum wheat. Durum wheat is also readily available if you prefer to make your own fresh pasta, the Italian way, from this ancient grain. The semolina refers to the mill of the durum wheat, not to a specific wheat type. The semolina grind of durum wheat is best for pasta and is the only kind of wheat allowed by law to be exported from Italy as dried Italian pasta.

Durum wheat is what is known as a hard wheat and it has a high protein concentration. The gluten found in durum wheat, like other ancient grains, is very different from modern bread wheat. The gluten found in durum wheat does not readily lend itself to bread making. However there is a Sicilian specialty, *Le pagnotte di Enna,* which is traditionally made with 100 percent durum wheat and is incredibly delicious. For those interested in making breads, rolls, and other non-pasta baked goods, there are finer grinds of durum flour that can be found with a little effort. Dining in places that use traditional ingredients and methods like durum flour to prepare their homemade pasta is one of the keys to successfully dining out.

Step Five: Sugar, ah, Honey, Honey

Sugar matters in terms of both type and quantity. Use raw forms and honey when possible.

Always use it surgically.

No high fructose corn syrup or anything that contains it.

No artificial sweeteners.

Not now, not ever.

'Nuff said.

Steps Six, Seven, and Eight:
Become a Grassroots Gourmet™, Days 1–30

Now that we know what we need to eat, it is time to briefly discuss how to eat, and just as importantly what not to eat. There are three simple principles that are easy to remember and even easier to execute. These are the core principles of becoming a Grassroots Gourmet™. These principles are covered much more extensively in *Eating Well, Living Better: A Grassroots Gourmet Guide to Good Health and Great Food.* Suffice to say, it is vital that we briefly touch upon them here as part of our overall program.

Avoid the call of the junk food/fast food siren. This is a difficult task because of the temptation of convenience. But as we have seen, the trappings of the modern Western diet that are offered up at the drive-throughs, vending machines, and supermarket snack food aisles subtly addict us in a modern incarnation of Circe's magic. It is not food, but a slow poison that is offered. We must steel ourselves like Odysseus to the mainmast. The good news is that after thirty days of freedom, you will no longer be tempted.

It is much like the addiction people suffer for cigarettes. In some ways, it can be even worse since you don't need to smoke cigarettes to live, but you do need to eat. That fact combined with the constant advertising, convenience, and salty, sweet, meat fried-concoctions can easily lead one into inducement. A simple, but highly effective strategy is simply to not buy junk food. If it is not in your house, your workplace, or your car you are much less likely to be tempted.

The advice for a fast-food place is a lot like the advice for avoiding bar fights. If you want to avoid a bar fight, don't go to a bar. For the fast food, pizza joints, and convenience shops: do not pull in, do not order home delivery, and do not stop at the 7-Eleven. After thirty days you will likely find that eating there will make you ill—perhaps the greatest reinforcement that you are on the correct path.

It is much like the response of former cigarette smokers who become nauseated by the smell of the cigarette that they once craved. If you are no longer patrolling the drive-through, raiding the pantry, or otherwise succumbing to the junk food/fast food siren's call of mass consumption then you must be procuring your own victuals. This brings us to the second of the three core Grassroots Gourmet™ principles, which should be familiar to anyone who has ever attended Sunday school: Thou shalt not commit adultery.

This, of course, means our food. When you are shopping try to avoid putting the processed, prepackaged, pre-prepared, and artificially preserved items in your cart. This will require additional effort and work. You may wish to specialty source your staples. If there is a local fishmonger to reliably provide fresh, wild-caught seafood it may be worth the trip. A farmer's market is a great opportunity to procure seasonal, fresh, and organic produce. Some farmer's markets also have vendors who can supply such items as cage-free or free-range organic eggs. You may also be able to source grass-fed, free-range beef. What you cannot source, you may be able to get shipped by finding the purveyors of the items you require on the Internet. Flours made from ancient grains are a good example.

You may also find yourself doing a bit more from scratch. This is not a bad thing, and when you have tasted the results you may never be able to go back to the mass-produced and usually bland commercial-brands. A great example is stock. A delicious, flavorful stock is the key to many great sauces, soups, stews, and scrumptious meals. Most commercial stocks are loaded with preservatives, insipid in flavor and loaded with salt. This can be a problem when cooking, because you are often reducing your stock and this can wind up making the whole meal taste over-salted.

A big batch of homemade stock is a kitchen staple that really requires minimal work. Pick a day when you will be home piddling around the house or just watching TV. Then simply pull out the chicken carcasses that you saved when you broke down the free-range, organic chickens. Add in carrots and celery bits, a few herbs, some peppercorns, onions, crushed garlic-clove, and perhaps a lemon that may have seen better days. Put it all in a pot and add a few quarts of water and let it simmer for a couple hours. Strain the liquid and you have enough stock for at least a month.

You just produced a kitchen staple finer in quality than anything you can buy, made out of basically leftovers. Such items are not just important in terms of the ingredients you use to infuse them with flavor and nutrition—what you don't add to them is just as important as well.

Remember: It doesn't matter where you get your appetite as long as you eat at home. No adultery.

Finally, we also want to utilize the concepts of timing and pro-portion. These two simple practices are so often overlooked when examining different dietary approaches. It is not just what you eat, but how you eat it that is important as well. The concept of pro-portion refers to the volume of food we put on our plate. A good general rule of thumb is to generously apportion servings of items like vegetables. Go with smaller servings of higher quality proteins. A grass-fed, pasture-raised steak of six or eight ounces makes for a perfectly satisfying meal. You don't need to consume half a side of mega-market industrial beef.

Hand-in-hand with proper proportioning is proper timing. It takes roughly twenty minutes to half an hour for the stomach to start to signal our brain that we have eaten something and we're getting full. So yes, if you shove four McMortem's, supersized fries and a small reservoir's worth of soft drink down your gullet in ten minutes you can still actually feel hungry. In about ten minutes more, you will no doubt start to feel all the effects of ingestion, none of them good.

If you start your meal with a small salad or appetizer, wait about fifteen minutes or so for the main course. Likewise if you are having a dessert, wait at least fifteen to twenty minutes after you have fin-ished the main entrée. You may enjoy a small dessert without feeling the need to consume the entire cake at one sitting. Utilizing such simple principles as proper timing and proportion we can construct titillating meals that satisfy with less. The value of our food is about quality, not just quantity.

And should you stray, say three My Belly Prayers and get back on the wagon.

The Belly Prayer
My bacterial buddies, which art in my belly,
Hallowed be thy fermentation.
Metabolic health do come.
If thy will be done in large intestine,
As it is in small.
Give us this day our non-modern wheat bread.
And forgive us our flatulence,
As we forgive those that smelt it and dealt it.
And lead us not into the drive-through,
But deliver us from HFCS.
For thine is the colon,
The pre-biotic, and the pro,
For soluble fiber and in-.
Amen.

Step Nine: The Value of Food

This is another concept that is covered extensively in *Eating Well, Living Better: A Grassroots Gourmet Approach to Good Health and Great Food*. Again, we will briefly touch upon the subject here. For reasons previously discussed, much of the marketing that appeals to our sense of food value plays upon our hardwired predilection to equate food quantity with food value.

It requires conscious effort to step back and evaluate the quality of the comestibles and utilize that variable as the predominant factor in determining its value. Because chicken is no longer just chicken, and a burger is no longer just a burger, and bread is not even just bread, examination of where the food was sourced, how it was produced and the degree of processing must now become our normal procedure.

This conscious interaction and effort is the only way to ascertain that the food we choose to eat is healthful. The government and its regulatory agencies can barely keep the food supply safe. Making sure what you eat supplies you with good health is our responsibility. Food safety does not mean a healthful diet—don't conflate the two.

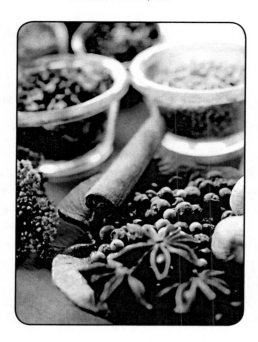

Spiced for Life (AKA Step Ten)

"So tell me what you want, what you really really want"
~"WANNABE," THE SPICE GIRLS[602]

The final cornerstone to the program is one of the most important practices. Utilizing both herbs and spices, it helps restore both taste and texture to our food. Research has confirmed what we intuitively know; when food pleases us, exquisitely satisfies us, we savor it. And in the process of doing so, we eat less and enjoy it more. Using herbs and spices to properly season quality ingredients produces these results.

By restoring such vitality back to our meals, we are also able to break the addictive and manipulative commercial use of sugar, salt, and fat. When preparing our foods, sugar, salt, and fat should be wielded by the chef in the manner that a surgeon uses a scalpel. The modern food industry uses sugar, salt, and fat to slay us comfortably numb like Jason Voorhees with a chainsaw at a frat party.

The use of herbs and spices is certainly nothing new. It is worth taking a moment to examine a brief history of herbs, spices, humanity, and food.

A Brief History of Herbs and Spices, or In Pursuit Of How to Make a Small Penis Splendid

The exact origins of humankind's first interactions with herbs and spices are irrevocably lost in the mists of time. Enclosed within those mists was a time when the relationship between a culinary application and a medical application were not as disparate as they are today. It was a time when the interconnection between what we consume and who we are was as intertwined as the serpents on the caduceus or the strands of our very DNA.

It is without a doubt that during this time, many thousands of years before the first written accounts, both herbs and spices were utilized for gastronomic, therapeutic, religious, and social purposes. Many accounts, books, programs, and courses of higher learning have attempted to recount the history of herbs and spices. Many of the historical facts and findings corroborate these modern theories and timelines. Many other facts and findings, like the characters in any good thriller, refuse to fold neatly and conveniently into place. The alluring mystery that surrounds the origins and early uses of herbs and spices permeates their contemporary aura like the half-remembered scent of that woman.

The history of herbs and spices, like any good spice collection, refuses to remain neatly organized and classified, constantly being reshuffled with the addition of previously unknown and unrecognized bits and pieces. All the while the old and stale are replaced with newer and more vibrant components. The history of humankind itself has been shaped by the relationship between civilization and the pursuit of herbs and spices. Herbs and spices have played a role in accumulation of individual fortunes, achievement of fame, successful romance, and promulgation of religion. They have likewise contributed to individual financial downfall, disgrace and disapprobation. On a grander stage their presence, or at times lack of, has shaped the courses of great civilizations and empires, and subsequently world history. Our modern world exists in its current form in no small part due to the global socioeconomic impact of the quest for herbs and spices.

The documented use of herbs and spices can easily be traced back to at least thirty-five hundred years ago. And like many food-related things, it involves gastronomy's paramour—alcohol. In the third millennium BCE the inhabitants of modern day Syria were using cumin and coriander seed to flavor their beer. Modern Belgian ales like *witbier* or *bière blanche* still use coriander to flavor the brew. Great ideas, like great a brew, are timeless.

The Ebers Papyrus is a document containing medical and other information from ancient Egypt dating back to around 1550 BCE. It lists many herbs and spices that are still commonly utilized today. During the heyday of the pharaohs, many of these herbs and spices were used for medical and other sundry applications as well as for consumption. Importantly, it lists the use of such non-native spices as cassia and cinnamon.

These two spices, often mislabeled and referred to as just cinnamon, are native to the tropical regions of India, Sri Lanka, and Southeast Asia. This indicates that at the time of the pharaohs trade routes existed between ancient Egypt and Asia.[603] The fact that these items made their way halfway around the globe over a millennium before the compass was invented is a testament to the esteem in which they were held, as well as the depth of the desire for them. These spices, now common in modern cookery, were used by the ancient Egyptians for embalming. They were critical to ensure that the Pharaoh would live eternally in the afterlife.

Today, Dr. Oz touts his "super-longevity prescription" with cinnamon as an integral ingredient in his "ultimate life-extending plan."[604] The interplay of herbs, spices, and the quest for immortality proves there is truly "nothing new under the sun (Ecclesiastes 1:9)."[605] Pepper, another native to India, was found stuffed into the nostrils of the mummy of Ramses II. He was entombed in 1213 BCE.

Even more revealing was what was found inside a simple clay jar recovered from the Syrian Desert. It seems the house of an unfortunate guy named Puzurum caught fire in what was then the town of Terqa. Fortunately for posterity, the heat of the fire acted like a kiln on a particular clay jar that was located in his home. The firing of the clay jar sealed and preserved its contents. All of this occurred around 1721 BCE and remained buried until very recently. When this particular jar was opened, cloves were found.[606] This is extremely significant because until about 1775, cloves existed on only a handful of Indonesian islands.[607]

These islands known as the Moluccas, or Maluku Islands, consist of five small islands: Ternate, Tidore, Moti, Makian, and Bacan. In a time before iron, when the world and particularly the ocean was an unknown and dangerous place, people explored and braved the edges of world's end. To brink and boundary they traveled driven by their need for herbs and spice, a need for flavor and taste; for religion and ceremony; for medicine and healing; for sex, and magic.

And in the days to come the world would continue to be twisted by that greatest shaper of human fortune, the common underpinning of all things spicy—desire. By remaining the only source of cloves, nutmeg, and mace for millennia, these Spice Islands would help shape the destiny of the world right up until our modern epoch. The desire for these spices was an impetus in the formation of the Portuguese, Spanish, French, Dutch, and English empires—and the basis of their wars.

They would launch an age of exploration and discovery that resulted in a clash of continents and cultures. And it was not just Europe and Asia that clashed. When Columbus mistook the Caribbean for the East Indies he ignited a mad dash of competition among these European powers to stake a claim in the previously unrecognized New World. And in this savage and unrestrained rapacity, some flourished while others died.

The success of the Spanish in exploiting the natives, their gold, their goods, and their land proved an irresistible seductress to the other powers of the time. The allure of Empire created economic upheaval and the formation of such entities as the Dutch East India Trading Company and its English version, the Governor and Company of Merchants of London trading into the East Indies. An entity commonly referred to as the East India Trading Company. In a very real sense, without spices there would be no Captain Jack Sparrow, savvy?

This European love of exotic spices can easily be traced to ancient Rome. Within the remains of a Roman army camp located in what is now Germany were found traces of coriander seeds and black pepper, neither indigenous to the region.[608] Dating from the time of the Roman occupation of England, then known as Britannia, are records regarding the purchase of black pepper from India. There have also been recovered remnants of Indian black pepper from the Roman ruins at Hadrian's Wall. Even at the farthest, most remote outposts of the Empire the Romans demanded their spices. In examining the genetics of mankind it is clear that the axiom,

"Where armies go, genes flow," universally holds true. With respect to the Romans, it seems that where they went their way of life, including their use of spices, left an equally indelible imprint upon the native peoples.

According to a document known as the *Periplus of the Erythraean Sea*, a direct sailing route from the Red Sea to India had been discovered in the first century BCE by a Greek known as Hippalus.[609] Shortly after Augustus annexed Egypt and her holdings in 30 BCE the Romans effectively executed a campaign in which they destroyed a number of Middle Eastern and African port towns that housed any competition to their ownership of the spice trade; the Roman imprint not infrequently resembled the heel of the boot. This was the first time in history a European power went to war over spices; it would not be the last.[610]

By the mid-first century AD, the Romans routinely sailed huge fleets of over one hundred ships from the Red Sea to India and as far south as modern-day Mozambique. Some of these cargo ships could displace over one thousand tons, over twice the tonnage of the Spanish galleons that would haul the wealth of the New World to the Old. With the fall of Rome on August 24, 410 AD, it would be over fifteen hundred years before Vasco de Gama reopened the waterways between Europe and India. Ironically, when Alaric first besieged Rome in 408 AD he was paid not only five thousand pounds of gold and thirty thousand pounds of silver, but three thousand pounds of pepper as well to leave. It was a telling tribute and foreshadowing as to the value and power of herbs and spices.

Following the fall of Rome, exotic herbs and spices did not disappear from the European continent but they did become substantially scarcer. The trade routes of the herbs and spices of India and Asia were now controlled by the Islamic powers of Arabia. These passageways not only remained viable but thrived under Arabic management. A consequence of the Arabic control of the flow of these goods for the Europeans was that some herbs and spices became extremely expensive.

During this time of fragmentation in Europe, some spices even became a form of accepted currency. Traces of this policy existed until the modern era; up until 1937 the King of England received rent from the mayor of Launceston that consisted of one hundred shillings and one pound of pepper. The law of international commerce dictates that as availability decreases, price and exclusivity increase. During the Middle Ages possession of an abundance of herbs and spices, especially the rare, exotic, and expensive ones, became associated with those social classes of economic means. In particular during this period, this would have been the nobility and aristocracy as well as the church.

The more direct spice routes of the ancient world eventually resurfaced to traverse their course to Europe through Italy. This made several Italian states, among them Venice, extremely wealthy. During this time in Northern Europe, the Vikings raided, explored, and settled from Northern Europe to Spain and Byzantium. The Viking Age opened up extraordinary trading—along with pirating and plundering across the entire region. Once again a profundity of herbs and spices began to bloom.

And that was a good thing for men such as William the Troubadour, also known as Duke William IX of Aquitaine (1071-1126). Spices such as pepper "... laid on thick (upon) ... two fat capons, white bread, (and served with) good wine ..."[611] served to fortify the good Duke. And indeed it seems he was in need of strong fortification. Being the world's first troubadour means being the world's first rock star. This means groupies and relentless fornication.

For as William tells the tale, as only a troubadour can, trouble began shortly after entering the city of Auvergne. Once inside the city walls, he was accosted by two ladies of noble bearing. For some unknown reason, they thought him an illiterate mute and shanghaied him away. And who was he to argue. Clearly, if they believed him a mute he had uttered not a word at all. These mistresses of mayhem confined the poor lad for a week as their *hostage*.

He lamented, or bragged depending on your point of view, about his *sacrifice* as a *hostage*. He surrendered himself to a ménage-à-trois with his captors. There are graphic details of the escapades in which he bedded the daring damsels 188 times over the course of the week. That works out to just over 26 times a day, which of course only has 24 hours. Math genius not required here, vivid imagination with a smidge of gullibility definitely encouraged.

And were it not but for the bracing quality of the spice, William confided that he would have nearly "broke my tool and burst my harness ...."[612] But then herbs and spices have always served as a bridge between those two instinctual obsessions, food and sex. Throughout recorded history and likely before, herbs and spices served not only culinary and medicinal usage, but played a predominant role as perfumes and aphrodisiacs.

This was perhaps highlighted nowhere better than in the book known as *The Perfumed Garden of Sensual Delight* by Cheikh Nefzaoui. Building upon the wealth of anecdotal evidence provided by such luminaries as William the Troubadour, this book was believed to have been written in its original Arabic somewhere between 1410 and 1434. This was the medieval equivalent of Internet porn, adult video on demand, *Fifty Shades of Grey*, and do-it-yourself Viagra all rolled into one big herbal and spice manual. It was a medieval blockbuster.

Within its lusty pages, the sheik extols the erotic virtues and potencies of various herb and spice combinations the equivalent of steroid-infused, nitrous-enhanced love potions. He advises that the prudent use of herbs and spices can enhance the act of lovemaking even more so than melted camel-hump fat, leather, leeches, or even hot pitch. Hard to believe there are more erotic activities than a smear of melted camel-hump fat upon the object of one's desire, but the sheik swore by it.

And as gratifying as a weenie-leeching sounds, he recommends that even more enjoyment can be had by chewing a little cubeb-pepper or cardamom and applying that directly to the head of the penis prior to intercourse, an act that gives new meaning to sharing a properly peppered salami. Using the same technique with a different blend consisting of cubeb-pepper, the spice pyrether, ginger, and cinnamon would cause a woman to desire cohabitation.

But then the focus and the economics of porn have never been in couple's therapy. They've always been much more phallocentric. The economics have been, and continue to be, for remedies to treat conditions of phallic insufficiency—something in which *The Perfumed Garden* has Cialis beaten hands down. In chapter eighteen, "Prescriptions for Increasing the Dimension of Small Members and for Making Them Splendid," the sheik notes that this topic:

"is of the first importance both for men and women. For men, because from a large and vigorous member there spring the affection and love of the woman; for the woman, because it is by such members that their amorous passions get appeased, and the greatest pleasure is procured for them. This is evident from the fact that many men, solely by reason of their insignificant member, are, as far as coition is concerned, objects of aversion to the women, who likewise entertain the same sentiment with regard to those whose members are soft, nerveless, and relaxed. Their whole happiness consists in the use of robust and strong members."[613]

With the future happiness of the entire human race resting precipitously upon their personal promontory, is it any wonder men spared no expense and traveled to the ends of the known world—and still do so—in order to carry a bigger club?

But identifying the problem is only half the battle. The sheik also proposes several remedies. Among them is rubbing the penis with tepid water until it "gets red and extended"[614] and then applying a mixture of honey and ginger prior to coitus—a medieval flavor-injector of sorts. An alternate mixture consists of a powder made of pepper, lavender, galanga (a relative of ginger), and musk mixed with honey and preserved ginger. Perhaps this serves as the source of the expression "to touch one gingerly." Both these herbal solutions seem preferable to other remedies which include leather and hot pitch, an oil made from leeches or eating poultry that are fed a strict diet of boiled donkey dong, corn, and onion.

But perhaps the most amazing fact is not these claims made on behalf of the herbs and spices, but the fact that there just may be some truth to them. Studies performed by Dr. Alan Hirsch examined the effects of different scents on sexual arousal by measuring penile blood flow. In a preliminary study a significant increase was found in response to the aroma of cinnamon buns.

However, in the final analysis the winner was a forty percent increase in penile blood flow that was found in response to a combination of lavender and pumpkin-pie scents. This was followed by the fragrance of doughnuts, clocking in at a 31.5 percent increase.[615] Perhaps Homer Simpson has known something all along, at least among male listeners of classic rock in Chicago; the volunteers were recruited from listeners of classic rock stations in Chicago. One of the caveats was that many of the all-male volunteers who found such scents enticing didn't have sex all that often. Hard to believe, and sad, but true.

Of note, among those volunteers who actually *had* frequent sex, the *Oriental spice* elicited the greatest response. A common ingredient in both pumpkin pie and Oriental spice is cinnamon. A murine study which was initially designed to assess the potential toxicity of cinnamon, *Cinnamomum zeylanicum,* and Indian long pepper, *Piper longum,* found no significant toxicity at high or chronic doses.

What they did find was that while the control group, which

received no spices, had significant weight gain, the groups receiving spices had none. That is, unless you count the significant increase in the weight of the reproductive organs of those mice receiving spice.[616] Now that, no doubt, is the finding that would bring a smile to the sheik's face. And perhaps explains the popularity of Dr. Oz's "super-*long*evity prescription" in his "ultimate life-*extending* plan."

With the onset of the Crusades, the floodgates completely gave way. By the middle of the Middle Ages, herbs and spices had leant a global nature to cuisine. That was long before modern television programming brought us wonderful international fusion cuisine such as Southern style deep-fried sushi.

Much like said sushi, this period of history has been a victim of our contemporary culture. The creation of urban myth-like speculation regarding the use of spices during the Middle Ages actually arose in the early nineteenth century. And like most urban myths, it has no basis in fact. The conventional wisdom holds that the food of the Middle Ages, like the food of ancient Rome, was heavily spiced and flavored. This may or may not have been true.

The definitive tome *De re coquinaria, On the Subject of Cooking*, was compiled in the 4th or early fifth century AD from an original likely written in the second century AD. This has erroneously been attributed to Marcus Gavius Apicius. He was a gourmand of legendary proportions who lived in the first century AD and is often referred to simply as Apicius.

Many of these recipes contain various herbs and spices. Pepper is among the most common, being found in 349 of the 468 recipes that comprise the work. A significant majority of these recipes contain many different herbs and additional spices. However, like many of the cookbooks of this period and before, while many ingredients were listed, quantities were oft missing. Trying to recapture the flavor profiles without knowing the full measure of ingredients would be like trying to reconstruct a plane crash without the black box. Since the majority of the imported spices would have been extremely expensive, it is reasonable to extrapolate that they would not have been frivolously utilized.

The cookbooks and records from the Middle Ages likewise often list ingredients without corresponding quantities. It was assumed during the 1800s that the *raison d'être* for all the elaborate use of herbs and spices was to cover up the forced consumption of foul and rotting meat and produce. The modern arrogance is to assume that without modern transportation and refrigeration that is of course all they had to eat.

Despite the modern hubris, the fact remains that a majority of food during this time period was locally produced. There is ample fact to support the argument that the bulk of the food consumed during this period was actually fresher than the preponderance of what is purchased in a modern megamart. This would have included animal proteins as well. As a matter of course, we now routinely pay more to acquire food prepared in exactly the same manner.

Then, as now, there were no doubt unscrupulous purveyors who would try to adulterate and pass off substandard fare. This is not a situation unique to any particular time period. This has occurred throughout the history of all food pathways and in all locations. Indeed, one need only look toward the recent modern usage of dyes to color beef a bolder and more attractive red and the use of harsh chemical agents to eliminate fishy smells from seafood to realize that some shylock will always try to make a buck at someone else's expense.

However, just as today, there were strict laws in the Middle Ages and significant consequences for trying to pass off fetid grub. In 1366, John Russell of Billingsgate was found guilty of selling thirty-seven pigeons that were "putrid, rotten, stinking and abominable ."[617] He was sentenced to the pillory while his stock of fetid pigeons burned beneath him. While the decomposed flesh blackened under his nose, he would have been publicly pelted with garbage, rotten eggs, mud, carcass parts, and excrement. He was quite literally in a shit storm that sent a very clear signal that tampering with the public health was as serious an offense then as it is now. Perhaps we should strive to hold people so accountable the next time GMO wheat miraculously appears growing in some farmer's field.

The final hole in the spices-for-fouled-flesh hypothesis is that the people who could afford spices in the first place were also the people who could afford to purchase meat and fish from more reputable sources. Therefore this explanation for spice usage makes little sense from an economic perspective.

So, if not to cover up off-putting flavors, why use herbs and spices?

Is there a reason beyond simply enhancing the flavor and texture of food?

How did all this get started in the first place?

Observations on Usage and Benefits of Herbs and Spices

The quantities as well as the number of different herbs and spices used in a recipe increases as one travels from cooler climates to warmer and more tropical climes.[618]

There has been some suggestion that the increased consumption of the spices and spice combinations increases perspiration and thus helps cool the body more effectively in these more tropical zones. However, the vast majority of herbs and spices used do not cause this physiologic response.[619] In addition, the additional effect from the consumption of those spices that do cause this response is insignificant compared to the body's innate cooling mechanisms. The spice effect in this instance is a bit like pissing in the ocean and expecting the tide to rise.

Herbs and spices add flavor, taste, color, and texture. They can add micronutrients and trace elements. And they bring antimicrobial activity. They are nature's preservatives acting to reduce the spoilage of particularly vulnerable comestibles like meat, fish, and seafood.

Throughout history, and in many areas of the world today, food-borne illness remains a significant affliction. An examination of the top thirty herbs and spices in terms of usage, from around the world, demonstrated that all of these have some degree of bactericidal or bacteriostatic properties. These thirty herbs and spices inhibited at least 25 percent of the most common food-borne pathogens. Fifteen of the thirty were effective on at least 75 percent of the bacteria tested.

Garlic, onion, allspice, and oregano inhibited or killed every bacterium they were tested on. Using these herbs and spices in combination yields an even greater efficacy as they have a synergistic effect when used together.[620] The piperine found in black pepper, one of the world's most commonly used spices, is effective against *Clostridium botulinum*, the bacteria responsible for botulism.

But piperine also increases the rate at which bacteria absorb the phytotoxins of other herbs and spices, a turbo booster of sorts.[621] The practice of flavoring foods with herbs and spices would have allowed foodstuffs to last longer and be safer to eat. This would have conferred a survival advantage to anyone preferring such edibles, especially those staples easily susceptible to spoilage such as the highly desirable protein sources like meat, fish, and seafood.

Thus early on in the history of humankind a preference for foods seasoned with herbs and spices may have led to the development of a type of *Darwinian Gastronomy*.[622] The end result of this evolutionary process combined with the historical socioeconomic influences mentioned in the previous chapter is our modern global cuisine. It is the result of the melding of food safety, health, and wellness. Today, the global cuisine runs the gamut of known flavor profiles, textures, and tastes and continues to breed new ones as cross-pollination and fusion occurs.

When it comes to herbs and spices, one of the most common questions is "What's the difference?" Therefore, before we proceed any further, it is useful to define exactly what is meant by a spice and what is meant by an herb. Both herbs and spices contain unique oleoresins and essential oils. It is these compounds, unique to the individual species, that give various herbs and spices their inimitable attributes.

These phytochemicals are generally not requisite for the plant to be able to perform photosynthesis. Because of this they are generally classified as secondary compounds. Although they may not be necessary for the plant to be able to perform photosynthesis they may still be essential for plant survival. This is because many of these compounds have been developed by the plants over eons to protect them from local pathogens. In much the same way that an Iberian ham gets its unique nutty flavor because the swine consume a diet rich in acorns, we can take advantage of the protective effects these compounds offer by consuming them. You are, quite literally, made of the stuff that you consume.

Generally, an *herb* refers to the use of the fresh or dried leaves of a plant. *Spices* are generally regarded as the flowers, buds, seeds, bark, or roots of plants. Another important attribute in defining spices is the fact that they tend to be used in dried form. It is, however, possible for a plant to be both an herb and spice. The plant known as *Coriandrum sativum* provides the herb known as cilantro when the leaves are used. When the seeds are harvested it is referred to as coriander. Not only are the uses different; the flavor profiles are distinct. Do not make the mistake of substituting ground coriander seed for fresh cilantro; you may wind up with a bitter face looking like Coach Gruden sucking on a lemon.

Millennia ago herbs and spices provided a pathway for better health and the survival of the human species. Along the way they infused our food with vibrancy and flavor, delivering us pleasure in the experience of sustenance. Now, as victims of the Western diet, we find ourselves starving in the midst of abundance, victims of the dark side of plenty.

We consume mass quantities of artificially preserved, overly processed, prepackaged, and pre-prepared foods that often lack vitality. In place of taste they offer only endless layers of sugar, salt, and fat. This has become the norm. It is time to use wholesome, quality ingredients along with herbs and spices to break these gastronomic shackles and learn to taste again.

Spiced for Life: Days 4–30 plus

No matter whether it is a spice or an herb, we will utilize both as a cornerstone in building a healthful foundation for delicious eating. You'll find entirely new culinary worlds to explore while at the same time avoiding the trappings of the modern Western diet. You are likely already familiar with the herbs and spices of a number of different flavor profiles.

Think of Asian cuisine and certain flavors come immediately to mind; most likely they contain spices like star anise and cinnamon among others. Think of Mexican cuisine and it may bring to mind the refreshing bite of cilantro and the heat of chili peppers. Italian food may sing of thyme, oregano, and basil. There are many excellent books that cover the composition of different flavor profiles from around the world.

When you are out dining and traveling, inquire about the herbs, spices, and seasonings that are used in meals you find particularly pleasing. Experiment and build a spice cabinet and herb garden that caters to the tastes you enjoy. These spices are the tools in your toolbox. They are the colors for your canvas. Mix them as they please your palate. Play with them as it suits your tastes. One of the rewarding aspects of building your own spice blends and flavor profiles, or tweaking readily available ones, is that you can make them uniquely suited to your preferences. If you like little more heat, you can add a little more chili powder. Prefer a smoky flavor, then maybe it is smoked paprika instead of regular. The potential is truly limitless.

Incorporating the spice blends as a regular part of your diet does more than just enhance the tastes and textures of your foods. Spices and herbs add important, healthful nutrients to the diet. They are great sources of trace minerals, anti-inflammatory compounds, antioxidants, antimicrobials, vitamins, and fiber.

Many herbs and spices are rich in antioxidant compounds. Among these are various anthocyanins and quercetin, compounds that are believed to give red wine its healthful benefit. These compounds and other antioxidants like kaempferol can help protect against degenerative diseases like Alzheimer-type dementia, certain types of cancers, and the effects of aging.[623] Herbs and spices can also enhance your body's own antioxidant capacity through turbocharging enzymes such as superoxide dismutase and catalase.

They are a great source of copper, manganese, dietary fiber, vitamin K, vitamin C, vitamin A, vitamin B complex, calcium, iron, potassium, zinc, selenium, and magnesium, and some even provide omega-3 fatty acids. The insoluble fiber helps promote gastrointestinal health and can also help relieve constipation. By binding to the bile salts that are produced by our own bodies and facilitating their excretion, insoluble dietary fiber helps to promote a favorable lipid profile and aids our body in removing toxins. Both copper and iron are necessary for healthy red blood cells. Zinc is a trace element that is needed by many enzymes throughout the body. Many herbs and spices are known for their ability to reduce inflammation, improve cardiovascular health, reduce the risk of certain cancers, and improve digestion.

Many, if not most, of the herbs and spices available have been used as both medicine and food for centuries all around the globe. In the Indian subcontinent, certain spices like turmeric have been shown to have powerful anti-inflammatory and antioxidant properties. It plays an important role in Ayurvedic medicine, which originates from this area.

Turmeric contains the extremely powerful antioxidant curcumin, which acts to help prevent damage to the liver that in some instances can lead to cirrhosis. It also helps the body eliminate compounds such as heterocyclic amines. These potentially carcinogenic compounds are the result of a variety of cooking processes. Curcumin has also been shown to directly inhibit the growth of skin cancers such as melanoma. It also slows the spread of breast cancer into the lungs.

Such powerful antioxidants may aid in reducing one of the dreaded diseases of modern civilization and the result of aging and inflammation—Alzheimer-type dementia. But some of the success relies on utilizing spices in combination. Together there is a synergistic effect. Common fresh-ground black pepper contains piperine. It also originates from the Indian subcontinent and can be found in many foods along with turmeric. There is more than just a savory and delightful taste combination between these two spices.

Piperine is necessary for the absorption of curcumin in the gastrointestinal tract. In addition to its own impressive antioxidant and antibacterial activity, piperine promotes digestive health. Derived from the freshly ground black pepper, the outer layer of the peppercorn stimulates the breakdown of fat cells thereby increasing your energy level.

Because of the powerful anti-inflammatory activity of many herbs and spices, they may relieve joint pain. Other herbs and spices have been shown to be useful for insomnia, anxiety, and muscle spasms. They can aid in digestion and help relieve nausea and vomiting, indigestion and diarrhea. Some spices, such as cinnamon, have been shown to reduce blood pressure and help in glucose metabolism. Herbs and spices rich in anthocyanins and chalcone polymers are powerful antioxidants. These compounds improve blood flow and can help prevent ulcer formation.

Other herbs and spices contain compounds with strong antibacterial and antifungal activity. Many of these have been used for centuries for medicinal purposes, including treatment of respiratory conditions such as congestion, asthma, coughs, bronchitis, sinusitis, sore throats, and laryngitis. Many are believed to have detoxifying properties. Such spices and herbs as oregano, thyme, and basil can be great sources of folate, iron, vitamin A, vitamin C, and vitamin K. With the powerful anti-inflammatory and antioxidant properties they can act to promote cardiovascular health, relieve arthritis and prevent such diseases as Alzheimer-type dementia and malignant tumors.

Hot chili peppers are rich in vitamin C. In addition to anti-inflammatory properties such spices contain antimicrobial and antiviral properties as well. Herbs and spices can act to help induce satiety and at the same time help crank up the metabolism. Simultaneously it helps you feel good while eating less, literally. The capsaicin found in chili peppers help us secrete our own endogenous opioids; the same compounds that are believed to give runners their natural high.

Fresh herbs should be bright and vibrant. They are easy to grow, and it is easy to have some of your favorite fresh herbs always readily available with just a windowsill planter. Dried herbs can store for several months. Being dried, they can concentrate certain flavors and compounds and can be a little more potent. However, herbs like basil, which contain many volatile components, can lose vitality and quickly become less than useful. Always purchase your dried herbs and spices from a reputable provider. Regardless of whom you purchase them from, after several months you may need to discard unused and washed-out dried herbs.

Spices will last longer, but ultimately fade as well. As with herbs, spices that contain volatile oils will have a shorter shelf life than those that do not. An easy way to extend the life of your spices is to buy whole spices where possible and grind them as you need them. This is also useful when you want to lightly toast the spices to alter their flavor profile. A simple spice grinder or an inexpensive coffee-bean grinder can be an indispensable kitchen ally in your utilization of spices; not to mention an aid in creating your own favorite blends.

You have likes and dislikes, favorites and items you might not care so much for. That's okay; that's the point. Take the Bruce Lee approach: Give everything a try, pick what you like, keep what is useful, and discard what isn't. This is all about you and charting your course. The spices, the recipes, the ingredients are your vessel.

Studies have shown that a properly seasoned and spiced meal leaves people more satisfied and with greater feelings of satiety than a boring meal made from the same ingredients. Combined with proper timing and portion control you will achieve a greater satisfaction while actually consuming less food. That helps you maintain the proper weight and leads to overall better health. Adhere to the Grassroots Gourmet™ principles and you can sail anywhere you like.

The quality ingredients, the proper balance, and the correct ratios along with spices and herbs supply you not only with a firm nutritional foundation; they properly prepare the ground for our microbial minions. It is quite likely that the beneficial effects of herbs and spices are related to their direct and indirect effects on the composition of our gut microbiome.[624,625,626] That is the intestinal revolution and the inflammatory solution.

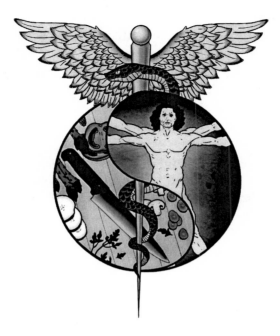

Moving Forward

The constituents of the modern Western diet are defined by the four P's: (over) processed, (artificially) preserved, prepackaged, and pre-prepared. These horsemen of dietary Armageddon leave behind in their wake a bland offering of wheats, sweets, meats, and greasy treats served between layers upon layers of sugar, salt, and fat.

They have not only affected us directly, but they have modified us indirectly through alterations in our gut microbiome. By altering this microenvironment the neighborhood we exist in is fundamentally changed. Our gut microbiome is the nexus where our environment meets our genetics. For those who consume the modern Western diet this sea of tranquility has become a sea of monsters. It has become a roiling sea of continuous, chronic low-grade inflammation. We emerge from this wasteland with our genetic weaknesses transformed into the diseases of modern civilization.

The detrimental effects of the components of the modern Western diet are compounded by the *obesogenic* environment in which the diet exists. Such surroundings foment unrestricted access to energy-dense and nutrient-poor foods, and large portion sizes, all in the setting of reduced physical activity. The presence of high-fat, high-sugar, highly salted, highly refined, and ultimately highly addictive foods that are always available can lead to chronic overconsumption. Our hedonic system is activated and overwhelmed. The result is like any pleasure-producing drug—habit-forming behavior, habituation, and a vicious cycle of addiction.

Such deceptively decadent packaging bypasses the normal homeostatic appetite-regulatory mechanisms we employ to counter such threats. The result is we unconsciously head back to the drive-through time and again, like lambs to the slaughter. One consequence of these actions is that we take in more energy than we can possibly use.[627]

The corruption and abuse of the modern food industry's use of sugar, salt, and fat is a terrible triumvirate. The addition of salt enhances the palatability of the sugar and fat combination.[628] It is the reason sweet cakes contain small amounts of salt and many breads and savory baked goods contain sugar. We succumb to the power of this unholy trinity because of our inherent, hardwired flaws. We become a large, wormlike Pizza the Hutt.

The singular focus on weight reduction as the only means to restore our body to balance and homeostasis has been attempted in various forms *ad nauseam*. The repeated failure of isolated dietary modification is well documented. It is clear that an isolated dietary approach is largely unsuccessful over the long-term, no matter the type of diet attempted.[629] A one-size-fits-all approach to get all to fit into one size is inappropriate and fails to address the need for metabolic health.

It is essential to understand that the environment under any scenario does not adapt to our genes. The genes we are born with hold the keys to what we may become—our phenotype. Where the determination as to whether our phenotype blooms in glory or succumbs to disability and disease occurs is within our gut. It is our diet that determines that internal microenvironment. Our gut microbiome depends on our diet and our diet depends on both the quantity and quality of what we choose to consume.

Within any group of people eating the same food, there can be a tremendous variation in response between the individuals. There can also be significant intra-individual variation. We constantly change with what we eat. When we eat something the body releases insulin and a number of other hormones and begins to shift to an anabolic state. During the fasting state and while we sleep, glucagon, epinephrine, and other hormones are released and the body shifts to a catabolic, oxidative state.

This balancing act is partly mediated by insulin sensitivity, leptin action, and the hypothalamic response.[630] These in turn are affected by emotional states, sleep, physical activity, disease states, and what and how we eat. The quantity and quality of what we choose to ingest directly impacts our bodies and our gut microbiome. This ultimately determines whether we exist in a state of health and wellness, of balance, or whether we are pushed from that point into a state of disease. There are genetic, psychological, and behavioral factors that interact with these physiological and metabolic systems and impact directly upon our food behavior.

It is incumbent upon us to re-examine what should be considered our dietary standard and how we should strive to return our bodies to such a state of homeostasis—a state of ease. It is doubtful that this can be accomplished through intensively trying to isolate single nutrients, vitamins, minerals, or other foodstuffs in separateness from the dietary whole. It is like trying to see the universe through a keyhole. Only by understanding the whole from whence we came may we shed the *dis-ease* impressed upon us by the modern Western diet.

Displacement and deficiency of omega-3 fatty acids are another hallmark of the modern Western diet. This can result in cognitive dysfunction, impaired vision, and other central nervous system abnormalities. Deficiency of omega-6 fatty acids can result in growth retardation, reproductive failure, fatty liver and scaly skin subject to transdermal water loss.[631] Combined essential-fatty-acid deficiencies lead to skin changes, decreased resistance to infections, altered mental status, structural CNS abnormalities, and impaired growth.

Such essential fatty acid deficiencies often coexist in the setting of protein-energy malnutrition (PEM). Certain genetic polymorphisms are more susceptible to others in such a setting. Your genetic blueprint may make you vulnerable to any number of the disabilities and diseases mentioned when the diet is inadequate. Yet when given adequate protein and essential fatty acids there is no disease. Your DNA has not changed. This is yet another example of genetics that do not cause a disease by their expression, but only when exposed to certain unfavorable environments that are a consequence of our diet.

This phenomenon was demonstrated in a study performed in Spain.[632] This study examined over seven thousand Spanish men and women as part of the ongoing PREDIMED inquiry into the various potential benefits to the Mediterranean diet. They looked at individuals with a genetic variant, the Transcription Factor 7-like 2 (TCF7L2-rs7903146) polymorphism, which predisposes people to an increased risk of glucose and lipid abnormalities as well as the development of type 2 diabetes. Just having this genetic variant significantly increases a person's risk of developing type 2 diabetes. But it doesn't guarantee it. The diabetes will only manifest in the right environment.

The study found that when people with this genetic variant embraced a traditional Mediterranean diet, their blood sugars, or blood glucose levels, were like that of someone without diabetes. They had no disease.

When such a dietary approach was rejected in favor of the modern Western diet, the fasting blood glucose levels were diagnostic of someone with type 2 diabetes. The same pattern was observed for total cholesterol, LDL cholesterol, and triglycerides. They developed disease.

This study had a very significant, hard end-point in terms of cardiovascular events. Those patients with the genetic variant who did not partake of the Mediterranean diet had roughly three times the risk of stroke. The participants' genetics did not change. The determinant of whether or not they developed disease was their dietary environment. This should give us hope.

Certain genetic markers that are associated with certain diseases do not always produce those diseases. We are learning that these diseases will not manifest unless the genes are exposed to a hazardous environment. It is not necessarily the gene that causes the disease, it is the environment that allows it to become manifest.

Two hundred years before it was a *Man versus Food* world, Jean Anthelme Brillat-Savarin famously wrote, "Tell me what you eat, and I shall tell you what you are."[633] That statement seems even more pertinent and true today than when it was originally written. And who we are, at least in the United States, is a nation that while living longer is not necessarily living healthier.

Through advances in modern medicine, engineering, sanitation, public health, and technology the average American is living longer than he or she did just decades ago.[634] Despite the gains in absolute years of average life expectancy, the healthy average life expectancy (HALE), one free from major disease and disability, is only sixty-eight years. That value places the US twenty-sixth among the thirty-four member countries of the Organization for Economic Co-operation and Development, for whom this variable was measured. This ranking is down thirteen spots from just a decade ago. All this, while across all measures, Americans spend more per capita on healthcare than residents in any other country.[635,636]

Our autumn years remain marred by the burden of chronic disease and disability. We may spend the last three decades[637] of our lives wandering about like Jacob Marley bound with chains of infirmary. These chronic ills of modern civilization now account for about half of the entire health-care burden of the United States.[638] They include many of the diseases that seem to increase in incidence and prevalence despite our best efforts. Diseases such as coronary artery disease, obesity, hypertension, diabetes, polycystic ovary syndrome, myopia, acne, gout, certain cancers, and autoimmune diseases.[639,640,641,642,643]

The largest single risk factor impacting the number of years we spend with chronic disease and disability is the composition of our diet. We spend about twice as much on food expenditures as we do on health care.[644] Despite the importance, despite the money spent, the standard American diet remains high in processed meats, trans-fats, sugars, refined carbohydrates, and added sodium; and low in vegetables, fruits, nuts, and seeds. The standard American diet is truly SAD. Of all the risk factors impacting the quality of our lives, the years lived free from disease and disability by any measure, none is more important than diet.

And it is not just about the mass quantities consumed. The composition of the diet is a more potent risk factor than obesity as measured by a high body mass index (BMI) equal to or greater than thirty. Quality matters. The end result of our modern Western diet is that while Americans may be living longer they are not necessarily doing so in good health.[645] To answer Brillat-Savarin's question, what we are is ill, and the cause is what we eat.

Yet it need not be so. Diets utilizing less processed and minimally adulterated foods, like those found in the preindustrial diet, have confirmed positive healthful outcomes[646]. Such diets have parallels in the diets of modern hunter-gatherers. This remains true even though such groups typically derive over half of their energy requirements from animal sources,[647] and anywhere from 28 percent to 58 percent of their daily energy requirements is derived from dietary fat,[648] with all due respect to Zooey Deschanel.

Over halfway across the globe, the classical diet of Crete is comprised of 35 percent to 40 percent fats. Yet the incidences of cardiovascular disease and other diseases of civilization are one-third of that seen in populations that consume the more modern Western diet.[649] The French paradox demonstrated rates of cardiovascular disease from one-third to one-half of that seen in Americans consuming the modern Western diet.[650] Approximately 37 percent to 42 percent of the dietary energy of the French diet comes from fats, with about 16 percent from saturated fat.[651] All these approaches consume more fat than the modern Western diet.[652]

We eat less fat, and less saturated fat, than many other societies around the world. Yet we suffer much more chronic disability and disease. Nonetheless the conventional wisdom continues to hammer home the over simplistic message that if we simply eat less fat we will become healthier. It is about natural, unprocessed, and varied choices. You don't have to be a gluten-free vegan. You certainly can be if you want but do it because it's the foods you love to eat, not as the result of some cockamamie Internet meme.

It is not that fats are bad and eating fats, even saturated fats, is the root cause of all our problems. It is the types of fats and unhealthy pro-inflammatory ratios we devour. The Japanese consume more sodium than the average American and live substantially longer. The Kuna Indians eat more salt than the average American and do not suffer hypertension, cardiovascular disease, or other diseases of modern civilization. It is not just the amount of sodium we consume; it is the sodium-to-potassium ratio and the ill effects of displacement reflected in that ratio. It is not the carbohydrates that cause our health-related problems, but the refined products that are devoid of any redeeming characteristics.

When foods are energy and nutrient dense, such as the naturally derived plant and animal sources, less volume is required to deliver needed amounts of energy and nutrients. Such a diet also supplies the raw materials that feed our microbial minions and keep them in a healthful harmony. A fatal flaw in the modern Western diet is that while it may be energy dense, it is nutrient poor. It fails to supply the proper fuel for our gut microbiome. The modern Western diet, with its innumerable chemicals and compounds, creates a toxic environment in which our normal gut flora cannot thrive. But by changing our diet we can change our internal environment and thus alter ourselves.

And therein is our window of opportunity. A study looked at individuals with certain genetic markers that make them susceptible to the development of metabolic syndrome—a precursor of type 2 diabetes. More than seven hundred overweight and obese people were studied for more than two years. There was a high-fat, with 40 percent of caloric intake from fat, group; and a low-fat, with 20 percent of caloric intake from fat, group. For individuals with one of those markers, the high-fat diet led to a statistically significant greater weight loss than the low-fat diet. Lower weight means less metabolic syndrome; that means less diabetes, disability and death.

In other words, a higher fat diet translated into less disability, disease, and risk of death for those with the right genes. For individuals without the certain genetic marker, it made no difference. Stop and think about that. Depending on your genetics, a higher fat diet could improve your health. This is the complete opposite of conventional wisdom and public perception. What this highlights is that it is about what is right for you, the individual. This life is not one size or one strategy fits all.

Since the Industrial Revolution and particularly in the last fifty to seventy-five years the modern Western diet has become dominated by refined carbohydrates in terms of macronutrient consumption. It has seen a displacement result in an increase in the omega-6 to omega-3–PUFA ratio along with an increase in trans-fatty acids. The carbohydrates that dominate the modern Western diet consist of a preponderance of high glycemic indices. There has been a decrease in the consumption of certain micronutrients, decreased fiber intake, a shift from a base-producing to an acidic diet, and an inversion of the normal sodium-to-potassium ratio.[653]

The short time period over which this has occurred does not allow for genomic adaption. Many of the polymorphisms that are now associated with certain disease states have likely been part of the original human genome. In other words, genes associated with the diseases of modern Western civilization do not manifest as such unless we expose ourselves to a conducive environment.

The traditional view makes us a victim of genetic inevitability. But we are captains of our own ships; we can be masters of our own fates. The faulty environment that brings disability and disease to our shores is one we sail to through the food we choose to eat.

The Maasai, a tribal group in Africa, consume a dairy-rich diet heavy in saturated fat and cholesterol. They consume about 600 mg per day of cholesterol compared to about 300 mg per day for the average American. Despite the high saturated-fat, high-cholesterol diet their serum total cholesterol is very low. They do not have a significant increase in blood pressure with age like that seen in those who consume the modern Western diet.

In addition to what has already been mentioned, the Maasai also have a very low incidence of coronary artery disease and other diseases of modern civilization. They are also as a general rule very physically fit.[654,655,656] The effect of diet must be taken in the context of physical activity and overall lifestyle. It is a lifestyle change we must master.

Dr. Mike's Grassroots Gourmet™ Program: An Intestinal Revolution and the Inflammatory Solution is the dietary keystone for health and wellness. But it should be combined with other practices that foster a healthy life full of happiness and enjoyment. After thirty days on the program you will have undergone a tremendously positive transformation. But where do you go from here?

As you move forward continue to apply the program, but remain flexible. Because life gets in the way, trying to be unyielding and rigid in adherence will only set you up for failure. A good rule of thumb is the 80/20 rule. If you can adhere to the ten steps of the program at least 80 percent of the time, if not more, you will achieve great long-term success.

If you have to occasionally travel, make the best possible choices. Plan ahead. Eat before you leave for the airport so you don't need to eat the airline food. Pack some snacks for that long car trip, try to find some decent place to eat off the highway in unfamiliar territory. And if you find yourself having to indulge in the modern Western diet because circumstances dictate it, or simply because it's a celebration: relax. A chili cheese dog with fries once in a blue moon does not condemn you to dietary damnation, although you may feel pretty crappy later. And when it does make you feel crappy later, when the food that you used to routinely consume as part of the modern Western diet now makes you a bit ill, that is a good sign.

Expand these positive results of your newfound metabolic health into other areas of your life. If you are a smoker, perhaps your thirty-day success with this can supply you the motivation to quit tobacco.

Perhaps it can supply you the motivation to engage in some physical activity—any physical activity. In addition to helping keep us at a healthy weight, physical activity and exercise have a myriad of short- and long-term health benefits. Life in our on-the-go, never-resting world can be quite stressful. Find positive ways that can help you reduce or at least effectively combat the stressors in your life.

Like the food we eat that sustains our body, our mind and our spirit, life is an experiential journey. Enjoy it. Lifestyle is not just what you eat, but what you do and, as Yoda might implore, what you do not. What and how we eat, how we feel, and how we move are inexorably linked in shaping our ultimate metabolic phenotype. As Metallica noted, "My lifestyle determines my deathstyle."[657]

We have detailed the thirty-day program. Now make it your own lifestyle. *Dr. Mike's Grassroots Gourmet™ Program: An Intestinal Revolution and the Inflammatory Solution* is briefly recapped below in ten easy-to-follow steps.

Detoxifying juice fast, days 1–3. It is recommended that you continue to juice at least once a day.

Probiotics, days 1–30. After the thirty-day program is complete, you should no longer require daily probiotics. However, feel free to use them as directed at your discretion.

Prebiotics, days 4–30. It is easy to make your diet rich in prebiotics by simply adding a healthy serving of fresh vegetables to your meals. Include fresh fruits for snacking and dessert and all your bases are covered. As with juicing, it is recommended that you continue this practice indefinitely.

No modern wheat, days 4–30. It is recommended that you continue to avoid all products containing modern wheat. Feel free to use other cereals, grains, and ancient wheat as desired.

No high fructose corn syrup or artificial sweeteners, days 4–30. As with the modern wheat, it is recommended that you never consume these again. When you have need to use sugar, use raw forms or substitutes that have redeeming characteristics like maple syrup, molasses or honey when possible.

Avoid the call of the junk food/fast food siren, days 4–30. This is pretty straightforward; no junk food or fast food. As with HFCS, these items should never pass between your lips again.

No adultery, days 4–30. As much as is possible, attempt to avoid the over-processed, artificially preserved, pre-prepared and prepackaged convenience items that make up such a large proportion of the modern Western diet. These are the four horsemen of the dietary Apocalypse and every attempt should be made to avoid them and their adulterated comestibles—forever.

Use timing and proportion, days 4–30. When constructing your meals utilize the principles of timing and proportion. You should practice these doctrines always.

Understand food value, days 4–30. When selecting what to eat get beyond equating value with quantity. Understand that because of the changes that have occurred to our food and our food pathways since the Industrial Revolution we must now carefully evaluate the quality of our food choices. *What* you are supersizing is more important than how much you get. As with timing and proportion, practice this always.

Be spiced for life, days 4–30. Utilize herbs and spices to add flavor, taste, and texture to your cuisine. Learn to taste again and break the modern Western diet's addictive abuse of sugar, salt, and fat. By doing this at every meal every day you will not only learn to taste again, you'll learn to live again.

We exist as part of the natural world, not in isolation against it. As part of Nature, we should enjoy the winds and tides of her natural rhythms and ratios. The only true measure of health will be the ratio between what we might have eaten and what we might have become on the one hand, and the things we have eaten and made of ourselves on the other.[658]

Acknowledgements

There are so many people to thank when a project like this comes to completion that invariably someone important will be left off the list. So perhaps it is best to begin with apologies to whoever remains unmentioned. All the innumerable contributions, in all the myriad ways are much appreciated. The responsibility for any oversight, and thus the blame, is mine and mine alone.

Another good place to begin is the beginning. So I must start with a tip of the hat to my good friends and troubadours, Wendy and Tim. If not for the full moon and the bright stars in the shadow of Chichén Itza—not to mention a margarita or two—this strange trip may never have been launched. May there be many more adventures outside our doors.

Special thanks has to go out to all those who have helped me keep a sharp eye and a warrior's heart for almost as many decades as I've been on this good Earth. To Soke Masaaki Hatsumi, for sharing his art, particularly with a grubby young *gaijin*. Kevin Millis, a repository of ancient skills and insights, for making the incomprehensible seem somehow achievable. To KT Cahill, for keeping us both sane—or at least as close as possible. To Mark Lithgow, for keeping the light of the true *Budoka* spirit shining and always offering an open door to a stranger in a strange land. To William Johnson, I could ask for no better companion to share the journey and the beatings; may our paths, and our blades, cross soon. To Susanne Williams, it is not the quantity of experience, but the intensity. To Dr. Glenn Morris, thanks for the magic, and the memories.

To all those friends and colleagues in the medical and healing communities who encouraged, reviewed and commented on this work as it progressed. Special thanks to Dr. Peggy Fleming, for keeping everything, including myself, in balance. To doctors John

McPherson, Arthur Moritz, and Amy Tucker—a heartfelt thanks for invaluable insight and observation.

I likewise owe a deep debt of gratitude to my good friends chefs Luca Paris, Susan Irby, Jennifer Booker, Joumana Accad, and Aine McAteer, for their valuable perception and unwavering support and belief in some radical idea, like that wholesome natural food that is good for you can be made into delicious meals. Thanks go out to Forbes Riley, always an inspiration for 'spicing' it up.

To Vicki Williams and Debbie Rose I thank you for the opportunity to present my thoughts to the public in the monthly columns that your publications afford. To Leticia Gomez, for making these dreams a written reality. To Josh Tolley, who has been an inspiration and a help in more ways than I can name; thank you for your friendship.

My final thoughts, as always, go to Jennifer, without whom nothing happens. Your support is the ship that we journey upon. You are the muse in the rigging and the wind in my black pirate sails.

References

(Editors) Carroll, R., & Prickett, S. (1997). *The Bible: Authorized King James Version* . New York: Oxford University Press.

Adabag, S., Lopez, F., Alonso, A., Mukamal, K., Buzkova, P., Rosenberg, M., et al. (2012). Risk of sudden cardiac death in obese individuals: The Atherosclerosis Risk in Communities (ARIC) study". *Rhythm Society 2012 Scientific Sessions* (pp. Abstract PO1-67.). Boston, MA.: Heart Rhythm Society.

Alas-Salvado, J., Farres, X., & Luque, X. (2008). Effect of Two Doses of a Mixture of Soluble Fibres on Body Weight and Metabolic Variables in Overweight or Obese Patients: a Randomized Tri al. *Br J Nutr* , 99 (6): 1380-1387.

Alderman, M. (2010, May 10). *Einstein on Salt: Is Less Sodium Always Better?* Retrieved January 23, 2013, from Einstein School of Medicine: http://www.einstein.yu.edu/video/?VID=162#top

Alpern, R., & Sakhaee, S. (1997). The Clinical Spectrum of Chronic Metabolic Acidosis: Homeostatic Mechanisms Produce Significant Morbidity. *Am J Kidney Dis* , 29:291-302.

American Cancer Society. (2004). *Cancer facts and figures 2004.* Atlanta, Georgia: American Cancer Society.

American Cancer Society. (2013). *Colorectal Cancer.* Retrieved November 17, 2013, from American Cancer Society: http://www. cancer.org/acs/groups/content/@epidemiologysurveilance/docu-ments/document/acspc-028323.pdf

Ames, B. N. (2001). DNA Damage for Micronutrient Deficiencies Is Likely to Be a Major Cause of Cancer. *Mutation Research/ Fundamental and Molecular Mechanisms of Mutagenesis* , 475 (1-2): 7-20.

Anderson, J., & Gilliland, S. (1999). Effect of fermented milk (yogurt) containing Lactobacillus acidophilus L1 on serum cholesterol in hypercholesterolemic humans. *J Am Coll Nutr.* , 18(1):43-50.

Anderson, J., Smith, B., & Gustafson, M. (1994). Health Benefits and Practical Aspects of High Fiber Diets. *Am J Clin Nutr* , 59 (supplement): 1442S-1247S.

Antonios, T., & MacGregor, G. (1996). Salt-More Adverse Effects. *Lancet* , 348:250-251.

Apfelbaum, M. (1992). Which Is the Nutritional Advantage of the Consumption of a Free-Cholesterol Butter? *Rev Prat* , 42:1925-1926.

Arnold, S. V., Smolderen, K. G., Buchanan, D. M., Li, Y., &

.Spertus, J. A. (2012). Perceived Stress in Myocardial Infarction Long-Term Mortality and Health Status Outcomes. *J Am Coll Cardiol.* , doi:10.1016/j.jacc.2012.06.044 .

Ask.com. (2013). *What Is the Weight of a Feather in Grams?* Retrieved July 4, 2013, from Ask.com: http://www.ask.com/question/what-is-the-weight-of-a-feather-in-grams

Associated Press. (2002, November 18). *Study: Atkins diet good for cholesterol.* Retrieved October 8, 2011, from USAToday.com: http://www.usatoday.com/news/health/2002-11-18-adkins_x.htm

Astorg, P., Arnault, N., Czernichow, S., Noisette, N., Galan, P., & Hercberg, S. (2004). Dietary Intakes and Food Sources of and-6 and and-3 PUFA in French Adult Men and Women. *Lipids* , 39:527-535.

Atchinson, J., Head, L., & Gates, A. (2010). Wheat As Food, Wheat As Industrial Substance; Comparative Geographies of Transformation and Mobility. *Geoforum* , 41:236-246.

Aywerx, J. (1999). PPAR gamma, the ultimate thrifty gene. *Diabetologia* , 42:1033-1049.

Bakhed, F., Ley, R., Sonnenberg, J., Peterson, D., & Gordon, J. (2005). Host-Bacterial Mutualism in the Human Intestine. *Science* , 307:1915-1920.

Baloch, U. K. (1999). *Wheat: post-harvest operations.* Pakistan: Pakistan agricultural research Council.

Barbeau, W., Bassaganya-Riere, J., & Hontacillas, R. (2007). Putting the Pieces of the Puzzle Together: a Series of Hypotheses on the Etiology and Pathogenesis of Type I Diabetes. *Med Hypotheses* , 68 (3): 607-619.

Barclay, A., Petocz, P., & McMillan-Price, J. (2008). Glycemic Index, Glycemic Load, and Chronic Disease: A Meta-Analysis of Observational Studies. *Am J Clin Nutr* , 87(3): 627-637.

Barona, J., Aristizabal, J. C., Blesso, C. N., Volek, J. S., & Fernandez, M. L. (2012). Grape Polyphenols Reduce Blood Pressure and Increase Flow-Mediated Vasodilation in Men with Metabolic Syndrome1. *The Journal of Nutrition* , 142 (9):1626-1632.

Bayer, R., Johns, M. D., & Galea, S. (2012). Salt and Public Health: Contested Science and the Challenge of Evidence-Based Decision Making. *Health Affairs* , 31 (12):2738-2746.

Befort, C. A., Nazir, N., & Perri, M. G. (2012). Prevalence of Obesity Among Adults From Rural and Urban Areas of the United States: Findings From NHANES (2005-2008). *Journal of Rural Health* , 28(4):392-7.

Bellows, L., & Moore, R. (2012, November). *Fat-Soluble Vitamins: A, D, E, and K.* Retrieved August 4, 2013, from Colorado State University: http://www.ext.colostate.edu/pubs/foodnut/09315.html

Benbeook, C. M., Butler, G., Latif, M. A., Leifert, C., & Davis, D. R. (2013). Organic Production Enhances Milk Nutritional Quality by Shifting Fatty Acid Composition: the United States-Wide, Eighteen-Month Study. *PLoS ONE* , DOI: 10.1371/journal.pone.0082429.

Berg, J., Tymoczko, J., & Stryer, L. (W H Freeman). *Biochemistry, 5th edition.* New York: 2002.

Bernardo, D., Garrote, J., & Fernanadez-Salazar, L. (2007). Is gliadin really safe for non--coeliac individuals? Production of interleukin 15 in biopsy culture from non--coeliac individuals challenged with gliadin peptides. *Gut* , 56 (6): 889-890.

Bernstin, A., & Willet, W. (2010). Trends in 24-h Urinary Sodium Excretion in the United States, 1957-2003: a Systematic Review. *Am J Clin Nutr* , 92:1172-1180.

Bertino, M., Beauchamp, G., Burke, D., & Engelman, K. (1982). Long-Term Reduction in Dietary Sodium Alters the Taste of Salt. *Am J Clin Nutr* , 36:1134-1144.

Bettage, A. (2009, January). *Cereal Knowledge Database: Club wheat: Functionally, the best sub-class and sub-species in soft wheat.* Retrieved December 31, 2011, from www.aacnet.org: http://www.aaccnet.org/CerScienceKnowledgedb/Summary/ABettge.asp

Bianconi, E., Piovesan, A., Facchin, F., Bersaudi, A., Casadei, R., Frabetti, F., et al. (2013). An estimation of the number of cells in the human body. *Ann Hum Biol* , 40(6):471.

Bibbins-Domingo, K., Cherow, G., Coxson, P., Moran, A., Lightwood, J., Pletcher, M., et al. (2010). Projected effect of dietary salt reductionson future cardiovascular disease. *NEJM* , 362(7):590-9.

Bible, T. H. (2007). *The Holy Bible: New Living Translation.* Caroil Stream, Illinois: Tyndale House.

BibleGateway.com. (2011). *Pslam 90.* Retrieved march 15, 2013, from BibleGateway.com: http://www.biblegateway.com/passage/?search=Psalm+90&version=NIV

Bier, D., Brosnan, J., & Flatt, J. (1999). Report of the IDECG Working Group on Lower and Upper Limits of Carbohydrate and Fat Intake. *Eur J Clin Nutr* , 53 (suppl):S177-178.

Billing, J., & Sherman, P. W. (1998). Antimicrobial Functions of Spices: Why Some Like It Hot. *The Quarterly Review of Biology* , Vol. 73, No.1; 3-49.

Birch, L. (1999). Development of Food Preferences. *Ann Rev Nutr* , 19:41-62.

Bleich, S. N., Wolfson, J. A., Vine, S., & Wang, C. (2014). Diet-Beverage Consumption and Caloric Intake Among US Adults, Overall and by Body Weight. *American Journal of Public Health* , 104 (3):e72-e78.

Blundell, J., & Macdiarmind, J. (1997). Passive Overconsumption. Fat Intake and Short-Term Energy Balance. *Ann NY Acad Sci* , 827:392-407.

Boaz, N. (2002). *Evolving Health: The Origins of Illness and How The Modern World is Making Us Sick.* New York: Wiley and Sons.

Bogh, M. K., Schmedes, A. V., Philipsen, P. A., Thieden, E., & Wulf, H. C. (2010). Vitamin D Production after UVB Exposure Depends on Baseline Vitamin D and Total Cholesterol but Not on Skin Pigmentation. *Journal of Investigative Dermatology* , 130: 546-553.

Bohn, T., Davidsson, L., Walczyk, T., & Hurrell, R. (2004). Phytic Acid Added to White-Wheat Bread Inhibits Fractional Apparent Magnesium Absorption in Humans. *Am J Clin Nutr* , 79 (3): 418-423.

Boughton, B. (2011, August 19). *Processed meat linked to increased stroke risk.* Retrieved from MedScape: http://www.medscape.com/viewarticle/791009

Bouton, M. (2007). *Learning and behavior: A contemporary synthesis.* Sunderland, MA: Sinauer Associates.

Boyles, S. (2013, December 10). *Endocrinology: Diabetes: Hearty Breakfast Aids A1c Control.* Retrieved December 11, 2013, from MedPage: http://www.medpagetoday.com/Endocrinology/Obesity/43351

Brand-Miller, J., Dickinson, S., Berkeley, A., & Allman-Farinelli, M. (2009). Glycemic Index, Glycemic Load, and Thrombogenesis. *Semin Thromb Hemost* , 35 (1): 111-118.

Brand-Miller, J., Thomas, M., Swan, V., Ahmad, Z., Petocz, P., & Colagiuri, S. (2003). Physiological Validation of the Concept of Glycemic Load in Lean Young Adults1. *The Journal of Nutrition* , 133 (9):2728-2732.

Brauser, D. (2013, March 15). *Proposed Subspecialty Combines Psychiatry, Cardiology.* Retrieved March 18, 2013, from Medscape: http://www.medscape.com/viewarticle/780867

Briefel, R., & Johnson, C. (2004). Secular Trends in Dietary Intake in the United States. *Ann Rev Nutr* , 24:401-431.

Brillat-Savarin, J. A. (2000). *Physiology of Taste, or Meditations on Transcendental Gastronomy (Translated by M.F. K. Fisher)*. New York, NY: Counterpoint Press.

Brillat-Savarin, J. A. (2009). *The Physiology of Taste*. New York: Alfred A. Knopf.

Brisman, J. (2002). Baker's Asthma. *Occupation and Environmental Medicine* , 59:498-502.

Brown, C. H. (2010). Development of Agriculture in Prehistoric Mesoamerica: The Linguistic Evidence. In J. E. Staller, & M. (. Carrasco, *Pre-Columbian Foodways: Interdisciplinary Approaches to Food, Culture, and Markets in Ancient Mesoamerica* (p. 101). New York: Springer Science.

Buffett, J., & Chapman, M. (Composers). (1988). Smart Woman (In A Real Short Skirt). [J. Buffet, Performer, & H. Water, Conductor]

Burnett, J. (2005). Brown Is Best. *History Today* , 55:52-54.

Burton-Freeman, B., Davis, P., & Schneeman, B. (2002). Plasma Cholecystokinin Is Associated with Subjective Measures of Satiety in Women. *Am J Clin Nutr* , 76:659-67.

Bushinsky, D. (1996). Metabolic Alkalosis Decreases Bone Calcium Efflux by Suppressing Osteoclast and Stimulating Osteoblasts. *Am J Physiol* , 271:F216-222.

Calderón-Montaño, J., Burgos-Morón, E., Pérez-Guerrero, C., & López-Lázaro, M. (2011). A review on the dietary flavonoid kaempferol. *Mini Rev Med Chem* , 11(4):298-344.

Campbell, B., Kreider, R., & Ziegenfuss, T. (2007). International Society of Sports Nutrition Position Stand: Protein and Exercise. *J Int Soc Sports Nutr* , 4:8.

Cani, P., Bibiloni, R., & Knauf, C. (2008). Changes in Gut Microbiotica Controlled Metabolic Endotoxemia-Induced Inflammation in High-and Fat Diet-Induced Obesity and Diabetes in Mice. *Diabetes* , 57 (6): 1470-1481.

Carey, O., Locke, C., & Cookson, J. (1993). Effect of Alterations of Dietary Sodium on the Severity of Asthma in Men. *Thorax* , 48:714-718.

Carnethon, M. R., D. De Chavez, P. J., Biggs, M. L., Lewis, C. E., Pankow, J. S., Bertoni, A. G., et al. (2012). Association of Weight Status With Mortality in Adults With Incident Diabetes. *JAMA* , 308(6):581-59.

Carrera-Bastos, P., Fontes-Villalba, M., O'Keefe, J. H., Lindeberg, S., & Cordain, L. (2011). The Western Diet and Lifestyle and Diseases of Civilization. *research reports And clinical cardiology* , (2) 15-35.

Cassidy, A., Mukamal, K. J., Liu, L., Franz, M., Eliassen, A. H., & Rimm, E. B. (2013). High Anthocyanin Intake Is Associated With a Reduced Risk of Myocardial Infarction in Young and Middle-Aged Women. *Circulation* , 127:188-196 doi: 10.1161/CIRCULATIONAHA.112.122408.

Cassidy, A., O'Reilly, E., Kay, C., Sampson, L., Franz, M., Forman, J., et al. (2011). Habitual intake of flavonoid subclasses and incident hypertension in adults. *Am J Clin Nutr.* , 93:338–347.

Casson, L. (1989). *The Periplus Maris Erythraei: Text With Introduction, Translation, and Commentary.* . Princeton, NJ: Princeton University Press.

Casteel, B. (2014). *Celiac Disease Linked to Increased Risk of Coronary Artery Disease: Study adds to mounting evidence about the role systemic inflammation may play in heart health.* Washington, DC: American College of Cardiology.

Castiglione, K., Read, N., & French, S. (1998). Food Intake Responses to Upper Gastrointestinal Lipid Infusions in Humans. *Physiol Behav* , 64:141-145.

CDC. (2011, August 17). *Healthy weight.* Retrieved December 10, 2012, from Centers for Disease Control: http://www.cdc.gov/healthyweight/assessing/index.html

Centers for Disease Control and Prevention. (2011, May 23). *2011 national diabetes fact sheet.* Retrieved July 13, 2013, from Centers for Disease Control and Prevention: http://www.cdc.gov/diabetes/pubs/estimates11.htm#1

Centers for Disease Control and Prevention. (2011, February 24). *Americans Consume Too Much Sodium.* Retrieved July 19, 2013, from Centers for Disease Control and Prevention: http://www.cdc.gov/features/dssodium/

Centers for Disease Control and Prevention. (2013, March 20). *high blood pressure.* Retrieved July 13, 2013, from Centers for Disease Control and Prevention: http://www.cdc.gov/bloodpressure/facts.htm

Centers for Disease Control and Prevention. (2011, July 11). *High Sodium, Low Potassium Diet Linked to Increased Risk of Death.* Retrieved July 17, 2013, from Centers for Disease Control and Prevention: http://www.cdc.gov/media/releases/2011/p0711_sodium-potassiumdiet.html

Centers for Disease Control and Prevention. (2013, June 5). *Sodium and Food Sources.* Retrieved July 15, 2013, from Centers for

Disease Control and Prevention: http://www.cdc.gov/salt/food.htm

Centers for Disease Control. (2012, May 1). *Inflammatory Bowel Disease (IBD)*. Retrieved October 16, 2013, from Centers for Disease Control and Prevention: http://www.cdc.gov/ibd/

Centers for Disease Control. (2003). *Summary Measures of Population Health: Report of Findings on methodologic and Data Issues.* Hyattsville, Md: U.S. Depsrtment of Health and Human Services.

Centers for Disease Control. (2004, February 6). *Trends in Intake of Energy and Macronutrients --- United States, 1971--2000.* Retrieved July 12, 2011, from CDC.gov: http://www.cdc.gov/mmwr/preview/mmwrhtml/mm5304a3.htm

Chalon, S. (2006). Omega-3 Fatty Acids and Monoamine Neurotransmission. *Prostag Leukot Essent Fatty Acids* , 75:259-269.

Chan, A., Downs, D., Tsai, C., Begley, B., Triplett, J., & Poppenga, R. (2002). *GENUS: Agrostemma.* Retrieved February 17, 2013, from Poisonous Plants of Pennsylvania: Commonwealth of PA - Department of Agriculture: http://cal.vet.upenn.edu/projects/poison/agbook/acer.htm

Charles, D. (2013, July 17). *In Oregon, The GMO Wheat Mystery Deepens.* Retrieved September 30, 2013, from NPR. org: http://www.npr.org/blogs/thesalt/2013/07/17/202684064/in-oregon-the-gmo-wheat-mystery-deepens

Chen, L., Caballero, B., Mitchell, D., Loria, C., Lin, P., Champagne, C., et al. (2010). Reducing Consumption of Sugar-Sweetened Beverages Is Associated with Reduced Blood Pressure: a Prospective Study among United States Adults. *Circulation* , 121:2398-2406.

Chen, L., Caballero, B., Mitchell, D., Loria, C., PH., L., & Champagne, C. (2010). Reducing Consumption of Sugar-Sweetened Beverages Is Associated with Reduced Blood Pressure. *Circulation* , 121:2398-2406.

Cherry, K. (2013). *The Conscious and Unconscious Mind.* Retrieved July 5, 2013, from About.com Psychology: http://psychology.about.com/od/theoriesofpersonality/a/consciousuncon.htm

Cherry, K. (2013). *What Is the Conscious Mind?* Retrieved July 5, 2013, from About.com Psychology: http://psychology.about.com/lr/psychoanalysis/755242/3/

Chiang, Y.-R., Ismail, W., Heintz, D., & Schaeffer, C. (2008). Study of Anoxic and Oxic Cholesterol Metabolism by Sterolibacterium denitrificans. *JOURNAL OF BACTERIOLOGY, ,* 905–914.

Chowdhury, R., Warnakula, S., Kunutsor, S., Crowe, F., Ward, H.

A., Johnson, L., et al. (2014). Association of Dietary, Circulating, and Supplement Fatty Acids With Coronary Risk: A Systematic Review and Meta-analysis. . *Annals of Internal Medicine.* , 160(6):398-406.

Chrpova, J., Skorpik, M., Prasilova, P., & Sip, V. (2003). Detection of Norin 10 Dwarfing Genes in Winter Wheat Varieties Registered in the Czech Republic. *Czech J. Genet Plant Breed* , 39(3):89-92.

Clark, A. L., Chyu, J., & Horwich, T. B. (2012). The Obesity Paradox in Men Versus Women With Systolic Heart Failure. *Ameriucan Heart Journal* , 110 (1) :77-82.

Cleave, T. (1974). *the saccharine disease.* Bristol, United Kingdom: John Wright and Sons, Ltd.

Cohen, L., Curhan, G., & Forman, J. (2012). Association of sweetened beverage intake with incident hypertension. *J Gen Intern Med.* , 27(9):1127-1134.

Colls, R., & Evans, B. (2010). rethinking "the obesity problem". *geography* , 95(2):99-105.

Confucius. (2013). *Danger Quotes.* Retrieved December 11, 2013, from BeainyQuote.com: http://www.brainyquote.com/quotes/keywords/danger.html

Connolly, C. (2003, August 10). *Public Policy Targeting Obesity.* Retrieved October 8, 2011, from WashingtonPost.com: http://www.washingtonpost.com/ac2/wp-dyn/A39239-2003Aug9?language=printer

Cordain, L. (1999). Cereal Grains: Humanity's Double Edge Sword. *World Rev Nutr Diet* , 84:19-73.

Cordain, L. (2002). The Nutritional Characteristics of a Contemporary Diet Based upon Paleolithic Food Groups. *J Am Neutraceutical Assoc* , 5:15-24.

Cordain, L. (2002). *The Paleo Diet.* New York: Wiley, Inc.

Cordain, L., Brand-Miller, J., Eaton, S., Mann, N., Holt, S., & Speth, J. (2000). Plant to Animal Subsistence Ratios and Macronutrient Energy Estimations and Worldwide Hunter-Gatherer Diets. *Am J Clin Nutr* , 71:682-692.

Cordain, L., Eades, M., & Eades, M. (2003). Hyperinsulinemic Disease of Civilization: More Than Just Syndrome X. *Comp Biochem Physiol Part A* , 136:95-112.

Cordain, L., Eaton, S. B., Sebastian, A., Mann, N., Lindeberg, S., Watkins, B. A., et al. (2005). Origins and evolution of the Western diet: health implications for the 21st century. *The American Journal of Nutrition* , (81):341-354.

Cordain, L., Eaton, S., & Brand-Miller, J. (2002). The Paradoxical Nature of Hunter-Gatherer Diets: Meat-based, yet Non-Atherogenic. *Eur J Clin Nutr* , 56 (supplement 1): S42-S52.

Cordain, L., Eaton, S., Brand-Miller, J., Lindeberg, S., & Jensen, C. (2002). An Evolutionary Analysis of the Etiology and Pathogenesis of Juvenile Onset Myopia. *Acta Opthamol Scand* , 80: 125-135.

Cordain, L., Eaton, S., Brand-Miller, J., Mann, N., & Hill, K. (2002). The Paradoxical Nature of Hunter-Gatherer Diets: Meat-based, yet Non--Atherogenic. *European Journal of Clinical Nutrition* , 56 (supplement): S42-52.

Cordain, L., Lindeberg, S., Hurtado, M., Hill, K., Eaton, S., & Brand-Miller, J. (2002). Acne Vulgaris: a Disease of Western Civilization. *Arch Dermatol* , 138:1584-1590.

Cordain, L., Miller, J., Eaton, S., & Mann, N. (2000). Macronutrient Estimations in Hunter-Gatherer Diets. *Am J Clin Nutr* , 72:1589-1590.

Cordain, L., Toohey, L., Smith, M., & Hickey, M. (2000). Modulation of Immune Function by Dietary Lectins in Rheumatoid Arthritis. *Bt J Nutr* , 83 (3): 207-217.

Cordain, L., Watkins, B., & Mann, N. (2001). Fatty Acid Composition and Energy Density of Foods Available to African Hominids. *World Rev Nutr Diet* , 90:144-161.

Cordain, L., Watkins, B., Florant, G., Kehler, M., Rogers, L., & Li, Y. (2002). Fatty Acid Analysis of Wild Ruminant Tissues: Evolutionary Implications for Reducing Diet-Related Chronic Diseas e. *European Journal of Clinical Nutrition* , 56: 181-191.

Corella, D., Carrasco, P., Sorli, J. V., Estruch, R., Rico-Sanz, J., Martinez-Gonzalez, A., et al. (2013). Mediterranean Diet Reduces the Adverse Effect of the TCF7L2-rs7903146 Polymorphism on Cardiovascular Risk Factors and Stroke Incidence: A randomized controlled trial in a high-cardiovascular-risk population. *Diabetes Care* , doi: 10.2337/dc13-0955.

Corti, R., Flammer, A. J., Hollenberg, N. K., & Luscher, T. F. (2009). Cocoa and Cardiovascular Health. *Circulation* , 119:1433-1441.

Coudray, C., Feillet-Coudray, C., Tressol, J., Gueux, E., Thien, S., Jaffrelo, L., et al. (2005). Stimulatory effect of inulin on intestinal absorption of calcium and magnesium in rats is modulated by dietary calcium intakes. *European Journal of Nutrition* , 44(5):293-302 .

Creamer, B., Shorter, R., & Bamforth, J. (1961). The turnover and shedding of epithelial cells: Part I The turnover in the gastro-intestinal tract. *Gut* , 2:110-116.

Crislip, M. (2009, January 16). *Probiotics.* Retrieved December 26, 2013, from Science-based Medicine: http://www.sciencebased-medicine.org/probiotics/

Cummins, A., & Roberts-Thomson, J. (2009). Prevalence of Celiac Disease in the Asia-Pacific Region. *J Gastroen Hepatol* , 24:1347-1351.

Dahl, L. (1972). Salt and Hypertension. *Am J Clin Nutrition* , 25(2):231-44.

Dalley, J., Laane, K., Theobald, D., Armstrong, H., Corlett, P., Chudasama, Y., et al. (2005). Time-Limited Modulation of Appetitive Pavlovian Memory by D1 and an MDA Receptors in the Nucleus Accumbens. *Proc Natl Acad Sci USA* , 102:6189-6194.

Dansinger, M. L., Gleason, J. A., Griffith, J. L., Selker, H. P., & Scaefer, E. J. (2005). Comparison of the Atkins, Ornish, Weight Watchers, and Zone Diets for Weight Loss and Heart Disease Risk Reduction: A Randomized Trial. *JAMA* , 293(1):43-53.

Das, S. R., Alexander, K. P., Chen, A. Y., Powell-Wiley, T. M., Diercks, D. B., Peterson, E. D., et al. (2011). Impact of Body Weight and Extreme Obesity on the Presentation, Treatment, and In-Hospital Outcomes of 50,149 Patients With ST-Segment Elevation Myocardial Infarction Results From the NCDR (National Cardiovascular Data Registry). *J Am Coll Cardiol* , 58(25):2642-2650.

Dawber TR, N. R. (1982). Eggs, serum cholesterol, and coronary heart disease. *American Journal of Clinical Nutrition* , 36:617-25.

Dawber, T., Kannel, W., Kagan, A., Donabedian, R., Mcnamara, P., & Pearson, G. (1967). Environmental Factors and Hypertension. In J. Stamler, R. Stamler, & T. (. Pullman, *The Epidemiology of Hypertension* (pp. 255 – 88). New York City: Grune and Stratton.

Dawson-Hughes, B. (2007). Protein Intake and Calcium Absorption: Potential Role of the Calcium Sensor Receptor. In P. Burckhardt, R. Heaney, & B. Dawson-Hughes, *Proceedings of the International Symposium on Nutritional Aspects of Osteoporosis* (pp. 217-227). Lausanne, Switzerland: Elsevier.

Day, L., Augustin, M., Batey, I., & Wrigley, C. (2006). Wheat-Gluten Uses and Industry Needs. *Trends Food Sci Technol* , 17:82-90.

De Araujo, I., & Rolls, E. (2004). Representation of the Human Brain of Food Texture and Oral Fat. *J Neurosci* , 24:3086-3093.

De Vincenzi, M., Vincentini, O., Di Nardo, G., Boirivant, M., Gazza, L., & Pogna, N. (2010). 2 Prolamin Peptides from Durum

Wheat Preclude Celiac Disease Specific T Cell Activation by Gluten Protein s. *EurJ Nutr* , 49 (4): 251-255.

Dehghan, M., Mente, A., Teo, K. K., Gao, P., Sleight, P., Dagenais, G., et al. (2012). Relationship Between Healthy Diet and Risk of Cardiovascular Disease Among Patients onDrug Therapies for Secondary Prevention : A Prospective Cohort Study of 31,546 High-Risk Individuals From 40 Countries. *Circulation* , 126:2705-2712.

Delgado-Lista, J., Lopez-Miranda, J., Cortes, B., Perez-Martinez, P., Lozano, A., Gomez-Luna, R., et al. (2008). Chronic Dietary Fat Intake Modifies the Postprandial Response and Hemostatic Markers to a Single Fatty Test Mea l. *Am J Clin Nutr* , 9:231.

Denton, D. (1984). *The Hunger for Salt. An Anthropological, Physiological and Medical Analysis.* New York: Springer.

Department Of Health and Human Services. (1988). *Surgeon General's Report on Nutrition and Health.* . Washington DC: Health and Human Services.

Depre, C., Vanoverschelde, J.-L. J., & Taegtmeyer, H. (1999). Glucose for the Heart. *Circulation* , 99:578-588.

Deschanel, Z. (2013). *Brainy Quote.* Retrieved December 7, 2013, from Brainy Quotes: http://www.brainyquote.com/quotes/quotes/z/zooeydesch540548.html

Devine, A., Criddle, R., Dick, I., Kerr, D., & Prince, R. (1995). A Longitudinal Study of the Effect of Sodium and Calcium Intakes on Regional Bone Density in Postmenopausal Women. *Am J Clin Nutr* , 62: 740-745.

Dewailly, E., Blanchet, C., Lemieux, S., Sauvé, L., Gingras, S., Ayotte, P., et al. (2001). n-3 Fatty acids and cardiovascular disease risk factors among the Inuit of Nunavik. *Am J Clin Nutr* , 74: 464-473.

Dictionary.com. (2013). *addiction.* Retrieved August 3, 2013, from Dictionary.com: http://dictionary.reference.com/browse/addiction?s=t

dictionary.com. (2013). *disease.* Retrieved December 14, 2013, from dictionary.com: http://dictionary.reference.com/browse/disease

Dilli, D., Aydin, B., Zenciroglu, A., Ozyazici, E., Beken, S., & Okumus, N. (2013). Treatment Outcomes of Infants With Cyanotic Congenital Heart Disease Treated With Synbiotics. *Pediatrics* , 132(4):e932-8.

Din, J., Newby, D., & Flapan, A. (2004). Omega-3 Fatty Acids and Cardiovascular Disease-Fishing for a Natural Treatment. *BMJ*

, 328:30-35.

Do, R., Xie, C., Zhang, X., Mannisto, S., H. K., Islam, S., et al. (2011). The Effect of Chromosome 9p21 Variants on Cardiovascular Disease May Be Modified by Dietary Intake: Evidence from a Case/Control and a Prospective Study. *PLoS Medicine* , 9(10):1-10.

Doherty, M., & Barry, R. (1981). Gluten-Induced Mucosal Changes in Subjects without Overt Small-Bowel Disease. *Lancet* , 1 (8219): 517-520.

Drago, S., El Asmar, R., & Pierro, M. (2006). Gliadin, Zonulin and Gut Permeability: Effects on Celiac and Non-Celiac Intestinal Mucosa and Intestinal Cell Lines. *Scand J Gastroenterol* , 41 (4): 408-419.

Drewnowski, A. (1997). Taste Preferences and Food Intake. *Ann Rev Nutr* , 17:237-253.

Drewnowski, A., & Almiron-Roig, E. (2010). Human Perceptions and Preferences for Fat-Rich Foods. In J. Montmayeur, & J. (. le Coutre, *Fat Detection: Taste, Texture, and Post Ingestive Effects* (p. Chapter 11). Boca Raton, Florida: CRC Press.

Drewnowski, A., & Bellisle, F. (2007). Is Sweetness Addictive? *Nutr Bull* , 32 (supplement 1): 52-60.

Dubnov, G., & Berry, E. (2003). Omega-6/Omega-3 Fatty Acid Ratio: the Israeli Paradox. *World Rev Nutr Diet* , 92:81-91.

Dubois, B., Peumans, W., & Van Damme, E. (1998). Regulation of Gelatinase B (MMP-9) in Leukocytes by Plant Lectins. *FEBS Lett* , 427 (2): 275-278.

Durtschi, A. (2001). *Nutritional Content of Whole Grains Versus Their Refined Flours.* Washington, DC: United States Department of Agriculture Economic Research Service.

Eaton, S. (1992). Humans, lipids and evolution. *Lipids* , (27): 814-820.

Eaton, S., Cordain, L., & Lindeberg, S. (2002). Evolutionary Health Promotion: a Consideration of Common Counter Arguments. *Prev Med* , 34 (2): 119-123.

Eaton, S., Konnor, M., & Shostak, M. (1988). Stone Agers in the Fast Lane: Chronic Degenerative Diseases in Evolutionary Perspective. *Am J Med* , 312:283-289.

Ebbeling, C. S.-L. (2012). Effects of Dietary Composition on Energy Expenditure During Weight-Loss Maintenance. . *JAMA* , 307 (24):2627-2634.

Edwards, L. (2010, September 23). *Estimate of flowering plant species to be cut by 600,000.* Retrieved Decenmber 2013, 9, from PhysOrg.com: http://phys.org/news204438872.html

Effects of Low-Sodium Diet Versus High Sodium Diet on Blood Pressure, Rennin, Aldosteronen, Catecholamines, Cholesterol and Triglyceride.. (2011). *Cochrane Database Syst Rev* , (11): CD004022.

Ehler, James T. (2012). *Food History timeline:50,000 BC to 1 BC.* Retrieved August 10, 2012, from Foodreference.com: http://www.foodreference.com/html/html/yearonlytimeline.html

Eknoyan, G. (2007). Adolphe Quetelet (1796–1874)—the average man and indices of obesity. *Nephrology Dialysis Transplantation* , Volume 23 (1):47-51.

Elliott, S., Keim, N., Stern, J., Teff, K., & Havel, P. (2002). Fructose, Weight Gain, and the Insulin Resistance Syndrome. *Am J Clin Nutr* , 76: 911-922.

Emken, E. (1984). nutritional biochemistry of trans and positional fatty acid isomers and hydrogenated oils. *Annu Rev Nutr* , (4): 339-376.

Escolar, E., Lamas, G. A., . Mark, D. B., Boineau, R., Goertz, C., Rosenberg, Y., et al. (2013). The Effect of an EDTA-based Chelation Regimen on Patients With Diabetes Mellitus and Prior Myocardial Infarction in the Trial to Assess Chelation Therapy (TACT). *Circulation* , http://circoutcomes.ahajournals.org/content/early/2013/11/19/CIRCOUTCOMES.113.000663.

Fabri, L. (2010). *Breaking of Bread the Jewish Understanding.* Retrieved December 9, 2013, from Congregation Netzar Torah Yeshua: http://messianicfellowship.50webs.com/bread.html

Fairfield, H. (2010, April 4). *Factory Food.* Retrieved July 17, 2013, from The New York Times: http://www.nytimes.com/imagepages/2010/04/04/business/04metrics_g.html?ref=business

Fanaro, S., Boehm, G., Garssen, J., Knol, J., Mosca, F., Stahl, B., et al. (2005). Galacto-oligosaccharides and long-chain fructo-oligosaccharides as prebiotics in infant formulas: a review. *Acta Paediatr Suppl.* , 94(449):22-26.

FDA. (2013, June 1). *Code of Federal Regulations Title 21.* Retrieved December 16, 2013, from US FDA: http://www.accessdata.fda.gov/scripts/cdrh/cfdocs/cfcfr/CFRSearch.cfm?fr=101.12

Feijó, F. M., Ballard, C., Foletto, K., Batista, B., Neves, A., Ribeiro, M., et al. (2013). Saccharin and aspartame, compared with sucrose, induce greater weight gain in adult Wistar rats, at similar total caloric intake levels. *Appetite* , 60 (1):203-207.

Feldman, M. (2001). Origin of Cultivated Wheat. In A. Bonjean, & W. (. Angus, *The World Wheat Book: a History of Wheat Breeding* (pp. 3-56). Paris, France: Lavoisier Publishing.

Feldman, M. (1995). Wheats. In J. Smartt, & N. (. Simmonds, *Evolution of Crop Plants* (pp. 185-192). Harlow, United Kingdom: Longman Scientific and Technical.

Fenster, M. (2013, March 28). *Enjoy A Blue Spring.* Retrieved August 3, 2013, from The Tampa Tribune: http://heweb.tbo.dc.publicus.com/he/life/health/enjoy-a-blue-spring-b82470817z1

Fenster, M. S. (2013, May 23). *Don't Pass on the Salt.* Retrieved July 14, 2013, from Pacific Standard: http://www.psmag.com/health/stop-worrying-about-salt-reduction-58334/

Fenster, M. S. (2012, January 4). *Don't Hold the Salt: Attempts to Curb Sodium Intake Are Misguided.* Retrieved july 14, 2013, from The Atlantic: http://www.theatlantic.com/health/archive/2012/01/dont-hold-the-salt-attempts-to-curb-sodium-intake-are-misguided/250712/

Fenster, M. S. (2012). *Eating Well, Living Better: A Grassroots Gourmet Guide to Good health and Great Food.* New York: Rowman and Littlefield .

Fenster, M. S. (2013, January 3). The obesity rate and the paradox: into the deeper and wider (part 2). *The Tampa tribune Hernando Today* , p. http://hernandotoday.com/article/20130103/ARTICLE/301039987.

Fenster, M. S. (2012, December 27). The obesity rate and the paradox: into the deeper and wider. *The Tampa Tribune Hernando Today* , pp. http://hernandotoday.com/lifestyles/hernando-sports/2012/dec/27/the-obesity-rate-and-the-paradox-into-the-deeper-a-ar-591277/.

Fenster, M. S. (2013, January 10). The skinny on obesity. *The Tampa Tribune Hernando Today* , p. http://hernandotoday.com/article/20130110/ARTICLE/301109987.

Filer, L. J. (1971). Salt in Infant Foods. *Nutr Rev* , 29(2):27-30.

Fine, B., Ty, A., Lestrange, N., & Levine, O. (1987). Sodium Deprivation Growth Failure in the Rat: Alterations and Tissue Composition and Fluid Spaces. *J Nutr* , 117:1623-1628.

Flegal, K. (1993). Defining obesity in children and adolescents: epidemiologic approaches. *Crit Rev Food Sci Nutr* , 33(4-5): 307-312.

Flegal, K., Kit, B., Orpana, H., & Graubard, B. (2013). Association of All-Cause Mortality with Overweight and Obesity using

Standard Body Mass Index Categories: A Systematic Review and Meta-analysis. *JAMA.* , 300 (1) pp 71-82.

Fokkema, M., Brouwer, D., Hasperhoven, M., Martini, I., & Muskeit, F. (2000). Short-Term Supplementation of Low-Does Gamma-Linolenic Acid (GLA), Alpha-Linolenic Acid (ALA), or GLA Plus ALA Does Not Augment LCP Omega-3 Status of Dutch Vegans to an Appreciable Extent. *Prostag Leukot Essent Fatty Acids* , 63:287-292.

Ford, E. S., Zhao, G., Tsai, J., & Li, C. (2011). Low-Risk Lifestyle Behaviors and All-Cause Mortality: Findings From the National Health and Nutrition Examination Survey III Mortality Study . *The American Journal of Public Health* , 101: 1922-1929.

Forsythe, C., Phinney, S., & Fernandez, M. (2008). Comparison of Low-Fat and Low Carbohydrate Diets on Circulating Fatty Acid Composition and Markers of Inflammation. *Lipids* , 43 (1): 65-77.

Fowler, S., Williams, K., Resendez, R., Hunt, K., Hazuda, H., & Stern, M. (2008). Fueling the obesity epidemic? Artificially sweetened beverage use and long-term weight gain. *Obesity* , 16 (8):1894-1900.

Fraga, M., Ballestar, E., Paz, M., Ropero, S., Setien, F., Ballestar, M., et al. (2005). Epigenetic Differences Arise during the Lifetime of Monozygotic Twins. *Proc Natl Acad Sci USA* , 102: 10604-10609.

Frassetto, L., Morris, R., & Sebastian, A. (1997). Potassium Bicarbonate Reduces Urinary Nitrogen Excretion in Postmenopausal Women. *J Clin Endocrinol Metab* , 82:254-259.

Frassetto, L., Todd, K., Morris, R., & Sebastian, A. (1998). Estimation of Net Endogenous Non-Carbonic Acid Production in Humans from Diet Potassium and Protein Content. *Am J Clin Nutr* , 68:576-583.

Freedman, D. A., & Petitti, D. B. (2001). Salt and Blood Pressure: Conventional Wisdom Reconsidered. *Eval Rev* , 25(3):267-87.

Freeman, M., Hibbeln, J., Wisner, K., Davis, J., Mischoulon, D., Peet, M., et al. (2006). Omega-3 Fatty Acids: Evidence Basis for Treatment and Future Research in Psychiatry. *J Clin Psychiatry* , 1954-1967.

Friedman, M. (1998). Fuel Partitioning and Food Intake. *Am J Clin Nutr* , 67:513S-518S.

Fuentes, F., Lopez-Miranda, J., Perez-Martinez, P., Jimenez, Y., Marin, C., Gomez, P., et al. (2008). chronic affects of a high-fat diet enriched with virgin olive oil and a low-fat diet enriched with alpha-linolenic acid on postprandial endothelial function and healthy men. *Br J Nutr* , 100:159-165.

Gadsby, P. (2004, October). *The Inuit Paradox*. Retrieved July 14, 2010, from Discover Magazine: http://discovermagazine.com/2004/oct/inuit-paradox/article_view?b_start:int=2

Galen (trnaslated by Brock, A. (2013). *On the Natural Faculties*. Retrieved February 19, 2013, from The Internet Classic Archive: http://classics.mit.edu/Galen/natfac.mb.txt

Gani, O. (2008). Are Fish Oil Omega-3 Long Chain Fatty Acids and Their Derivatives Peroxisome Proliferator Activated Receptor Agonists? *Cardiovasc Diabetol* , 7:6.

Gardener, H., Rundek, T., Markert, M., Wright, C., Elkind, M., & Sacco, R. (2012). Diet soft drink consumption is associated with an increased risk of vascular events in the Northern Manhattan Study. *J Gen Intern Med.* , 27(9):1120-1126.

Gardner, M. N., & Brandt, A. M. (2006). "The Doctors' Choice Is America's Choice". *Am J Public Health.* , 96(2): 222–232.

Geiss, L. S., Li, Y., Kirtland, K., Barker, L., Burrows, N. R., & Gregg, E. W. (2012, November 16). Increasing Prevalence of Diagnosed Diabetes — United States and Puerto Rico, 1995–2010. *CDC Morbidity and Mortality Weekly Report (MMWR)* , pp. 61(45);918-921.

George, J., Majeed, W., Mackenzie, I. S., MacDonald, T. M., & Wei, L. (2013). Association between cardiovascular events and sodium-containing effervescent, dispersible, and soluble drugs: nested case-control study. *British Medical Journal* , 347:f6954 .

German, J. B., & Dillard, C. J. (2004). Saturated fats: what dietary intake? *Am J Clin Nutr* , 80 (3): 550-559.

Gibson, A., & Sinclair, A. (1981). Are Eskimos Obligate Carnivores? *Lancet* , 1:1100.

Gilbertson, T., Yu, T., & Shah, B. (2010). Gustatory Mechanisms for Fat Detection. In M. JP, & l. C. (Editors), *Fat Detection: Taste, Texture, and Post Ingestive Effects* (p. Chapter 3). Boca Raton, Florida: CRC Press.

Ginor, M. A. (1999). *Foie Gras: A Passion*. New York: John Wiley and Sons, Inc.

Glossman, H. H. (210). Origin of 7-Dehtdrocholesterol (Provitamin D) in the Skin. *Journal of Investigative Dermatology* , 130: 2139-2141.

Godfrey, K., & Barker, D. (2000). Fetal Nutrition and Adult Disease. *Am J Clin Nutr* , 17:1344S-1352S.

Goldfield, G., Lorello, C., & Doucet, E. (2007). Methylphenidate

Reduces Energy Intake and Dietary Fat Intake and Adult: a Mechanism of Reduced Reinforcing the Value of Food? *Am J Clin Nutr* , 86:308-315.

Goldsmith, S. (2010, March 10). *Brooklyn Dem Felix Ortiz wants to ban use of salt in New York restaurants.* Retrieved October 8, 2011, from NYDailynews.com: http://articles.nydailynews.com/2010-03-11/local/27058674_1_salt-restaurants-fast-food

Goncharov, A., Bloom, M., Pavuk, M., Birman, I., & Carpenter, D. (2010). Blood pressure and hypertension in relation to levels of serum polychlorinated biphenyls in residents of Anniston, Alabama. *J of Hypertension* , 2053-60.

Gotshall, R., Mickleborough, T., & Cordain, L. (2000). Dietary Salt Restriction Improves Pulmonary Function in Exercise-Induced Asthma. *Med Sci Sports Exerc* , 32:1815-1819.

Gould, S. (2002). *The Structure of Evolutionary Theory.* Cambridge, MA: Harvard University Press.

Grant, W. (2009). In Defense of the Sun: an Estimate of Changes in Mortality Rates in the United States Is Mean Serum 25-Hydroxy Vitamin D Levels Were Raised to 45 Ng/ML by Solar Ultraviolet-to Be Irradiance. *Dermatoendocrinol* , 1 (4): 207-214.

Graudal, N., & Jurgens, G. (2011). The Sodium Phantom. . *BMJ* , 343:d6119.

Graudel, N., Hubeck-Graudel, T., & Jurgens, G. (2011). Effects of Low-Sodium Diet Versus High Sodium Diet on Blood Pressure, Rennin, of the Austrian, Catecholamines, Cholesterol and Triglycerid e. *Cochrane Database Syst Rev* , (11): CD004022.

Griffin M, N. A. (2010). Plaque area at carotid and common femoral bifurcations and prevalence of clinical cardiovascular disease. *International Angiology* , Jun;29(3):216-25.

Grimes, D. (2006). Are Statins Analogues of Vitamin D? *Lancet* , 83-85.

Grobbee, D., & Hoffman, A. (1986). The Sodium Restriction: Lower Blood Pressure? . *British Medical Journal (Clinical Research Edition)* , 293 (6538): 27 – 9.

Gross, L. S., Li, L., Ford, E. S., & Liu, S. (2004). Increased Composition of Refined Carbohydrates and the Epidemic of Type II Diabetes in United States: an Ecological Assessment. *Am J Clin Nutr* , 79:774 -- 779.

Guallar, E., Stranges, S., Mulrow, C., Appel, L. J., & Miller III, E. R. (2013). Enough Is Enough: Stop Wasting Money on Vitamin and

Mineral Supplements. *Annals of Internal Medicine*, 159(12):850-851.

Gurven, M., & Kaplan, H. (2007). Longevity among Hunter-Gatherer's: a Cross-Cultural Examination. *Popul Dev Rev*, 33:321-365.

Gyamfi, B. E., & Kersh, R. (2011). Child and adolescent fast-food choice and the influence of calorie labeling: a natural experiment. *International Journal of Obesity*, 35:493-500.

Handelman, G. J., Nightingale, Z. D., Lichtenstein, A. H., Schaefer, E. J., & Blumberg, J. B. (1999). Lutein and zeaxanthin concentrations in plasma after dietary supplementation with egg yolk. *Am J Clin Nutr*, 70:247–51.

Hargrove, J. L. (2007). Does the History of Food Energy Units Suggest a Solution to the "Calorie Confusion"? *Nutrition Journal*, 6: 44-55.

Hargrove, J. L. (2006). History of the Calorie Nutrition. *The Journal of Nutrition*, and 36:2957-2961.

Harris, S. J. (1964, January 9). Strictly Personal . *New Castle News*, p. 4.

Hastorf, C., & Weismantal, M. J. (2007). Food: Where Opposites Meet. In K. C. Twiss, *The Archeology of Food and Identity* (pp. 308-331). Carbondale, IL: Southern Illinois University Press.

HealthFinder.gov. (2013, October 15). *Crohn's and Colitis May Be Tied to Risk of Heart Attack, Stroke.* Retrieved October 16, 2013, from HealthFinder.gov: http://www.healthfinder.gov/News/Article.aspx?id=681075

Henney, J. E., Taylor, C. L., & Boon, C. S. (2010). *Strategies to Reduce Sodium Intake in the United States.* Washington, DC: The National Academies Press.

Henry, D. (1990, November 7). Salt Talks: for 90% of Americans, Salt Doesn't Matter Much. *Associated Press.*

Herodotus. (2011, June 3). *Histories II,2.92.* Retrieved July 30, 2012, from Project Gutenberg: http://www.gutenberg.org/wiki/Egypt_%28Bookshelf%29

Holick, M. (2007). Vitamin D Deficiency. *New England Journal of Medicine*, 357 (3): 266-281.

Hollenberg, Norman K.Martinez, G., McCullough, M., Meinking, T., Passan, D., Preston, M., et al. (1997). Aging, Acculturation, Salt Intake, and Hypertension in the Kuna of Panama. *Hypertension*, 29: 171-176 .

Holliday, M. (1986). Body Composition and Energy Needs during Growth. In F. Falkner, & J. (. Tanner, *Human Growth: a*

Comprehensive Treatise (2nd edition, volume 2) (pp. 101-117). New York: Plenum Press.

Home Depot. (2013). *8 in.x 2-1/4 in. x 4in. Clay Brick.* Retrieved July for, 2013, from Home Depot.com: http://www.homedepot.com/p/8-in-x-2-1-4-in-x-4-in-Clay-Brick-RED0126MCO/100323015#. UdWVu-znbGg

Hoogwerf, B. J., & Huang, J. C. (2012). *Cardiovascular Disease Prevention Lipid-Lowering Strategies and Reduction of Coronary Heart Disease Risk.* Cleveland, Ohio (page 12): The Cleveland Clinic.

Hsu, C.-K., Liao, J.-W., Chung, Y.-C., Hsieh, C.-P., & Chan, Y.-C. (2004). Xylooligosaccharides and Fructooligosaccharides Affect the Intestinal Microbiota and Precancerous Colonic Lesion Development in. *J. Nutr. June* , 134: 1523-1528.

Huffington Post. (2011, May 25). *FDA Approved: The Maximum Amount Of Defects Allowed In Your Food.* Retrieved January 2, 2014, from Huffington Post: http://www.huffington-post.com/2010/10/26/fda-approved-rat-hairs-an_n_773608. html#s165326&title=Pizza_Sauce_30

Hunt, J., Johnson, L., & Fariba-Roughead, Z. (2009). Dietary Protein and Calcium Interact to Influence Calcium Retention: a Controlled Feeding Study. *Am J Clin Nutr* , 89:1357-1365.

IMDB. (2013). *Boromir.* Retrieved November 22, 2013, from IMDB: http://www.imdb.com/character/ch0000140/quotes

IMDB. (2013). *Wall Street.* Retrieved November 22, 2013, from IMDB: http://www.imdb.com/title/tt0094291/quotes

I-Min Lee, E. J. (2012). Effect of physical inactivity on major non-communicable diseases worldwide: an analysis of burden of disease and life expectancy. *The Lancet* , Volume 380, Issue 9838, Pages 219 - 229.

Inaizumi, M., Takeda, M., Suzuki, A., Sawano, S., & Fushiki, T. (2001). Preference for High-Fat Food in Mice: Fried Potatoes Compared with Boiled Potatoes. *Appetite* , 36:237-238.

Iwasawa, H., & Yamazaki, M. (2009). Differences in Biological Response Modifier-like Activities According to the Strain and Maturity of Bananas. *Food Sci. Technol. Res.* , 15 (3): 275 – 282.

Jackson, P. (Director). (2002). *The Lord of the Rings: The Two Towers* [Motion Picture].

Jakobsen, M., Dethlefsen, C., & Joensen, A. (2010). Intake of Carbohydrates Compared with Intake of Saturated Fatty Acids and Risk of Myocardial Infarction: Importance of the Glycemic Inde x.

Am J Clin Nutr , 91 (6): 1764-1768.

Jala, D., Smits, G., Johnson, R., & Conchol, M. (2010). Increased Fructose Associates with Elevated Blood Pressure. *Journal of the American Society of Nephrology* , 21:1416-1418.

Janakiram, N. B., & V. Rao, C. (2009). Role of Lipoxins and Resolvins as Anti-Inflammatory and Proresolving Mediators in Colon Cancer . *Current Molecular Medicine* , 9(5):565-79.

Jansson, B. (1986). Geographic Cancer Risk and Intracellular Potassium/Sodium Ratios. *Cancer Detect Prev* , 9:171-194.

Jenkins, D., Wolever, T., & Collier, G. (1987). Metabolic Effects of a Low Glycemic Diet. *Am J Clin Nutr* , 46:968-975.

Jens, R., Hetfield, J., & Ulrich, L. (Composers). (2003). Frantic. [Metallica, Performer]

Joelving, F. (2012, September 17). *Salt intake tied to higher blood pressure in kids.* Retrieved January 17, 2013, from Reuters: http://www.reuters.com/article/2012/09/17/us-salt-intake-tied-to-higher-blood-pres-idUSBRE88G0EY20120917.

Johri, R., & Zutshi, U. (1992). An Ayurevedic formulation"Trikatu"and its constituents. *Journal of Ethnopharmacology* , 37:85-91.

Joseph C Ratliff, G. M. (2008). Eggs modulate the inflammatory response to carbohydrate restricted diets in overweight men . *Nutrition & Metabolism* , Volume 5, Number 1 (2008), 6, DOI: 10.1186/1743-7075-5-6.

JSTOR. (2013). *Supreme Court of the United States. Food and Drugs Act. Adulteration of Foodstuffs. United States v. Lexington Mill & Elevator Co. Decided Feb. 24, 1914.* Retrieved December 19, 2013, from Public Health Reports (1896-1970): http://www.jstor.org/stable/4570603

Julie A. Mattison, J. A., Roth, G. S., Beasley, T. M., Tilmont, E. M., Handy, A. M., Herbert, R. L., et al. (2012). Impact of caloric restriction on health and survival in rhesus monkeys from the NIA study. *Nature* , 489:318-321.

Jun Wu, P. B.-H. (2012). Beige Adipocytes Are a Distinct Type of Thermogenic Fat Cell in Mouse and Human. *Cell* , Volume 150, Issue 2, 366-376, 12 July 2012.

Kadohisa, M., Verhagen, J., & Rolls, E. (2005). The Primate Amygdala: Neuronall Representations of the Viscosity, Fat Texture, Temperature, Grittiness and Tastes of Foods. *Neuroscience* , 132: 33-48.

Kankova, K. (2008). Diabetic Threesome (Hyperglycemia, Renal Function and Nutrition) and Advanced Glycation and Products: Evidence for the Multiple-Hit Agenda? *Proc Nutr Soc* , 67 (1): 60-74.

Karell, K., Louka, A., Moodie, S., Ascher, H., Clot, F., Greco, L., et al. (2003). HLA types in celiac disease patient not caring in the DQ A1*05-DQ B1*02 (DQ 2) heterozygote dimer: Results from the European genetics cluster of celiac disease. *Human Immunology* , 64:469-477.

Karlsson, F. H., Nookaew, I., Tremaroli, V., Fagerberg, B., Petranovic, D., Backhed, F., et al. (2012, December for). Symptomatic Atherosclerosis Associated with an Altered Gut Metagenome. *Nature* , 3:1245.

Kastorini, C., Milionis, H., Esposito, K., Giugliano, D., Goudevenos, J., & Panagiotakos, D. (2011). The effect of Mediterranean diet on metabolic syndrome and its components: a meta-analysis of 50 studies and 534,906 individuals. *J Am Coll Cardiol.* , 57(11):1299-313. doi: 10.1016/j.jacc.2010.09.073.

Kaunitz, H. (1956). Cause and Consequences of Salt Consumption. *Nature* , 178:1141-1144.

Kell, 1. B. (2010). Towards a unifying, systems biology understanding of large-scale cellular death and destruction caused by poorly liganded iron: Parkinson's, Huntington's, Alzheimer's, prions, bactericides, chemical toxicology and others as examples. *Archives of Toxicology,* , 84(11):825-889.

Kelly, G. (2008). Inulin-Type Prebiotics-A Review: Part 1. *Alt Med Rev* , 13(4):315-329.

Kersetter, J., Gaffney, E., & O'Brien, O. (2007). Dietary Protein Increases Intestinal Calcium Absorption and Improves Bone Balance: an Hypothesis. In P. Burckhardt, R. Heaney, & B. (. Dawson-Hughes, *Proceedings of the International Symposium on Nutritional Aspects of Osteoporosis* (pp. 204-216). Lausanne, Switzerland: E$lsevier.

Kersh, R., & Monroe, J. (2002). The Politics Of Obesity: Seven Steps To Government Action. *Health Affairs* , 21(6):142-153.

Kessler, D. (2009). *The End of Overeating: Taking Control of the Insatiable American Appetite.* New York: Rodale press.

Khaneja, R., Perez-Fons, L., Fakhry, S., Baccigalupi, L., Steiger, S., To, E. ,., et al. (2010). Carotenoids found in Bacillus. *J Appl Microbiol* , 108(6):1889-902.

Khare, C. (1965). *Indian Herbal Remedies: Rational Western Therapy, Ayurvedic, and Other Traditional Usage.* New York:

Springer Scince.

Kidwell, B. (2002, October 8). *All Grass, No Grain.* Retrieved July 14, 2013, from Progressive Farmer Magazine: http://www.progressivefarmer.com/farmer/magazine/article/0.14730,355103,00.html

King, S. (2013, January 28). *The Best Selling Drugs of All Time; Humira Joins The Elite.* Retrieved October 25, 2013, from Forbes.com: http://www.forbes.com/sites/simonking/2013/01/28/the-best-selling-drugs-of-all-time-humira-joins-the-elite/

Kinney, N., & Antill, R. (1996). Role of Olfaction in the Formation of Preference for High-Fat Foods in Mice. *Physiol Behav* , 59:475-478.

Kitamura, M. (2013, February 6). *Swapping Animal Fats for Plant Oils May Be 'Misguided'.* Retrieved August 17, 2013, from Bloomberg.com: http://www.bloomberg.com/news/2013-02-05/substituting-vegetable-oils-for-animal-fats-may-be-misguided-.html

Klein, E. A., Thompaon, I. M., Tangen, C. M., Crowley, J. J., Lucia, M. S., Goodman, P. J., et al. (2011). Vitamin E and the Risk of Prostate Cancer: The Selenium and Vitamin E Cancer Prevention Trial (SELECT). *Journal of the American Medical Association* , 306(14):1549-1556.

Koren, O., Spor, A., Felin, J., Fak, F., Stombaugh, J., Tremaroli, V., et al. (2011). Human Oral, Gut, and Plaque Microbiota in Patients with Atherosclerosis. *Proceedings of the National Academy Of Sciences, USA* , 108 (supplement 1): 4592-4598.

Koy, M. K., & Goldman, J. D. (2012, September). *Potassium Intake of the U.S. Population: What We Eat in America, NHANES 2009-2010.* Retrieved July 17, 2013, from Food Surveys Research Group: http://www.ars.usda.gov/SP2UserFiles/Place/12355000/pdf/DBrief/10_potassium_intake_0910.pdf

Kris-Etherton, P., Harris, W., & Appel, L. (2002). Fish Consumption, Fish Oil, Omega-3 Fatty Acids, and Cardiovascular Disease. *Circulation* , 106:2747-2757.

Kumar, M. V., Sambaiah, K., & Lokesh, B. R. (2000). Hypocholesterolemic effect of anhydrous milk fat ghee is mediated by increasing the secretion of biliary lipids. *The Journal of Nutritional Biochemistry* , 11(2):69-75.

Kummerow FA, K. Y. (1977). The influence of egg consumption on the serum cholesterol level in human subjects. *American journal of Clinical Nutrition* , 30:664-73.

Kurlansky, M. (2002). *Salt: A World History.* New York: Penguin Books.

Kuti, J. O., & Torres, E. S. (1996). Potential Nutritional and Health Benefits of Tree Spinach. In J. (. Janick, *Progress in New Crops* (pp. 516-520). Arlington, Va.: ASHS Press.

Larsson, S. C., Orsini, N., & Wolk, A. (2011). Dietary Potassium Intake and Risk of Stroke: A Dose-Response Meta-Analysis of Prospective Studies. . *Stroke* , doi: 10.1161/STROKEAHA.111.622142.

Larsson, S. C., Virtamo, J., & wolk, A. (2012). Chocolate consumption and risk of stroke: A prospective cohort of men and meta-analysis. *Neurology* , doi: 10.1212/WNL.0b013e31826aacfa.

Larsson, S. C., Virtamo, J., & Wolk, A. (2011). Red meat consumption and risk of stroke in Swedish men. *Am J Clin Nutr* , 94:417-421.

Last, A., & Wilson, S. (2006). Low-Carbohydrate Diets. *Am Fam Physician* , 73:1942-1948.

Lavie, C. J., De Schutter, A., Patel, D. A., Romero-Corral, A., Artham, S. M., & Milani, R. V. (2012). Body Composition and Survival in Stable Coronary Heart Disease:Impact of Lean Mass Index and Body Fat in the "Obesity Paradox. *Journal of the American College of Cardiology* , 60(15):1374-1380.

Lavie, C. J., McAuley, P. A., Church, T. S., Milani, R. V., & Blair, S. N. (2014). Obesity and Cardiovascular Diseases-Implications Regarding Fitness, Fatness and Severity in the Obesity Paradox. *Jornal of the American College of Cardiology* , doi: 10.1016/j.jacc.2014.01.022.

Lavie, C. J., Milani, R. V., & Ventura, H. O. (2009). Obesity and Cardiovascular Disease: Risk Factor, Paradox, and Impact of Weight Loss. *Journal of the American College of Cardiology* , 53(21):1925-1932.

Layman, D. K. (2013). *Bad Cholesterol-Not Really.* Retrieved August 10, 2013, from Qivana: http://www.qivanaproducts.com/bad-cholesterol-not-really-2/

Lecerf, J., & de Lorgeril, M. (2011). Dietary Cholesterol: from Physiology to Cardiovascular Risk. *Br J Nutr* , 106 (1): 6-14.

Lee, J., O'Keefe, J., & Bell, D. (2008). Vitamin D Deficiency and Important, Common, and Easily Treatable Cardiovascular Risk Factor? *J Am Coll Cardiol* , 52 (24): 1949-1956.

Lee, J., O'Keefe, J., Lavie, C., Marchioli, R., & Harris, W. (2008). Omega-3 Fatty Acids for Cardio Protection. *Mayo Clin Proc* , 83:324-332.

Lemann, J. (1999). Relationship between Urinary Calcium and Net Acid Excretion As Determined by Dietary Protein and Potassium: a Revie w. *Nephron* , 81 (supplement 1): 18-25.

Lemogoum, D., Ngatchou, W., Janssen, C., Leeman, M., Van bortel, L., Boutouyrie, P., et al. (2012). Effects of Hunter-Gatherer Subsitence Mode on Arterial Distensibility in Cameroonian Pygmies. *Hypertension* , doi:10.1161/HYPERTENSIONAHA.111.187757.

Leonard, B. (2007). Inflammation, Depression and Dementia: Are They Connected? *Neurochem Res* , 32:1749-1756.

Leonard, W. R., Snodgrass, J., & Robertson, M. L. (2010). Evolutionary Perspectives on Fat Ingestion and Metabolism in Humans. In J.-P. Montmayeur, & J. (. le Coutre, *Fat Detection: Taste, Texture, and Post-Ingestive Effects* (pp. 1 -- 14). Boca Raton, Florida: CRC Press.

Leonard, W., & Robertson, M. (1997). Comparative Primate Energetics and Hominid Evolution. *Am J Phys Anthropol* , 102:265-281.

Leonard, W., Robertson, M., Snodgrass, J., & Kuzawa, C. (2003). Metabolic Correlates of Hominid Brain Evolution. *Comp Biochem Physiol Part A* , 136:5-15.

Leonardi, M., Gerbault, P., Thomas, M. G., & Burger, J. (2012). The evolution of lactase persistence in Europe. A synthesis of archaeological and genetic evidence. *International Dairy Journal* , 22 (2): 88-97.

Lerner Research Institute . (2011, April 6). *Common dietary fat and intestinal microbes linked to heart disease.* Retrieved December 2013, 16, from ScienceDaily: http://www.sciencedaily.com/releases/2011/04/110406131814.htm

Levi, J., Segal, L. M., St. Laurent, R., Lang, A., & Rayburn, J. (2012). *F as in Fat: How Obesity Threatens America's Future.* Princeton, NJ: The Robert Wood Johnson Foundation.

Lewis, K., Lutgendorff, F., & Phan, V. (2010). Enhanced Translocation of Bacteria across Metabolically Stressed Epithelia Is Reduced by Butyrate. *Inflamm Bowel Dis* , 16 (7): 1138-1148.

Lewsi, C. E., McTigue, K., Burke, L. E., Poirier, P., Eckel, R. H., Howard, B. V., et al. (2011, June 8). *Mortality, Health Outcomes, and Body Mass Index in the Overweight Range:A Science Advisory From the American Heart Association.* Retrieved October 7, 2011, from Circulation:American Heart Association: http://circ.ahajournals.org/content/early/2009/06/08/CIRCULATIONAHA.109.192574.full.pdf+html

Ley, R., Turnbaugh, P., Klein, S., & Gordon, J. (2006). Microbial Ecology: Human Gut Microbes Associated with Obesity. *Nature* , 444:1022-1023.

Lichtenstein, A. (2003). Dietary fat and cardiovascular disease risk: quantity or quality? *J Womens Health* , 12 (2): 109-114.

Lichtenstein, A., Kennedy, E., Barrier, P., Danford, D., Ernst, N., Grundy, S., et al. (1998). Dietary Fat Consumption and Health. *Nutr Rev* , 56 (5 part 2):S 3-28.

Lindeberg, S. (2010). *Food and Western Disease: Health and Nutrition from an Evolutionary Perspective.* Chichester, United Kingdom: Wiley-Blackwell.

Lindseth, G., & Lindseth, P. (1995). The Relationship of Diet to Airsickness. *Aviat Space Environ Med* , 66: 537-541.

Linus Pauling Institute. (2012, January 27). *Essential Fatty Acids.* Retrieved August 4, 2013, from Oregon State University: http://lpi. oregonstate.edu/infocenter/othernuts/omega3fa/

Liu, S., Manson, J., Buring, J., Stampfer, M., Willett, W., & Ridker, P. (2002). Relation between a Diet with a High Glycemic Load and Plasma Concentrations of High Sensitive C- Reactive Protein in Middle-Aged Women. *Am J Clin Nutr* , 75:492-498.

Livepositively.com. (2013). *Coca-Cola.* Retrieved August 3, 2013, from Livepositively.com: https://parks.livepositively.com/ parks/NutritionConnectionFacts.pdf

Lohi, S., Mustalahti, K., Kaukinen, K., Laurila, K., Collin, P., Rissanen, H., et al. (2007). Increasing Prevalence of Celiac Disease over Time. *Aliment Pharmacol Therapy* , 26:1217-1225.

Lopez-Jimenez, F., & Sahakyan, K. (2012, August 27). Normal weight individuals with belly fat at highest CVD risk . Munich, Germany: European Society of Cardiology Meeting.

Loscalzo, J. (2013). Gut Microbiota, the Genome, and Diet in Atherogenesis. *New England Journal of Medicine* , 368 (17): 1647 -- 1649.

Losowsky, M. (2008). A History of Coeliac Disease. *Digestive Diseases* , 26:112-120.

Ludwig, D. (2002). The Glycemic Index: Physiological Mechanisms Relating Obesity, Diabetes, and Cardiovascular Disease. *JAMA* , 287:2414-2423.

Lui, S., & Willett, W. (2002). Dietary Glycemic Load and Atherothrombotic Risk. *Curr Atheroscler Rep* , 4:454-461.

Lussana, F., Painter, R., Ocke, M., Buller, H., Bossuyt, P., &

Roseboom, T. (2008). Prenatal Exposure to the Dutch Famine Is Associated with a Preference for Fatty Foods and a More Atherogenic Lipid Profile. *Am J Clin Nutr* , 88:1648-1652.

MacGregor, G., & DeWardener, H. (1998). *Salt, Diet, and Health.* Cambridge, England: Cambridge University Press.

Macko, S. A., Engel, M. H., Andrusevich, V., Lubec, G., O'Connrll, T. C., & Hedges, R. E. (1999). Documenting the diet in ancient human populations through stable isotope analysis of hair. *Phil. Trans. R. Soc Lond. B* , vol. 354 (1379): 65-76.

Madsen, T., Skou, H., & Hansen, V. (2001). C-Reactor Protein, Dietary n-3 Fatty Acids, and the Extent of Coronary Disease. *Am J Cardiol* , 88:1139-1142.

Magistretti, P. J., Pellerin, L., & Martin, J.-L. (2000). *Brain Energy Metabolism:An Integrated Cellular Perspective* . Retrieved August 3, 2013, from Neuropsychopharmacology: The Fifth Generation of Progress: http://www.acnp.org/g4/gn401000064/ch064.html

Manabe, Y., Matsumura, S., & Fushiki, T. (2010). Preference for High-Fat Food in Animals. In J. Montmayeur, & J. (. le Coutre, *Fat Detection: Taste, Texture, and Post Ingestive Effects* (p. Chapter 10). Boca Raton, FL: CRC Press.

Mann, G., Shaffer, R., & Rich, A. (1965). Physical Fitness and Immunity to Heart-Disease and the Masai. *Lancet* , 2: 1308-1310.

Mann, G., Shaffer, R., Anderson, R., & Sandstead, H. (1964). Cardiovascular Disease in the Maasai. *J Atheroscler Res* , 4:289-312.

Mann, G., Spoerry, A., Gray, M., & Jarashow, D. (1972). Atherosclerosis in the Masai. *Am J Epidemiol* , 95:26-37.

Margolskee, R., Dyer, J., Kokrashvilli, Z., Salmon, K., Ilegems, E., Daly, K., et al. (2007). T1r3T1r3T1r3T1r3 and Gustducin in Gut Sense of Sugars to Regulate Expression of Sodium-Glucose Co-1. *Proc Natl Acad Sci USA* , 104:15075-15080.

Maria Luz Fernandez, M. C. (2010). Revisiting Dietary Cholesterol Recommendations: Does the Evidence Support a Limit of 300 mg/d? . *Current Atherosclerosis Reports* , Volume 12, Number 6 (2010), 377-383, DOI: 10.1007/s11883-010-0130-7 .

Marni, J. (2010, December 20). A reversal on carbs. *The Los Angeles Times* , pp. http://articles.latimes.com/2010/dec/20/health/la-he-carbs-20101220.

Marshall, R. (Director). (2011). *Pirates of the Caribbean: On Stranger Tides* [Motion Picture].

Martin, C. (2012, July 24th). *World's Worst Jumbo Junk Food.*

Retrieved September 14th, 2013, from The Sun: http://www.thesun.co.uk/sol/homepage/features/2988347/Worlds-worst-jumbo-junk-food.html?offset=1

Mason, S. (2013, July 15). *UCLA researchers find link between intestinal bacteria and white blood cell cancer.* Retrieved July 20, 2013, from UCLA newsroom: http://newsroom.ucla.edu/portal/ucla/ucla-researchers-find-link-between-245945.aspx

Massey, L., & Whiting, S. (1995). Dietary Salt, Urinary Calcium, and Kidney Stone Risk. *Nutr Rev* , 53:131-139.

Mattison, J. A., Roth, G. S., Beasley, T. M., Tilmont, E. M., Handy, A. T., Herbert, R. L., et al. (2012). Impact of caloric restriction on health and survival in rhesus monkeys from the NIA study. *Nature* , 489:318–321.

Mayer, J. D., Roberts, R. D., & Barsade, S. G. (2008). Human Abilities: Emotional Intelligence. *Annual Review of Psychology* , (59): 507-36.

Mayer, J. (1969). *White House Conference on Food Nutrition and Health: Final Report.* . Washington DC: Government printing office.

Mbalilak, i. J., Masesa, Z., Strømme, S., Høstmark, A., Sundquist, J., Wändell, P., et al. (2010). Daily energy expenditure and cardiovascular risk in Masai, rural and urban Bantu Tanzanians. *Br J Sports Med.* , 44(2):121-126.

McCullough, M., Chevaux, K., Jackson, L., Preston, M., Martinez, G., HH, S., et al. (2006). Hypertension, the Kuna, and the epidemiology of flavanols. *J Cardiovasc Pharmacol.* , 47 Suppl 2:S103-9; discussion 119-21.

McCullough, M., Peterson, J., Patel, R., Jacques, P., Shah, R., & Dwyer, J. (2012). Flavonoid intake and cardiovascular disease mortality in a prospective cohort of US adults. *Am J Clin Nutr* , 95:454–464.

McKay, B. (2002, July 23). Governments Standard Lumps Hunks, Athletes with Truly Obese. *Wall Street Journal* , p. http://online.wsj.com/news/articles/SB1027369796834182760.

McLaughlin, R. (2010). *Rome and the Distant East: Trade Routes to the Ancient Lands of Arabia, India and China.* Continuum US: New York.

McNamara, R., Jandacek, R., Rider, T., Tao, P., Cole-Strauss, A., & Lipton, J. (2010). Omega-3 fatty acid deficiency increases constitutive pro-inflammatory cytokine production in rats: relationship with central serotonin turnover. *Prostaglandins Leukot Essent Fatty*

Acids. , 83(4-6):185-91.

Meadows, S., & Hakonson, T. (1982). Contributions of Tissue to Body Mass in Elk. *Journal of wildlife management* , 46:838-841.

Medina-Remón, A., Zamora-Ros, R., Rotchés-Ribalta, M., Andres-Lacueva, C., Martínez-González, M., Covas, M., et al. (2011). Total polyphenol excretion and blood pressure in subjects at high cardiovascular risk. *Nutr Metab Cardiovasc Dis.* , 21(5):323-31. .

Mensink, R., Zock, P., Kestor, A., & Katan, M. (2003). Effects of Dietary Fatty Acids and Carbohydrates on the Ratio of Serum Total to HDL Cholesterol and on Serum Lipids and Apolipoproteins: a Meta-Analysis of 60 Controlled Trials. *Am J Clin Nutr* , 77:1146-1155.

Mercedes R. Carnethon, P., Peter John D. De Chavez, M., Mary L. Biggs, P., Cora E. Lewis, M., James S. Pankow, P., Alain G. Bertoni, M. M., et al. (2012). Association of Weight Status With Mortality in Adults With Incident Diabetes . *JAMA.* , 308(6):581-590. doi:10.1001/jama.2012.9282 .

Merriam-Webster. (2013). *Dictionary.* Retrieved July 4, 2013, from m-w.com: http://www.merriam-webster.com/dictionary/

Micha, R., Wallace, S., & Mozaffarian, D. (2010). Red and Processed Meat Consumption and Risk of Incident Coronary Heart Disease, Stroke, and Diabetes Mellitus: A Systematic Review and Meta-Analysis. *Circulation* , 121(21):2271-2283.

Michaelsson, G., Gerden, B., & Hagforsen, E. (2000). Psoriasis Patients with Antibiotics to Gliadin Can Be Improved by a Gluten-Free Diet. *Br J Dermatol* , 142 (1): 44-51.

Mickelborough, T., Gotshall, R., Kluka, E., Miller, C., & Cordain, L. (2001). Dietary Chloride As a Possible Determinant of the Severity Exercise-Induced Asthma. *Eur J Appl Physiol* , 85:450-456.

Miller, M. (1945). Low Sodium Chloride Intake in the Treatment of Insomnia and Tension States. *JAMA* , 129:262-266.

Milton, K. (1987). Primate Diets and Got Morphology: Implications for Human Evolution. In M. Harris, & E. (. Ross, *Food and Even Lose in: toward a Theory of Human Food Habits* (pp. 93-116). Philadelphia, Pennsylvania: Temple University Press.

Mintz, M. (2013, November 23). *The New Cholesterol Guidelines and Diabetes.* Retrieved November 28, 2013, from Medscape: http://boards.medscape.com/forums/?128@@.2a5af828!comment=1

Molla MT, M. J. (2003). *Summary Measures of Population Health: Report of findings on methodologic and data issues.* Hyattsville, MD.:

National Center for Health Statistics.

Molodecky, N. A., & Kaplan, G. G. (2010). Environmental Risk Factors for Inflammatory Bowel Disease. *Gastroenterology and Hepatology* , 6 (5):339-346.

Montagu, J. (1994). Length of life in the ancient world: a controlled study. *Journal of the Royal Society of Medicine* , (87) 25-26.

Montonen, J., Jarvinen, R., Knekt, P., Heliovaara, M., & Reunanen, A. (2007). Consumption of Sweetened Beverages and Intakes of Fructose and Glucose Predict Type II Diabetes Occurrence. *J Nutr* , 137:1447-1454.

Morris, M. J., Na, E. S., & Johnson, A. K. (2008). Salt Craving: the Psychobiology of Pathogenic Sodium Intake. *Physiol Behav* , 94 (5): 709-721.

Morris, R., Sebastian, A., Forman, A., Tanaka, M., & Schmidlin, O. (1999). Normotensive Salt Sensitivity: Effects of Race and Dietary Potassium. *Hypertension* , 33:18-23.

Motoi, H., & Kodama, T. (2003). Isolation and Characterization of Angiotensin I Angiotensin I-Converting Enzyme Inhibitory Peptide from Wheat. *Nahrung* , 47:354-358.

Mozaffarian, D. (2008). Fish and and-3 Fatty Acids for the Prevention of Fatal Coronary Heart Disease and Sudden Cardiac Death. *Am J Clin Nutr* , 87:1991S-1996S.

Murray, C. J., Abraham, J., Ali, M. K., Alverado, M., Atkinson, C., Baddour, L. M., et al. (2013). The State of US Health, 1990-2010:Burden of Diseases, Injuries, and Risk Factors. *The Journal of the American Medical Association* , doi:10.1001/jama.2013.13805.

Mursu, J., Robien, K., Harnack, L. J., Park, K., & Jacobs Jr., D. R. (2011). Dietary Supplements and Mortality Rate in Older Women:The Iowa Women's Health Study . *Archives of Internal Medicine* , 171(18):1625-1633.

Muskiet, F. A. (2010). Pathophysiology and Evolutionary Aspects of Dietary Fats and Long-Chain Polyunsaturated Fatty Acids Across the Lifecycle. In J.-P. Montmayeur, & J. (. le Coutre, *Fat Detection: Taste, Texture, and Post Ingestive Effects* (pp. 15 -- 53). Boca Raton, Florida: CRC Press.

Muskiet, F., & Kuipers, R. (2010). Lessons from Shore-based Hunter-Gatherer Diets in East Africa. In S. Cunnane, & K. (. Stewart, *Human Brain Evolution: the Influence of Fresh Water and Marine Food Reserves* (pp. 77-104). Hoboken, New Jersey: John Wiley & Sons.

Myese, P. (1993). Intermediary Metabolism of Fructose. *Am J Clin Nutr* , 58 (supplement): 754S- 765S.

Nainggolan, L. (2010, April 21). *IOM recommends FDA set new standards for salt in foods.* . Retrieved January 23, 2013, from the-heart.org: : http://www.theheart.org/article/1068389.do

National Center for Complementary and Alternative Medicine. (2013, May 28). *Oral Probiotics: An Introduction.* Retrieved December 25, 2013, from National Center for Complementary and Alternative Medicine: http://nccam.nih.gov/health/probiotics/introduction.htm

National Osteoporosis Foundation. (1998). osteoporosis: review of the evidence for prevention, diagnosis, and treatment and cost-effectiveness analysis. *Osteoporosis* , 8 (supplement): S1 -- 88.

Nationmaster.com. (2011). *Health Statistics.* Retrieved October 7, 2011, from Nationmaster.com: http://www.nationmaster.com/graph/hea_lif_exp_at_bir_tot_yea-life-expectancy-birth-total-years

Neel, J. (1999). Diabetes Mellitus: a "Thrifty" Genotype Rendered Detrimental It "Progress"? *Bull World health Organ* , 77:694-703.

Neese, R., & Williams, G. (1994). *Why we get Sick. The New Science of Darwinian Medicine.* New York: Times Books.

Nefzaoui, C. (1886). *The Perfumed Garden of the Cheikh Nefzaoui.* London: Kama Shastra Society of London and Benares.

Nelsen, D. A. (2002). Gluten-Sensitive Eneropathy (Celiac Disease): More Common Than You Think. *American Family Physician* , 66(12):2259-2266.

Nelson, G., Schmidt, P., & Kelly, D. (1995). Low-Fat Diets Do Not Lower Plasma Cholesterol Levels in Healthy Men Compared to High Fat Diets with Similar Fatty Acid Composition at Constant Caloric Intake. *Lipids* , 30:969-976.

Ness, G., & Chambers, C. (2000). Feedback and hormonal regulation of hepatic 3-hydroxy-3-methylglutaryl coenzyme A reductase: the concept of cholesterol buffering capacity. *Proc Soc Exp Biol Med.* , 224(1):8-19.

Ness, G., Zhao, Z., & Wiggins, L. (1994). Insulin and Glucagon Modulate Hepatic 3 Hydroxy to 3 Methylglutaryl-Coenzyme a Reductase Activity by Affecting Immunoreactive Protein Levels. *J Biol Chem* , 269 (46):29168-29172.

Neufeld, E., Stonik, J., Demosky, S. J., Knapper, C., Combs, C., Cooney, A., et al. (2004). The ABC A1 Transporter Modulates Late Endocytic Trafficking: Insights from the Correction of the Genetic

Defect in Tangier Disease. *J Biol Chem* , to 79:15571-15578.

Nicholls, S. (2013). Standards and classification: A perspective on the 'obesity epidemic'. *Social science & medicine* , 87:9-15.

Niness, K. R. (1999). Inulin and Oligofructose: What Are They? *J. Nutr.* , 129(7):1402S-1406s .

Novotny, J., & etal. (2012). Low calorie cranberry juice lowers blood pressure in healthy adults. *American Heart Association's High Blood Pressure Research Meeting* (p. HBPR 2012; Abstract 299). Wasington, DC: American Heart Association.

NYC.gov. (2008). *National Salt Reduction Initiative.* Retrieved January 23, 2013, from NYC.gov: http://www.nyc.gov/html/doh/html/cardio/cardio-salt-initiative.shtml

NYC.gov. . (2008). *National Salt Reduction Initiative.* Retrieved January 23, 2013, from NYC.gov: http://www.nyc.gov/html/doh/html/cardio/cardio-salt-initiative.shtml

O'Mahony, R., Al-Khtheeri, H., Weerasekera, D., Fernando, N., Vaira, D., & Holton, J. (2005). Bactericidal and anti-adhesive properties of culinary and medicinal plants against Helicobacter pylori. *World Journal of Gatroenterology* , 11(47):7499-7507.

O'Dea, K. (1984). Marked Improvement in Carbohydrate and Lipid Metabolism in Diabetic Australian Aborigines after Temporary Reversion to Traditional Lifestyle. *Diabetes* , 33 (6): 596-603.

O'Donnell, M. J., Yusef, S., Mente, A., Gao, P., Mann, J. F., & Teo, K. (2011). Urinary Sodium and Potassium Excretion and Risk of Cardiovascular Events. . *Journal of The American Medical Association* , 306(20):2262-2264.

OECD health data 2012. (2012). *OECD health data 2012—frequently requested data.* Retrieved July 13, 2013, from OECD health data 2012: http://www.oecd.org/health/health-systems/oecdhealth-data2012-frequentlyrequested-data.htm.

O'Keefe, S. (2000). An Overview of Oils and Fats, with a Special Emphasis on Olive Oil. In K. Kiple, & K. (. Ornelas, *The Cambridge World History or Food Volume 1* (pp. 375 -- 397). Cambridge, United Kingdom: Cambridge University Press.

Heads, T. T. (Performer). (1980). Once-In-A-Lifetime.

Ordovas, J., Corella, D., Cupples, L., Demissie, S., Kelleher, A., Coltell, O., et al. (2002). Polyunsaturated Fatty Acids Modulate the Effects of the APOA-1 G-A Polymorphism on HDL-Cholesterol Concentrations in a Sex-Specific Manner: The Framingham Study. *Am J Clin Nutr* , 75:38-46.

Oretega, F. B., Lee, D.-c., Katzmarzyk, P. T., Ruiz, J. R., Sui, X., Church, T. S., et al. (2012). The intriguing metabolically healthy but obese phenotype: cardiovascular prognosis and role of fitness. *European Heart Journal*, doi: 10.1093/eurheartj/ehs174.

Orpana, H. M., Berthelot, J.-M., Kaplan, M. S., Feeny, D. H., McFarland, B., & Ross, N. A. (2010). BMI and Mortality: Results From a National Longitudinal Study of Canadian Adults. *Obesity*, 18(1):214-218.

Oz, M. (2013). *Dr. Oz's Super-Longevity Prescription*. Retrieved July 6, 2013, from www.doctoroz.com: http://www.doctoroz.com/episode/dr-ozs-super-longevity-prescription

Painter, J. (2006, July 31). *Scientific American*. Retrieved September 14, 2013, from How to Food Manufacturers Calculate the Calorie Count of Packaged Foods?: http://www.scientificamerican.com/article.cfm?id=how-do-food-manufacturers

Pak, C., Fuller, C., Sakhaee, K., Preminger, G., & Britton, F. (1985). Long-Term Treatment of Calcium Nephrolithiasis with Potassium Citrate. *J Urol*, 134:11-19.

Patterson, R., Kristal, A., Peters, J., Neuhouser, M., Rock, C., Cheskin, L., et al. (2000). Changes in Diet, Weight, and Serum Lipid Levels Associated with Olestra Consumption. *Arch Intern med*, 19:141-147.

Patty W Siri-Tarino, Q. S. (2010). Meta-analysis of prospective cohort studies evaluating the association of saturated fat with cardiovascular disease. *The American Journal of Clinical Nutrition*, vol. 91 no. 3 535-546.

Pella, D., Dubnov, G., & Singh, R. (2003). Effects of an Indo-Mediterranean Diet on the Omega-6/Omega-3 Ratio in Patients at High Risk of Coronary Artery Disease: the Indian Parado x. *World Rev Nutr Diet*, 92:74-80.

Peng, L., Li, Z., & Green, R. (2009). Butyrate Enhances the Intestinal Barrier by Facilitating Tight Junction Assembly Via Activation of AMP-Activated Protein Kinase in Caco-2 Cell Monolayers. *J Nutr*, 139:1619-1625.

Pengiran-Tengah, C., Lock, R., Unsworth, D., & Wills, A. (2004). Multiple Sclerosis and Occult Gluten Sensitivity. *Neurology*, 64 (12): 2326-2327.

Penn State College of Agricultural Sciences. (2002). *Herb and Spice History*. UniversityPark, Pa: Penn State College of Agricultural Sciences.

Pérez-Castrillón, J. L., Vega, G., Abad, L., Sanz, A., Chaves, J., Hernandez, G., et al. (2007). Effects of Atorvastatin on Vitamin D Levels in Patients With Acute Ischemic Heart Disease. *Am J Cardiol* , 99:903-905.

Perez-Fons, L., Steiger, S., Khaneja, R., Bramley, P. M., Cutting, S. M., Sandmann, G., et al. (2011). Identification and the Developmental Formation of Carotenoid Pigments in the Yellow/Orange Bacillus Spore Former s. *Biochimica et Biophysica Acta* , 1811:177-185.

Petrou, S., Ordway, R., Kirber, M., Dopico, A., Hamilton, J., Walsh, J. J., et al. (1995). Direct Effects of Fatty Acids and Other Charged Lipids on Ion Channel Activity in Smooth Muscle Cells. *Prostag Leukotr Essent fatty Acids* , 52:173-178.

Pflughoeft, K., & Versalovic, J. (2012). Human Microbiome in Health and Disease. *Annu Rev Pathol* , 7:99-122.

Picard, C., Fioramonti, J., Francios, A., Robinson, T., Neant, F., & Matuchansky, C. (2005). Review article: bifidobacteria as probiotic agents – physiological effects and clinical benefits. *Alimentary Pharmacology & Therapeutics* , 22(6):495–512.

Pollack, A. (2013, June 18). A.M.A. Recognizes Obesity as a Disease. *New York Times* , p. B1.

Pollan, M. (2002, March 31). *Power Steer.* Retrieved July 14, 2013, from New York Times: http://www.nytimes.com/2002/03/31/magazine/power-steer.html?pagewanted=all&src=pm

Population Reference Bureau. (2006, March no. 8). The Future of Human Life Expectancy: Have We Reached the Ceiling or is the Sky the Limit? *Research Highlights in the Demography and Economics of Aging* , pp. 1-4.

Porcelli, M., & Gugelchuk, G. (1995). A Trek to the Top: A Review of Acute Mountain Sickness. *J Am Osteopath Assoc* , 95:718-720.

Preidt, R. (2014, April 17). *Low Birth Weight, Lack of Breast-Feeding Tied to Inflammation Risk in Adulthood.* Retrieved April 18, 2014, from Health Day: http://consumer.healthday.com/women-s-health-information-34/breast-feeding-news-82/briefs-emb-4-14-birth-weight-breastfeeding-baby-s-health-prsb-cifar-release-batch-1134-686836.html

Preminger, G., Sakhaee, K., Skurla, C., & Pak, C. (1985). Prevention of Recurrent Calcium Stone Formation with Potassium Citrate Therapy in Patients with Distal Renal Tubular Acidosis. *J Urol* , 134:20-23.

Purslow, L., Sandhu, M., Forouh, i. N., Young, E., Luben, R.,

Welch, A., et al. (2008). Energy intake at breakfast and weight change: prospective study of 6,764 middle-aged men and women. *Am J Epidemiol.* , 167(2):188-92.

Rabinovitz, H. R., Boaz, M., Ganz, T. a., Jakubowicz, D., Matas, Z., Madar, Z., et al. (2013). Big breakfast rich in protein and fat improves glycemic control in type 2 diabetics. *Obesity: A Research Journal* , DOI: 10.1002/oby.20654.

Rakhimova, M., Esslinger, B., & Schulze-Krebs, A. (2009). In Vitro Differentiation of Human Monocytes into Dendritic Cells by Peptic-Tryptic Digest of Gliadin Is Independent of Genetic Predisposition in the Presence of Celiac Disease. *J Clin Immunol* , 29 (1): 29-37.

Ramsden, C. E., Zamaora, D., Boonseng, L., Majchrzak-Hong, S., Faurot, K. R., Suchindran, C. M., et al. (2013). Use of dietary linoleic acid for secondary prevention of coronary heart disease and death: evaluation of recovered data from the Sydney Diet Heart Study and updated meta-analysis. *BMJ* , 346:e8707 (doi: http://dx.doi.org/10.1136/bmj.e8707).

Ramsden, C. E., Zamora, D., Leelarthaepin, B., Majchrzak-Hong, S. F., Faurot, K. R., Suchindran, C. M., et al. (2013). Use of Dietary Linoleic Acid for Secondary Prevention of Coronary Heart Disease and Death:Evaluation of Recovered Data from the Sydney Diet Heart Study and Updated Meta-Analysis. *British Medical Journal* , 346:e8707 doi: 10.1136/bmj.e8707 .

Ramsden, C., Faurot, K., & Carrera-Bastos, P. (2001). Dietary Fat Quality and Coronary Heart Disease Prevention: a Unified Theory Based on Evolutionary, Historical, Global, and Modern Perspectives. *Curr Treat Options Cardiovasc Med* , 11 (4): 289-301.

Rapp, J. R. (1982). Dahl Salt-Susceptible and Salt-Resistant Rats: A Review. *Hypertension* , 4:753-763.

Rappaport, S. (2003). In Vivo Approaches to Quantifying and Imaging Brain Arachidonic and Docosahexaenoic Acid Metabolis m. *J Pediatr* , 143:S26-S34.

Rappaport, S., Rao, J., & Igarashi, M. (2007). Brain Metabolism of Nutritionally Essential Poly-Unsaturated Fatty Acids Depends on Both the Diet and the Live r. *Prostag Leukot Essent Fatty Acids* , 77:251-261.

Ravnskov, U. (2002). Hypothesis out-of-Date. The Diet-Heart Idea. *J Clin Epidemiol* , 55:1057-1063.

Ravnskov, U. (1998). The questionable role of saturated and

polyunsaturated Fatty Acids and Cardiovascular Diseas e. *J Clin Epidemiol* , 51:443-460.

Ravnskov, U., Allen, C., Atrens, D., Enig, M., Groves, B., Kauffman, M., et al. (2002). Studies of Dietary Fat and Heart Disease. *Science* , 295:1464-1465.

Rawlins, M., & Culyer, A. (2004). National Institute for Clinical Excellence and Its Value Judgments. *BMJ* , 329(7459):224-7.

Read, P. P. (1974). *Alive: The Story of the Andes Survivors.* New York, New York: Avon books (HarperCollins).

Reaven, G. (1995). Pathophysiology of Insulin Resustance in Human Disease. *Physiol Rev* , 75:473-486.

Reaven, G. (2005). The Insulin Resistance Syndrome: Definition and Dietary Approaches to Treatment. *Annu Rev Nutr* , 25:391-406.

Reed, D., McGee, D., Yano, K., & Hankin, J. (1985). Diet, Blood Pressure, and Multicolinearity. *Hypertension* , 405-10.

Reichelt, K., & Jensen, D. (2004). Ig a Antibodies against Gliadin and Gluten and Multiple Sclerosis. *Acta Neurol Scand* , 110 (4): 239-241.

Renaud, S., & de Lorgeril, M. (1992). Wine, alcohol, platelets, and the French paradox for coronary heart disease. *Lancet* , 339(8808):1523-1526.

Richardson, A., & Ross, M. (2003, november). *Physical Signs of Fatty Acid Deficiency.* Retrieved August 4, 2013, from Food and Behaviour Research: http://www.fabresearch.org/uploads/1493/FACTSHEET%20002-PFADS%202003-11.pdf

Rister, R. (2011, May 5). *Eating Less Salt Does Not Necessarily Cut High Blood Pressure and Heart Disease Risks.* Retrieved December 17, 2011, from SteadyHealth.com: http://www.steadyhealth.com/articles/Eating_Less_Salt_Does_Not_Necessarily_Cut_High_Blood_Pressure_and_Heart_Disease_Risks_a1787.html)

Ritz, E. (2005). Salt—friend or foe? *Nephrol Dial Transplant* , doi:10.1093/ndt/gfi256.

Robbins, C. S., Hilgendorf, I., Weber, G. F., Theuri, I., Iwamoto, Y., Figueiredo, J.-L., et al. (2013). Local proliferation dominates lesional macrophage accumulation in atherosclerosis. *Nature Medicine* , doi:10.1038/nm.3258.

Roberts, C., & Liu, S. (2009). Effects of Glycemic Load on Metabolic Health and Type II Diabetes Mellitus. *J DiabetesSci Technol* , 3 (4): 697-704.

Robertson, J. (2003). Dietary Salt and Hypertension: a Scientific

Issue or a Matter of Faith? *J Eval Clin Pract* , 9 (1):1 – 22.

Rohrmann, S., Overvad,K, Bueno-de-Mesquita, H., Jakobsen, M., Egeberg, R., Tjønneland, A., et al. (2013). Meat consumption and mortality--results from the European Prospective Investigation into Cancer and Nutrition. *BMC Med* , 11:63. doi: 10.1186/1741-7015-11-63.

Rolls, E. (2004). smell, taste, texture, And temperature multimodal representations of the brain, and their relevance to the control of appetite. *Nutr Rev* , 62:S193-S204.

Romero-Corral, A. S., Sierra-Johnson, J., Korenfeld, Y., Boarin, S., Korinek, J., Jensen, M. D., et al. (2009). Normal weight obesity: a risk factor for cardiometabolic dysregulation and cardiovascular mortality. *European Heart Journal* , doi:10.1093/eurheartj/ehp487.

Rose, M. (2008, July 4). *Blueberries: History, Culture and Uses.* Retrieved March 8, 2013, from Dave's Garden: http://davesgarden.com/guides/articles/view/1333/

Rosen, C. J., Adams, J. S., Bikle, D. D., Black, D. M., Demay, M. B., Manson, J. E., et al. (2012). The Nonskeletal Effects of Vitamin D: An Endocrine Society Scientific Statement. *Endocrine Reviews* , 33:456-492.

Ross, A. C., Taylor, C. L., Yaktine, A. L., & Del Valle, H. B. (2011). *DRIDIETARY REFERENCE INTAKES : Calcium Vitamin D.* Washington, DC: THE NATIONAL ACADEMIES PRESS.

Rozin, P., & Schiller, D. (1980). The nature and acquisition of a prefernce for chili pepper by humans. *Motivation and Emotion* , 77-100.

Rubin MD., A. L. (2011). *Vitamin D For Dummies.* Hoboken, NJ: Wiley Publishing Company.

Rubio-Tapia, A., Kyle, R., Kaplan, E., Johnson, D., Page, W., Erdtmann, F., et al. (2009). Increased Prevalence and Mortality in Undiagnosed Celiac Disease. *Gastroenterology* , 137:88-93.

Rule, D., Broughton, K., Shellito, S., & Maiorano, G. (2002). Comparison of Muscle Fatty Acid Profiles and Cholesterol Concentrations of Bison, Beef Cattle, Elk, and Chicken. *Journal of Animal Science* , 80: 1202-1211.

Saad, M., Khan, A., Sharma, A., Michael, R., Riad-Gabriel, M., Boyadjian, R., et al. (1998). Physiological insulinemia acutely modulates plasma leptin. *Diabetes* , 47:544–549.

Sacks, F., Svetkey, L., Vollmer, W., Appel, I., Bray, G., & Harsha, D. (2001). Effects on Blood Pressure of Reduce Dietary Sodium and the Dietary Approaches to Stop Hypertension (Dash) Diet. . *New England Journal of Medicine* , 344 (1): 3 – 10 .

Sagan, C., & Druyan, A. (1992). *Shadows of Forgotten Ancestors.* New York: Random House.

Sahakyan, K. (2012). Normal weight individuals with belly fat at highest CVD risk. *European Society of Cardiology* (pp. http://www. escardio.org/about/press/press-releases/esc12-munich/Pages/ weight-obesity-cardiovascular-mortality-risk.aspx). Munich: European Society of Cardiology.

Saja, K., Chatterjee, U., Chatterjee, B., & Sudhakaran, P. (2007). Activation Dependent Expression of MMPs in Peripheral Blood Mononuclear Cells Involves Protein Kinase A. *Mol Cell Biochem* , 296 (1-2): 185-192.

Sakakeeny, L., Roubenoff, R., Obi, M., Fontes, J. D., Benjamin, E. J., Bujanover, Y., et al. (2012). Plasma Pyridoxal-5-Phosphate Is Inversely Associated with Systemic Markers of Inflammation in a Population of U.S. Adults. *The Journal of Nutrtition* , doi: 10.3945/ jn.111.153056.

Salas-Salvadó, J., Bulló, M., Babio, N., Martínez-González, M., Ibarrola-Jurado, N., Basora, J., et al. (2011). Reduction in the incidence of type 2 diabetes with the Mediterranean diet: results of the PREDIMED-Reus nutrition intervention randomized trial. *Diabetes Care.* , 34(1):14-9. doi: 10.2337/dc10-1288. .

Salcedo, G., Danchez-Monge, G., Garcia-Casado, G., Aremntia, A., Gomez, L., & Barber, D. (2004). The Cereal Alpha Amylase/ Trypsin Inhibitor Family Associated with Bakers' Asthma and Food Allerg y. In E. Mills, & P. Shewry, *Plant Food Allergens* (pp. 70-86). Oxford, United Kingdom: Blackwell Science Ltd.

Samra, R. A. (2010). Fats and Satiety. In J. Montmayeur, & l. C., *Fat Detection: Taste, Texture, and Post Ingestive Effects.* (p. Chapter 15). Boca Raton, Fl: CRC Press.

Schaeffer, O. (1971). When the Eskimo Comes to Town. *Nutrition Today* , 6:8-16.

Schiffman, S., & Dackis, C. (1975). Taste of Nutrients: Amino Acids, Vitamins and Fatty Acids. *Percept Psychophys* , 17:140-146.

Schmidt, C. (2005, October 20). *Happy 120th? Science Pushes Human Longevity.* Retrieved October 10, 2011, from National Geographic.com: http://news.nationalgeographic.com/ news/2005/10/1020_051020_human_lifespan.html

Scholz-Ahrens, K. E., Ade, P., Marten, B., Weber, P., Timm, W.,

Açil, Y., et al. (2007). Prebiotics, Probiotics, and Synbiotics Affect Mineral Absorption, Bone Mineral Content, and Bone Structure. *J. Nutr.* , 137(3): 838S-846S .

Schusdziarra, V., Hausmann, M., Wittke, C., Mittermeier, J., Kellner, M., Naumann, A., et al. (2011). Impact of breakfast on daily energy intake - an analysis of absolute versus relative breakfast calories. *Nutrition Journal* , doi:10.1186/1475-2891-10-5.

Sebastian, A., Frassetto, L., Sellmeyer, D., Merriam, R., & Morris, R. (2002). Estimation of the Net Acid Load of the Diet of Ancestral Preagricultural Homo Sapiens and Their Hominid Ancestors. *Am J Clin Nutr* , 76:1308-1316.

Sebastian, A., Harris, S., Ottaway, J., Todd, K., & Morris, R. (1994). Improve Mineral Balance and Skeletal Metabolism and Postmenopausal Women Treated with Potassium Bicarbonate. *New England Journal of Medicine* , 330:1776-1781.

Seidell, J. (1998). Dietary Fat and Obesity: an Epidemiologic Perspective. *Am J Clin Nutr* , 67:546S-550S.

Serhan, C., Hong, S., Gronert, K., Colgan, S., Devchand, P., Mirick, G., et al. (2002). Resolvins: a family of bioactive products of omega-3 fatty acid transformation circuits initiated by aspirin treatment that counter proinflammation signals. *J Exp Med.* , 196(8):1025-37.

Sesso, H. D., Christen, W. G., Bubes, V., Smith, J. P., MacFadyen, J., Schvartz, M., et al. (2012). Multivitamins in the Prevention of Cardiovascular Disease in Men: The Physicians' Health Study II Randomized Controlled Trial. *JAMA.* , 308(17):1751-1760.

Shaffer, P. (1921). Antiketogenesis II. The ketogenic antiketogenic balance in man. *J Biol Chem* , 47: 463-473.

Shah, A., Al-Shareef, A., Ageel, A., & Qureshi, S. (1988). Toxicity Studies in Mice of Comment Spices Cinnamomum Zeylanicum Bark and Piper Longum Fruits. *Plant Foods for Human Nutrition* , (52) 3:231 -- 239.

Sharma, A. (2013). *How BMI Obfuscates Public Health and Clinical Approaches to Obesity*. Retrieved December 14, 2013, from Dr. Sharma's Obesity Notes: http://www.drsharma.ca/how-bmi-obfuscates-public-health-and-clinical-approaches-to-obesity.html

Sharma, A., Kribben, A., Schattenfroh, S., Cetto, C., & Distler, A. (1990). Salt Sensitivity in Humans Is Associated with Abnormal Acid-based Regulation. *Hypertension* , 16:407-413.

Sherman, P. W., & Billing, J. (1999, June). Darwinian Gastronomy:

Why We Use Spices. *BioScience* , 49(6):453-463.

Sheu, W., Lee, I., Chen, W., & Chan, Y. (2008). Effects of xylo-oligosaccharides in type 2 diabetes mellitus. *J Nutr Sci Vitaminol* , 54(5):396-401.

Shewry, P. (2009). Wheat. *Journal of Experimental Botany* , 60 (6):1537-1553.

Sigelman, C. K., & Rider, E. A. (2009). *Life-Span Human Development.* Belmont, California: WWadsworth, Cengage Learning.

Silk, D., Davis, A., Vulevic, J., Tzortzis, G., & Gibson, G. (2009). Clinical trial: the effects of a trans-galactooligosaccharide prebiotic on faecal microbiota and symptoms in irritable bowel syndrome. *Aliment Pharmacol Ther.* , 29(5):508-518. .

Simopoulos, A. (2001). Evolutionary Aspects of Diet and Essential Fatty Acids. *World Rev Nutr Diet* , 88:18-27.

Simopoulos, A. P. (1999). Essential fatty acids in health and chronic disease. *The American Journal of Nutrition* , 70 (3):560S-569S.

Simopoulos, A. P. (2004). Omega-6/Omega-3 Essential Fatty Acid Ratio and Chronic Diseases. *FOOD REVIEWS INTERNATIONAL* , 20(1):77-90.

Simopoulos, A. (2001). The Mediterranean Diets: What Is so Special about the Diet of Greece? The Scientific Evidence. *J Nutr* , 131:3065S-3073S.

Simopoulus, A. (2002). Omega-3 Fatty Acids in Inflammation and Autoimmune Disease. *J Am Coll Nutr* , 21:495-505.

Singh, N. (2010). Blockade of Dendritic Cell Development by Bacterial Fermentation Products Butyrate and Propionate through a Transporter (Slc 5a8)-Dependent Inhibition of Histone Deacetylases. *J Biol Chem* , 285 (36): 27601-27608.

Singh, R., Barden, A., Mori, T., & Beilin, L. (2001). Advanced Glycation and Products: A Review. *Diabetologia* , 44:129-146.

Sir, i. P., & Krauss, R. (2005). Influence of Dietary Carbohydrate and Fat on LDL and HDL Particle Distributions. *Curr Atheroscler Rep* , 7 (6): 455-459.

Siri-Tarino, P., Sun, Q., Hu, F., & Krauss, R. (2010). Meta-Analysis of Prospective Cohort Studies Evaluating the Association of Saturated Fat with Cardiovascular Disease. *Am J Clin Nutr* , 91 (3): 535-546.

Skaper, S. (2008). Signaling Pathways with Small Molecule Mimetics and Modulators to Achieve Neuroprotection and Regeneration. *CNS Neurol Disord Drug Targets* , 7:45.

Skylas, D., Mackintosh, J., Cordwell, S., Basseal, D., Walsh, B., Harry, J., et al. (2000). Proteome Approach to the Characterization of Protein Composition in the Developing and Mature Wheat Grain Endosperm. *Journal of Cereal Science* , 32:169-188.

Smalley, J., & Blake, M. (2003). Sweet Beginnings: Stalk Sugar and the Domestication of Maize. *Current Anthropology* , 44(5):675-703.

Smilowitz, J., German, J., & Zivkovic, A. (2010). Food Intake and Obesity: The Case of Fat. In J. Montmayeur, & J. (. le Coutre, *Fat Detection: Taste, Texture, and Post Ingestive Effects* (p. Chapter 22). Boca Raton, Fl: CRC Press.

Smith, W., Crombie, I., Tavendale, R., Gulland, S., & Tunstall-Pedoe, H. (1988). Urinary Electrolyte Excretion, Alcohol Consumption, and Blood Pressure in the Scottish Heart Health Study. *BMJ,* , 297 (6644): 329 – 30.

Sobel, J. (2007). Using a Model of the Food and Nutrition System for Examining Whole-Grain Foods from Agriculture to Health. In J. Sobel, *Whole Gr and Health* (pp. 17-25). Oxford, United Kingdom: Blackwell Publishing.

Sofi, F., Whittaker, A., Cesari, F., Gori, A., Fiorillo, C., Becatti, M., et al. (2013). Characterization of Khorasan Wheat (Kamut) and Impact of a Replacement Diet on Cardiovascular Risk Factors: Crossover Dietary Intervention Study. *Eur J Clin Nutr* , 67 (2): 190-195.

Spaenij-Dekking, L., Kooy-Winkelaar, Y., Van Aeelen, P., Drijfhout, J., Jonker, H., Van Soest, L., et al. (2005). Natural Variation in Toxicity of Wheat: Potential for Selection of Nontoxic Fridays for Celiac Disease Patients. *Gastroenterology* , 129:797-806.

Spence, J. D., Jenkins, D. J., & Davignon, J. (2012). Egg yolk consumption and carotid plaque. *Atherosclerosis* , doi:10.1016/j.atherosclerosis.2012.07.032.

Staller, J. E. (2010). Ethnohistoric Sources on Foodways, Feasts, and Festivals in Mesoamerica. In J. Staller, & M. (. Carrasco, *Pre-Columbian Foodways: Interdisciplinary Approached to Food, Culture, and Markets in Ancient Mesoamerica* (p. 64). New York: Spinger Science.

Stanford School of Medicine. (2013). *Stanford Research into the Impact of Tobacco Advertising*. Retrieved December 10, 2013, from www.stanford.edu: http://tobacco.stanford.edu/tobacco_main/slogans.php

Stanhope, J., Sampson, V., & Prior, I. (1981). The Tokelau Island Migrant Study: Serum Lipid Concentration into Environments. *J*

Chronic Dis , 34 (2-3): 45-55.

Stanhope, K., & Havel, P. (2010). fructose composition: recent results and their potential implications. *Annals of the New York Academy of Science* , March: 1190 (1): 15 to 24.

Stanhope, K., Bremer, A., Medici, V., Nakajima, K., Ito, Y., Nakano, T., et al. (2011). Consumption of fructose and high fructose corn syrup increase postprandial triglycerides, LDL-cholesterol, and apolipoprotein-B in young men and women. *J Clin Endocrinol Metab* , 96 (10):e1596-1605.

Stolarz-Skrzypek, K., Kuznetsova, T., Thijs, L., Tikhonoff, V., Se-idlerová, J., & T, R. (2011). Fatal and Nonfatal Outcomes, Incidence of Hypertension, and Blood Pressure Changes in Relation to Urinary Sodium Excretion. *JAMA* , 305(17):1777-1785.

Stone, N. J., Robinson, J., Lichtenstein, A. H., Merz, C. N., . Lloyd-Jones, D. M., Blum, A. C., et al. (2013). 2013 ACC/AHA Guideline on the Treatment of Blood Cholesterol to Reduce Atherosclerotic Cardiovascular Risk in Adults. *Journal of the American College of Cardiology* , doi:10.1016/j.jacc.2013.11.002.

Stone, O. (Director). (1987). *Wall Street* [Motion Picture].

Storck, J., & Teague, W. (1952). *Flour for man's bread, a history of milling.* Minneapolis: University of Minnesota Press.

Sturm, R., & Hattori, A. (2013). Morbid obesity rates continue to rise rapidly in the United States. *Int J Obes* , 37(6):889-91.

Sundram, K., Ismail, A., Hayes, K. C., Jeyamalar, R., & Pathana-than, R. (1997). Trans (Elaidic) Fatty Acids Adversely Affect the Lipoprotein Profile Relative to Specific Saturated Fatty Acids in Humans. *the Journal of Nutrition* , 127: 514S–520S.

Swithers, S. E. (2013). Artificial Sweeteners Produce the Coun-terintuitive Effect of Inducing Metabolic Derangements. *Trends in Endocronology and Metabolism* , 1-11.

Takahashi, M., Fukunaga, H., Fukudome, S.-I., & Yoshikawa, M. (2000). Behavioural and Pharmacological Studies on Gluten exor-phin A5, a Newly Isolated Bioactive Food Protein Fragment in Mice. *Japanese Journal of Pharmacology* , 84:259-265.

Tang, W., Wang, Z., Levison, B., Koeth, R., Britt, E., Fu, X., et al. (2013). Intestinal Microbial Metabolism of Phosphatidylcholine in Cardiovascular Risk. *New England Journal of Medicine* , 368 (17): 1575-1584.

Tannahill, R. (1973). *Food in History.* New York, NY: Stein and Day Publishers.

Tarini, J., & Wolever, T. (2010). The Fermentable Fibre Insulin Increases Postprandial Serum Short-Chain Fatty Acid and Reduces Free-Fatty Acid and Ghrelin in Healthy Subjects. *Appl Physiol Nutr Metab* , 35 (1): 9-16.

Taubes, G. (2007). *Good Calories, Bad Calories* . New York: Alfred Knopf Publishers.

Taubes, G. (2012, June 2). Salt, We Misjudged You. *The New York Times* , p. SR8.

Taubes, G. (2001). The Soft Science of Dietary Fat. *Science* , 291:2535-2541.

Taylor, R., Ashton, K., Moxham, T., Hooper, L., & Ebrahim, S. (2011). Reduced dietary salt for the prevention of cardiovascular disease. . *Cochrane Database Syst Rev.* , Jul 6;(7):CD009217. doi: 10.1002/14651858.CD009217.

Teff, K. L., Grudziak, J., Townsend, R. R., Dunn, T. N., Grant, R. W., Adams, S. H., et al. (2009). Endocrine and Metabolic Effects of Consuming Fructose-and Glucose-Sweetened Beverages with Meals in Obese Men and Women: Influence of Insulin Resistance on Plasma Triglyceride Response s. *J Clin Endocrinol Metab* , 94 (5): 1562-1569.

Teff, K., Elliott, S., Tschop, M., Kieffer, T., Rader, D., Heiman, M., et al. (2004). Dietary fructose reduces circulating insulin and leptin, attenuates postprandial suppression of ghrelin, and increases triglycerides in women. *J Clin Endocrinol Metab* , 89:2963–2972.

Thai-Van, H., Bounaix, M., & Fraysse, B. (2001). Meniere's Disease:Pathophysiology and Treatment. *Drugs* , 61:1089-1102.

The Holy Bible. (1984). *The Holy Bible: New International Version; Ecclesiastes 1:9.* Colorado Springs, Colorado: International Bible Society.

The Institute of Medicine of the National Academies. (2002). Dietary Fats: Total Fat and Fatty Acids. In T. I. Academies, *Dietary Reference Intakes for Energy, Carbohydrate, Fiber, Fat, Fatty Acids, Cholesterol, Protein and Amino Acids* (pp. 335-432). Washington, DC: The National Academy Press.

The World's Healthiest Foods. (2013). *Should your foods be colorful?* Retrieved December 22, 2013, from The World's Healthiest Foods: http://whfoods.org/genpage.php?tname=dailytip&dbid=128

Thomas, F., Bean, K., Pannier, B., Oppert, J., Guize, L., & Benetos, A. (2005). Cardiovascular mortality in overweight subjects: the key role of associated risk factors. *Hypertension* , 46:654-659.

Thorn, G., Forsham, P., Frawley, T., Wilson, D., Renold, A., Fredrickson, D., et al. (1951). Advances in the Diagnosis and Treatment of Adrenal Insufficiency. *Am J Med* , 10:595-611.

Tinbergen, N. (1961). *The Study of Instinct.* New York: Oxford University Press.

Toepel, U., Knebel, J., J., H., le Coutre, J., & Murray, M. (2009). The Brain Tracks the Energetic Value in Food Images. *NeuroImage* , 44:967-974.

Topping, D. (2007). Cereal Complex Carbohydrates and Their Contribution to Human Health. *Journal of Cereal Science* , 46:220-229.

Torres, S., & Nowson, C. (2008). Relationship between Stress, Eating Behavior, and Obesity. *Nutrition* , 23:887-894.

Torsoli, A. (2013, November 14). *Diabetes Kills One Person Every Six Seconds, Estimates Show.* Retrieved November 16, 2013, from Bloomberg News : http://www.bloomberg.com/news/2013-11-14/diabetes-kills-one-person-every-six-seconds-new-estimates-show.html

Tremaroli, V., & Backhed, F. (2012). Functional Interactions between the Gut Microbiota and Host Metabolism. *Nature* , 489:242-249.

Trowell, H. (1985). Dietary Fiber: a Paradigm. In H. Trowell, D. Burkitt, K. Heaton, & R. Doll, *Dietary Fibre, Fibre-Depleted Foods and Disease* (pp. 1-20). New York: Academic Press.

Trowell, H. (1980). From Normotension to Hypertension in Kenyans and Ugandans 1928-1978. *East Afr Med J* , 57:167-173.

Turner, J. (2005). *Spice: A History of Temptation.* New York: Vintage Books.

Tuyns, A. (1988). Salt and Gastrointestinal Cancer. *Nutr Cancer* , 11:229-232.

United States Department of Agriculture. (2005, August). *sweetener consumption in the United States.* Retrieved July 14, 2013, from United States Department of Agriculture Economic Research Service: http://www.ers.usda.gov/publications/sssm-sugar-and-sweeteners-outlook/sss243-01.aspx

United States Department of Agriculture. (2000). *USDA fact book.* Retrieved July 14, 2013, from United States Department of agriculture: http://www.usda.gov/factbook/chapter2.pdf

United States Department of Agriculture, Economic Research Service. (2005, August). *food consumption (per capita).* Retrieved

July 14, 2013, from US Department of Agriculture: http://www.ers. usda.gov/media/326278/sss24301_002.pdf

United States Department Of Labor. (2012, September 25th). *Consumer Expenditures -- 2011.* Retrieved July 13, 2013, from United States Department of Labor, Bureau of Labor Statistics -- Economic Releases: http://www.bls.gov/news.release/cesan.nr0.htm

United States Select Committee on Nutrition and Human Needs. (1977). *Eating in America: Dietary Goals for the United States.* Washington DC: Government printing office.

United States Select Committee on Nutrition and Human Needs. (1997). *Eating in America: Dietary Goals for the United States.* Washington DC: Government printing office.

University of Maryland Medical Center. (2011). *Omega-3 fatty acids.* Retrieved August 4, 2013, from University of Maryland Medical Center: http://umm.edu/health/medical/altmed/supplement/omega3-fatty-acids

Uribe, S., & (Translated Rivera, D. F. (2012, June 2). *Bread.* Retrieved December 9, 2013, from WebIslam: http://www.webislam. com/articles/66023-bread.html

USDA Center for Nutrition Policy and Promotion. (1997, May 17). *DIETARY GUIDANCE ON SODIUM:SHOULD WE TAKE IT WITH A GRAIN OF SALT?* . Retrieved December 17, 2011, from USDA Nutrition Insights: http://www.cnpp.usda.gov/publications/ nutritioninsights/insight3.pdf

USDA. (2010). *Report of the DGAC on the Dietary Guidelines for Americans, 2010 Part D. Section 6: Sodium, Potassium, and Water.* Retrieved August 25, 2013, from Report of the DGAC on the Dietary Guidelines for Americans, 2010: http://www.cnpp.usda.gov/ Publications/DietaryGuidelines/2010/DGAC/Report/D-6-Sodium-PotassiumWater.pdf

van den Broeck, H., de Jong, H. C., Salentijin, E. M., Dekking, L., Bosch, D., Hamer, R. J., et al. (2010). Presence of celiac disease epitopes in modern and old hexaploid wheat varities: wheat breeding may have contributed to increased prevalance of celiac disease. *Theor Appl Genet* , 121:1527-1539.

Van Herpen, T., Goryunova, S., van der Schoot, J., Mitreva, M., Salentijin, E., Vorst, O., et al. (2006). Alpha-Gliadin Genes from the A, B, and D Genomes of Wheat Contain Different Sets of Celiac Disease Epitopes. *BMC Genomics* , 7:1-13.

Van Wymelbelke, V., Himaya, A., Louis-Sylvestre, J., & Fantino,

M. (1998). Influence of Medium-Chain and Long-Chain Triacylglycerols on the Control of Food Intake in Men. *Am J Clin Nutr* , 68:226-234.

Vandepoele, K., & Van de Peer, Y. (2005). Exploring the Plant Transcriptome through Phylogenetic Profiling. *Plant Physiology* , 137(1): 31-42.

Varbo, A., Benn, M., Tybjaeg-Hansen, A., & Nordestgaard, B. (2013). Elevated Remnant Cholesterol Causes Both Low-Grade Inflammation and Ischemic Heart Disease While Low-Density Lippoprotein Cholesterol Causes Ischemic Heart Disease Without Inflammation. *Circulation* , doi: 10.1161/?CIRCULATIONAHA.113003008.

Vieth, R. (2006). What Is the Optimal Vitamin D Status for Health? *Prog Biophys Mol Biol* , 92 (1): 26-32.

Vogel, K., Johnson, V., & Mattern, P. (1978). Protein and Lysine Contents of Endosperm and Bran of the Parents and Progenies of Crosses of Common Whea t. *Crop Science* , 18:751-754.

Vyas, A. (2014). Diet Drink Consumption and the Risk of Cardiovascular Events: A Report from the Women's Health Initiative. *American College of Cardiology* (p. Oral presentation March 30 at 8 a.m. EDT; Room 146 C.). Washington, DC: American College of Cardiology.

Walker, B. (2011, December 1). *FDA Proposes Regulating Salt in Food.* Retrieved December 17, 2011, from The New American: http://thenewamerican.com/usnews/politics/10007-fda-proposes-regulating-salt-in-food

Walker, K. M. (2013, June 21). *Hip Fractures.* Retrieved July 24, 2013, from Up to Date: http://www.uptodate.com/contents/hip-fractures-in-adults

Wan, Y., Poole, R., Huttly, A., Toscano-Underwood, C., Feeney, K., Welgham, S., et al. (2008). Transcriptome Analysis of the Grain Development in Hexaploid Wheat. *BMC Genomics* , 9:121-137.

Wang, Z., Klipfell, E., Bennett, B., Koeth, R., Levison, B., DuGar, B., et al. (2011). Gut Flora Metabolism of Phosphatidylcholine Promotes Cardiovascular Disease. *Nature* , 472 (7341): 57-63.

Girls, T. S. (Performer). (1996). Wannabe.

Warwick, Z., Hall, W., Pappas, T., & Schiffman, S. (1993). Taste and Smells of Fish and Enhance the Satiating Effect of Both a High-Carbohydrate and a High-Fat Meal in Humans. *Physiol Behav* , 53:553-563.

Welch, I., Sepple, C., & Read, N. (1998). Comparisons of the

Effects on Satiety and Eating Behavior of Infusion of Lipid into the Different Regions of the Small Intestine. *Gut* , 29:306-311.

Wells, H. (2013). *Ratios*. Retrieved December 9, 2013, from Brady quote.com: http://www.brainyquote.com/quotes/keywords/ratio.html

Wells, R., & Preston, R. (1998). Effects of Repeated Urea Dilution Measurement on Feedlot Performance and Consistency of Estimated Body Composition and Steers a Different Breed Types. *Journal of animal science* , 76:2799-2804.

Westman, E. C. (2002). Is dietary carbohydrate essential for human nutrition? *The American Journal of Clinical Nutrition* , 75 (5): 951-953 .

Whitaker, J. (1975). *Feedlot Empire: Beef Cattle Feeding in Illinois and Iowa, 1840-1900*. Ames, Iowa: The Iowa State University Press.

WHO. (2013, March). *Overweight and Obesity*. Retrieved December 12, 2013, from World Health Organization: http://www.who.int/mediacentre/factsheets/fs311/en/

Whole Grains Council. (2013, March 21). *Health Study: Kamut Wheat Versus Modern Wheat*. Retrieved July 21, 2013, from Whole Grains Council: http://wholegrainscouncil.org/newsroom/blog/2013/03/health-study-kamut-wheat-vs-modern-wheat

Whole grains Council. (2012, January 12). *Research Sheds Light on Gluten Issues*. Retrieved September 15, 2013, from Whole Grains Council: http://wholegrainscouncil.org/newsroom/blog/2012/01/research-sheds-light-on-gluten-issues

Wilkes, H., & Wilkes, S. (1972). The Green Revolution. *Environment* , 14(8):32-39.

Willett, W. (1998). Is Dietary Fat a Major Determinant of Body Fat? *Am J Cli Nutr* , 67:556S-562S.

Williams, E. (2010). Salt Production and Trade in Mesoamerica. In J. E. Staller, & M. (. Carrasco, *Pre-Columbian Foodways: Interdisciplinary Approaches to Food, Culture, and Markets in Ancient Mesoamerica* (p. 182). New York: Springer Science.

Winslow, R. (2013, July 11). Longer, Not Healthier Lives. *Wall St. Journal* , p. A3.

Wise, R. (2004). Dopamine, Learning and Motivation. *Nat Rev Neurosci* , 5:483-494.

Wolever, T., & Jenkins, D. (1987). The Use of the Glycemic Index in predicting the Blood Glucose Response to Mixed Meals. *Am J Clin Nutr* , 43: 167-172.

Wood, S. (2013, November 19). *'Extraordinary' Chelation Effects in Diabetes Propel TACT into Spotlight Again.* Retrieved November 19, 2013, from Medscape: http://www.medscape.com/viewarticle/814643?src=wnl_edit_cfna#1

Wood, W. G., Eckertb, G. P., Igbavboaa, U., & Müllerb, W. E. (2010). STATINS AND NEUROPROTECTION: A PRESCRIPTION TO MOVE THE FIELD FORWARD. *Ann N Y Acad Sci.* , 1199: 69–76.

World Health Organization. (2012). *Global Health Expenditure.* Retrieved July 13, 2013, from World Health Organization: http://www.who.int/nha/expenditure_database/en/

Wrangham, R. (2009). *Catching Fire: How Cooking Made Us Human.* New York: Basic Books.

Wright, J. D. (2010, November). *Trends in Intake of Energy and Macronutrients in Adults From 1999-2000 Through 2007-2008.* Retrieved July 15, 2013, from Centers for Disease Control and Prevention: http://www.cdc.gov/nchs/data/databriefs/db49.htm

Wright, K. (1991). The origins and development of ground stone assemblages in late Pleistocene Southwest Asia. *Paleorient* , (17): 19-45.

Yajnik, C., & Yudkin, J. (2004). the Y-Y Paradox. *Lancet* , 363:163.

Yamamoto, M., Mouillet, G., Oguri, A., Gilard, M., Laskar, M., Eltchaninoff, H., et al. (2013). Effect of Body Mass Index on 30- and 365-Day Complication and Survival Rates of Transcatheter Aortic Valve Implantation (from the FRench Aortic National CoreValve and Edwards 2 [FRANCE 2] Registry). *American Journal of Cardiology* , 112(12):1932-1937.

Yan, L. (2013, March 20). *Dark Green Leafy Vegetables.* Retrieved December 22, 2013, from USDA.gov: http://www.ars.usda.gov/News/docs.htm?docid=23199

Yang, Q. (2010). Gain weight by "going diet?" Artificial sweeteners and the neurobiology of sugar cravings. *Yale J Biol Med* , 83 (2):101-108.

Yang, Q., Liu, T., Kuklina, E. V., Flanders, W. D., Hong, Y., & Gillespie, C. (2011). Sodium and Potassium Intake and Mortality Among US Adults: Prospective Data From the Third National Health and Nutrition Examination Survey. *Arch Intern Med.* , 171(13):1183-1191. doi:10.1001/archinternmed.2011.257.

Yang, Q., T, L., EV, K., WD, F., Y, H., C, G., et al. (2011). Sodium and potassium intake and mortality among US adults: prospective data from the Third National Health and Nutrition Examination Survey. *Arch Intern Med* , 171 (13);1183-1191.

Yang, Q., Zhang, Z., Gregg, E. W., Flanders, D., Merritt, R., & Hu, F. B. (2014). Added Sugar Intake and Cardiovascular Diseases Mortality Among US Adults. . *JAMA Intern Med.* , doi:10.1001/jamainternmed.2013.13563. .

Yi, W., Fischer, J., Krewer, G., & Akoh, C. (2005). Phenolic compounds from blueberries can inhibit colon cancer cell proliferation and induce apoptosis. *J Agric Food Chem.* , 53(18):7320-9.

Yusuf, S. (2013). *The Need for Balance in Evaluating the Evidence on Na and CVD.* Retrieved from Institute of Medicine: http://www.iom.edu/~/media/Files/Activity%20Files/Nutrition/ConsequencesSodiumReduction/2012-DEC-04/Presentations/13_Salim%20Yusuf.pdf

Zhang, X., Zhang, G., Zhang, H., Karin, M., Bai, H., & Cai, D. (2008). Hypothalamic IKKβ/NF-B and ER Stress Link Overnutrition to Energy Imbalance and Obesity. *Cell* , 135 (1):61-73.

Zhao, F., Su, Y., Dunham, S., Rakszegi, M., Bedo, Z., McGrath, S., et al. (2009). Variation in Mineral Micronutrient Concentrations in Grain of Wheat Lines of Diverse Origin. *Journal of Cereal Science* , 49 (2): 290-295.

Zohary, D., & Hopf, M. (2000). *Domestication of plants in the Old World.* Oxford: Oxford University Press.

Zulick, M. D. (2013). *Declaration of Independence (Preamble).* Retrieved July 4, 2013, from Zulick Home Page: http://users.wfu.edu/zulick/340/Declaration.html

Endnotes

Shut the Hell Up!
1   (Iwasawa & Yamazaki, 2009)
2   (Gardner & Brandt, 2006)

Discordance and Despair: The Diseases of Modern Civilization
3   (Wrangham, 2009) page 43
4   (Murray, et al., 2013)
5   (Torsoli, 2013)
6   (American Cancer Society, 2013)
7   (Murray, et al., 2013)
8   (Hollenberg, et al., 1997)
9   (McCullough, Peterson, Patel, Jacques, Shah, & Dwyer, 2012)
10   (McCullough, et al., 2006)
11   (Montagu, 1994)
12   (Creamer, Shorter, & Bamforth, 1961)
13   (Bianconi, et al., 2013)
14   (IMDB, 2013)

Survival of the Fittest: How the Greed for Sugar, Salt, and Fat Allowed Us to Conquer the World
15   (IMDB, 2013)
16   [2] (Buffett, J., & Chapman, M. Composers. 1988)
17   (Leonardi, Gerbault, Thomas, & Burger, 2012)
18   (Molodecky & Kaplan, 2010)
19   (Depre, Vanoverschelde, & Taegtmeyer, 1999)
20   (Magistretti, Pellerin, & Martin, 2000)
21   (Birch, 1999)
22   (Zhang, Zhang, Zhang, Karin, Bai, & Cai, 2008)
23   (Stanhope, et al., 2011)
24   (Yang, Zhang, Gregg, Flanders, Merritt, & Hu, 2014)
25   (Chen, Caballero, Mitchell, Loria, PH., & Champagne, 2010)
26   (Jala, Smits, Johnson, & Conchol, 2010)
27   (Jala, Smits, Johnson, & Conchol, 2010)
28   (Livepositively.com, 2013)
29   (Fenster M., 2013)
30   (Barona, Aristizabal, Blesso, Volek, & Fernandez, 2012)
31   (Dictionary.com, 2013)

32   (Kessler, 2009)
33   (Fowler, Williams, Resendez, Hunt, Hazuda, & Stern, 2008)
34   (Bleich, Wolfson, Vine, & Wang, 2014)
35   (Swithers, 2013)
36   (Cohen, Curhan, & Forman, 2012)
37   (Gardener, Rundek, Markert, Wright, Elkind, & Sacco, 2012)
38   (Vyas, 2014)
39   (Swithers, 2013)
40   (Feijó, et al., 2013)
41   (Yang, 2010)
42   (Westman, Is dietary carbohydrate essential for human nutri-
        tion?, 2002)
43   (Kurlansky, 2002)
44   (Kurlansky, 2002)
45   (Bishop, 2010)
46   (Freedman & Petitti, 2001)
47   (United States Select Committee on Nutrition and Human
        Needs, 1977)
48   (Rapp, 1982)
49   (Department Of Health and Human Services, Public Health
        Service, 1988)
50   (Dawber, Kannel, Kagan, Donabedian, Mcnamara, & Pearson,
        1967)
51   (Reed, McGee, Yano, & Hankin, 1985)
52   (Smith, Crombie, Tavendale, Gulland, & Tunstall-Pedoe,
        1988)
53   (Henry, 1990)
54   (NYC.gov, 2008)
55   (Nainggolan, 2010)
56   (Graudal & Jurgens, 2011)
57   (Bayer, Johns, & Galea, 2012)
58   (Bayer, Johns, & Galea, 2012)
59   (Alderman, 2010)
60   (Rawlins & Culyer, 2004)
61   (Grobbee & Hoffman, 1986)
62   (Robertson, 2003)
63   (Stolarz-Skrzypek, et al., 2011)
64   (O'Donnell, et al., 2011)
65   (Grauda, Hubeck-Graudal, & Jurgens, 2011)
66   (Yusuf, 2013)

67   (Taylor, Ashton, Moxham, Hooper, & Ebrahim, Reduced Dietary Salt for the Prevention of Cardiovascular Disease, 2011)
68   (Graudel, Hubeck-Graudel, & Jurgens, 2011)
69   (O'Donnell, Yusef, Mente, Gao, Mann, & Teo, 2011)
70   (Oparil, 2014)
71   (O'Donnell, et al., 2014)
72   (USDA, 2010)
73   (Cordain, et al., 2005)
74   (Larsson, Orsini, & Wolk, 28 July 2011.)
75   (Yang, et al., 2011)
76   (Taubes, 2012)
77   (Kurlansky, 2002)
78   (MacGregor & DeWardener, 1998)
79   (Freedman & Petitti, 2001)
80   (Bernstin & Willet, 2010)
81   (USDA Center for Nutrition Policy and Promotion, 1997)
82   (Henney, Taylor, & Boon, 2010)
83   (Fine, Ty, Lestrange, & Levine, 1987)
84   (Kaunitz, 1956)
85   (MacGregor & DeWardener, 1998)
86   (Morris, Na, & Johnson, 2008)
87   (Thorn, et al., 1951)
88   (Bertino, Beauchamp, Burke, & Engelman, 1982)
89   (Wise, 2004)
90   (Morris, Na, & Johnson, 2008)
91   (Depre, Vanoverschelde, & Taegtmeyer, 1999)
92   (Muskiet, 2010)
93   (Leonard & Robertson, 1997)
94   (Leonard, Robertson, Snodgrass, & Kuzawa, 2003)
95   (Milton, 1987)
96   (Wrangham, 2009)
97   (Cordain, Eaton, Miller, Mann, & Hill, 2002)
98   (Cordain, Miller, Eaton, & Mann, 2000)
99   (Cordain, Brand-Miller, Eaton, Mann, Holt, & Speth, 2000)
100   (Leonard, Snodgrass, & Robertson, 2010)
101   (Wrangham, 2009)
102   (Cordain, Watkins, & Mann, Fatty Acid Composition and Energy Density of Foods Available to African Hominids, 2001)
103   (Lussana, Painter, Ocke, Buller, Bossuyt, & Roseboom, 2008)

104   (Preidt, 2014)
105   (Holliday, 1986)
106   (Preidt, 2014)
107   (Cordain, Brand-Miller, Eaton, Mann, Holt, & Speth, 2000)
108   (Leonard, Snodgrass, & Robertson, 2010)
109   (Toepel, Knebel, J., le Coutre, & Murray, 2009)
110   (Richardson & Ross, 2003)
111   (University of Maryland Medical Center, 2011)
112   (Linus Pauling Institute, 2012)
113   (Cordain, Watkins, & Mann, 2001)
114   (Din, Newby, & Flapan, 2004)
115   (Lee, O'Keefe, Lavie, Marchioli, & Harris, 2008)
116   (Mozaffarian, 2008)
117   (Leonard B. , 2007)
118   (Skaper, 2008)
119   (Rappaport, Rao, & Igarashi, Brain Metabolism of Nutrition-
        ally Essential Poly-Unsaturated Fatty Acids Depends on Both
        the Diet and the Live r, 2007)
120   (Fokkema, Brouwer, Hasperhoven, Martini, & Muskeit, 2000)
121   (Rappaport, 2003)
122   (Chalon, 2006)
123   (Freeman, et al., 2006)
124   (Janakiram & V. Rao, 2009)
125   (Serhan, et al., 2002)
126   (Muskiet, 2010)
127   (Aywerx, 1999)
128   (Gani, 2008)
129   (Lecerf & de Lorgeril, 2011)
130   (Apfelbaum, 1992)
131   (Lecerf & de Lorgeril, 2011)
132   (Handelman, Nightingale, Lichtenstein, Schaefer, & Blum-
        berg, 1999)
133   (Lichtenstein, et al., 1998)
134   (Lichtenstein A. , 2003)
135   (Robbins, et al., 2013)
136   (Varbo, Benn, Tybjaeg-Hansen, & Nordestgaard, 2013)
137   (Stone, et al., 2013)
138   (Mintz, 2013)
139   (Rosen, et al., 2012)
140   (Bogh, Schmedes, Philipsen, Thieden, & Wulf, 2010)

141   (Glossman, 210)
142   (Grimes, 2006)
143   (Pérez-Castrillón, et al., 2007)
144   (Bellows & Moore, 2012)
145   (Manabe, Matsumura, & Fushiki, 2010)
146   (Inaizumi, Takeda, Suzuki, Sawano, & Fushiki, 2001)
147   (Gilbertson, Yu, & Shah, 2010)
148   (Petrou, et al., 1995)
149   (Schiffman & Dackis, 1975)
150   (Margolskee, et al., 2007)
151   (Manabe, Matsumura, & Fushiki, 2010)
152   (Kinney & Antill, 1996)
153   (Kadohisa, Verhagen, & Rolls, 2005)
154   (Gilbertson, Yu, & Shah, 2010)
155   (Dalley, et al., 2005)
156   (Drewnowski & Bellisle, Is Sweetness Addictive?, 2007)
157   (Goldfield, Lorello, & Doucet, 2007)
158   (Manabe, Matsumura, & Fushiki, 2010)
159   (Drewnowski, 1997)
160   (Welch, Sepple, & Read, 1998)
161   (Castiglione, Read, & French, 1998)
162   (Van Wymelbelke, Himaya, Louis-Sylvestre, & Fantino, 1998)
163   (Patterson, et al., 2000)
164   (Vyas, 2014)
165   (Samra, 2010)
166   (Friedman, 1998)
167   (Burton-Freeman, Davis, & Schneeman, 2002)
168   (Smilowitz, German, & Zivkovic, 2010)
169   (Warwick, Hall, Pappas, & Schiffman, 1993)
170   (Rolls, 2004)
171   (De Araujo & Rolls, 2004)
172   (IMDB, 2013)

The Pleasure Principle: Why We Love Sugar, Salt, and Fat

173   (Home Depot, 2013)
174   (Ask.com, 2013)
175   (Merriam-Webster, 2013)
176   (Merriam-Webster, 2013)
177   (Merriam-Webster, 2013)
178   (Zulick, 2013)

179   (Cherry, 2013)
180   (Cherry, The Conscious and Unconscious Mind, 2013)
181   (Tinbergen, 1961)
182   (Marshall, 2011)
183   (Mayer, Roberts, & Barsade, 2008)
184   (Leakey & Lewin, 1978)
185   (Butler & Hope, 1995)
186   (Smilowitz, German, & Zivkovic, 2010)
187   (Kessler, 2009)
188   (Kessler, 2009)
189   (Kessler, 2009)
190   (Inaizumi, Takeda, Suzuki, Sawano, & Fushiki, 2001)
191   (Drewnowski & Almiron-Roig, Human Perceptions and Pref-
        erences for Fat-Rich Foods, 2010)
192   (Blundell & Macdiarmind, 1997)
193   (Bouton, 2007)
194   (Samra, 2010)
195   (Drewnowski & Almiron-Roig, Human Perceptions and Pref-
        erences for Fat-Rich Foods, 2010)
196   (Torres & Nowson, 2008)
197   (Taflinger, 1996)
198   (Sagan & Druyan, 1992)

A Weakness Exposed: The Agricultural to the Industrial Revolution

199   (Confucius, 2013)
200   (Deschanel, 2013)
201   (Wright, 1991)
202   (Eaton, 1992)
203   (Feldman, 2001)
204   (Sofi F. , et al., 2013)
205   (Edwards, 2010)
206   (Sofi, et al., 2013)
207   (Stanford School of Medicine, 2013)
208   (King, 2013)
209   (Lindeberg, 2010)
210   (Alas-Salvado, Farres, & Luque, 2008)
211   (Tarini & Wolever, 2010)
212   (Cordain L. , The Nutritional Characteristics of a Contemporary Diet Based upon Paleolithic Food Groups, 2002)
213   (Anderson, Smith, & Gustafson, 1994)

214   (Topping, 2007)
215   (Fabri, 2010)
216   (Editors) Carroll & Prickett, The Bible: Authorized King James Version , 1997)
217   (Uribe & (Translated Rivera, 2012)
218   (Nelsen, 2002)
219   (Van Herpen, et al., 2006)
220   (Whole grains Council, 2012)
221   (Atchinson, Head, & Gates, 2010)
222   (Day, Augustin, Batey, & Wrigley, 2006)
223   (van den Broeck, et al., 2010)
224   (Salcedo, Danchez-Monge, Garcia-Casado, Aremntia, Gomez, & Barber, 2004)
225   (Brisman, 2002)
226   (Takahashi, Fukunaga, Fukudome, & Yoshikawa, 2000)
227   (Motoi & Kodama, 2003)
228   (Shewry, 2009)
229   (Wan, et al., 2008)
230   (Skylas, et al., 2000)
231   (Losowsky, 2008)
232   (Drago, El Asmar, & Pierro, 2006)
233   (Drago, El Asmar, & Pierro, 2006)
234   (Bernardo, Garrote, & Fernanadez-Salazar, 2007)
235   (Rakhimova, Esslinger, & Schulze-Krebs, 2009)
236   (Doherty & Barry, 1981)
237   (Cordain L. , Cereal Grains: Humanity's Double Edge Sword, 1999)
238   (Reichelt & Jensen, 2004)
239   (Pengiran-Tengah, Lock, Unsworth, & Wills, 2004)
240   (Barbeau, Bassaganya-Riere, & Hontacillas, 2007)
241   (Cordain, Toohey, Smith, & Hickey, 2000)
242   (Michaelsson, Gerden, & Hagforsen, 2000)
243   (Nelsen, 2002)
244   (De Vincenzi, Vincentini, Di Nardo, Boirivant, Gazza, & Pogna, 2010)
245   (Whole grains Council, 2012)
246   (Saja, Chatterjee, Chatterjee, & Sudhakaran, 2007)
247   (Dubois, Peumans, & Van Damme, 1998)
248   (van der Kuil, et al., 2010)
249   (Gadsby, 2004)

250   (Dewailly, et al., 2001)
251   (Kastorini, et al., 2011)
252   (Salas-Salvadó, et al., 2011)
253   (Medina-Remón, et al., 2011)
254   (Fuentes, et al., 2008)
255   (Delgado-Lista, et al., 2008)
256   (Simopoulos, 2001)
257   (Ramsden, Faurot, & Carrera-Bastos, 2001)
258   (The Institute of Medicine of the National Academies, 2002)
259   (Nelson, Schmidt, & Kelly, 1995)
260   (Stanhope, Sampson, & Prior, 1981)
261   (German & Dillard, 2004)
262   (Chowdhury, et al., 2014)
263   (Siri-Tarino, Sun, Hu, & Krauss, 2010)
264   (Micha, Wallace, & Mozaffarian, 2010)
265   (Rohrmann, et al., 2013)
266   (The Institute of Medicine of the National Academies, 2002)
267   (Kris-Etherton, Harris, & Appel, 2002)
268   (Simopoulus, 2002)
269   (Madsen, Skou, & Hansen, 2001)
270   (Benbeook, Butler, Latif, Leifert, & Davis, 2013)
271   (Simopoulos, 2001)
272   (Cordain, Eaton, & Brand-Miller, The Paradoxical Nature of Hunter-Gatherer Diets: Meat-based, yet Non-Atherogenic, 2002)
273   (Gurven & Kaplan, 2007)
274   (Eaton, Cordain, & Lindeberg, Evolutionary Health Promotion: a Consideration of Common Counter Arguments, 2002)
275   (Cordain, Watkins, Florant, Kehler, Rogers, & Li, 2002)
276   (Cordain L. , The Paleo Diet, 2002)
277   (Cordain, Watkins, Florant, Kehler, Rogers, & Li, 2002)
278   (Cordain, Watkins, Florant, Kehler, Rogers, & Li, 2002)
279   (Meadows & Hakonson, 1982)
280   (Rule, Broughton, Shellito, & Maiorano, 2002)
281   (Whitaker, 1975)
282   (Ritz, 2005)
283   (Centers for Disease Control and Prevention, 2011)
284   (O'Donnell, et al., 2014)
285   (Yang, et al., 2011)
286   (Centers for Disease Control and Prevention, 2011)

287   (Antonios & MacGregor, 1996)
288   (Massey & Whiting, 1995)
289   (Devine, Criddle, Dick, Kerr, & Prince, 1995)
290   (Gotshall, Mickleborough, & Cordain, 2000)
291   (Miller, 1945)
292   (Lindseth & Lindseth, 1995)
293   (Porcelli & Gugelchuk, 1995)
294   (Thai-Van, Bounaix, & Fraysse, 2001)
295   (Jansson, 1986)
296   (Tuyns, 1988)
297   (Carey, Locke, & Cookson, 1993)
298   (Frassetto, Todd, Morris, & Sebastian, 1998)
299   (Sebastian, Frassetto, Sellmeyer, Merriam, & Morris, 2002)
300   (O'Keefe, 2000)
301   (Carrera-Bastos, Fontes-Villalba, O'Keefe, Lindeberg, & Cordain, 2011)
302   (Cordain, Eades, & Eades, 2003)
303   (Reaven, Pathophysiology of Insulin Resustance in Human Disease, 1995)
304   (Cordain L. , Eaton, Brand-Miller, Lindeberg, & Jensen, 2002)
305   (Cordain, Lindeberg, Hurtado, Hill, Eaton, & Brand-Miller, 2002)

The Modern Western Diet: A Weakness Exploited and Explained
306   (Metallica, 1986)
307   (Hargrove, Does the History of Food Energy Units Suggest a Solution to the "Calorie Confusion"?, 2007)p.45
308   (Hargrove, History of the Calorie Nutrition, 2006)
309   (Painter, 2006)
310   (CDC, 2011)
311   (WHO, 2013)
312   (Colls & Evans, 2010)
313   (Flegal K. , 1993)
314   (McKay, 2002)
315   (Nicholls, 2013)
316   (Pollack, A.M.A. Recognizes Obesity as a Disease, 2013)
317   (World Health Organization, 2012)
318   (dictionary.com, 2013)
319   (Flegal, Kit, Orpana, & Graubard, Association of all-cause mortality with overweight and obesity using standard body

mass index categories: a systematic review and meta-analysis., 2013)

320   (Lavie, McAuley, Church, Milani, & Blair, 2014)
321   (Fenster, The obesity rate and the paradox: into the deeper and wider, 2012)
322   (Lavie, De Schutter, Patel, Romero-Corral, Artham, & Milani, 2012)
323   (Carnethon, et al., 2012)
324   (Clark, Chyu, & Horwich, 2012)
325   (Yamamoto, et al., 2013)
326   (Adabag, et al., 2012)
327   (Romero-Corral, et al., 2009)
328   (Sahakyan, 2012)
329   (Lavie, Milani, & Ventura, Obesity and Cardiovascular Disease: Risk Factor, Paradox, and Impact of Weight Loss, 2009)
330   (Das, et al., 2011)
331   (Lavie, McAuley, Church, Milani, & Blair, 2014)
332   (Sturm & Hattori, 2013)
333   (Mattison, et al., 2012)
334   (Nicholls, 2013)
335   (Sharma A. , 2013)
336   (Sharma A. , 2013)
337   (Ebbeling, 2012)
338   (Ebbeling, 2012)
339   (Cordain, et al., 2005)
340   (United States Department of Agriculture, Economic Research Service, 2005)
341   (O'Keefe, 2000)
342   (Emken, 1984)
343   (Sundram, Ismail, Hayes, Jeyamalar, & Pathanathan, 1997)
344   (FDA, 2013)
345   (Whitaker, 1975)
346   (Whitaker, 1975)
347   (Rule, Broughton, Shellito, & Maiorano, 2002)
348   (Cordain, Watkins, Florant, Kehler, Rogers, & Li, 2002)
349   (Wells & Preston, 1998)
350   (Pollan, 2002)
351   (Kidwell, 2002)
352   (Siri-Tarino, Sun, Hu, & Krauss, 2010)
353   (German & Dillard, 2004)

354   (Chowdhury, et al., 2014)

355   (Ravnskov, 1998)

356   (Ravnskov, Hypothesis out-of-Date. The Diet-Heart Idea, 2002)

357   (Ravnskov, et al., 2002)

358   (Seidell, 1998)

359   (Willett, 1998)

360   (Taubes, The Soft Science of Dietary Fat, 2001)

361   (Astorg, Arnault, Czernichow, Noisette, Galan, & Hercberg, 2004)

362   (Renaud & de Lorgeril, 1992)

363   (Ramsden, et al., 2013)

364   (Ramsden, et al., 2013)

365   (Kitamura, 2013)

366   (Mensink, Zock, Kestor, & Katan, 2003)

367   (Mensink, Zock, Kester, & katan, 2003)

368   (Mensink, Zock, Kestor, & Katan, 2003)

369   (The Institute of Medicine of the National Academies, 2002)

370   (The Institute of Medicine of the National Academies, 2002)

371   (Kris-Etherton, Harris, & Appel, 2002)

372   (Simopoulus, 2002)

373   (Madsen, Skou, & Hansen, 2001)

374   (Freeman, et al., 2006)

375   (McNamara, Jandacek, Rider, Tao, Cole-Strauss, & Lipton, 2010)

376   (Din, Newby, & Flapan, 2004)

377   (Lee, O'Keefe, Lavie, Marchioli, & Harris, 2008)

378   (Mozaffarian, 2008)

379   (Leonard B. , 2007)

380   (Skaper, 2008)

381   (Cordain L. , The Paleo Diet, 2002)

382   (Simopoulos, 2001)

383   (Cordain, Eaten & Brand-Miller, The Paradoxical Nature of The Hunter-Gatherer Diets: Meat-based yet non atherogenic, 2002)

384   (Simopoulos, Evolutionary Aspects of Diet and Essential Fatty Acids., 2001)

385   (Pella, Dubnov, & Singh, 2003)

386   (Dubnov & Berry, 2003)

387   (Cordain, Watkins, Florant, Kehler, Rogers, & Li, 2002)

388   (Cordain L. , The Paleo Diet, 2002)
389   (Layman, 2013)
390   (Berg, Tymoczko, & Stryer, W H Freeman)
391   (Lecerf & de Lorgeril, 2011)
392   (Apfelbaum, 1992)
393   (Lecerf & de Lorgeril, 2011)
394   (Lichtenstein, et al., 1998)
395   (Lichtenstein A. , 2003)
396   (Dalby, 2003)
397   (Cleave, 1974)
398   (United States Department of Agriculture, 2000)
399   (United States Department of Agriculture, 2005)
400   (Stanhope & Havel, 2010)
401   (Saad, et al., 1998)
402   (Teff, et al., 2004)
403   (Myese, 1993)
404   (Elliott, Keim, Stern, Teff, & Havel, 2002)
405   (Teff, et al., 2009)
406   (Livepositively.com, 2013)
407   (Jala, Smits, Johnson, & Conchol, 2010)
408   (Stanhope, et al., 2011)
409   (Chen, Caballero, Mitchell, Loria, PH., & Champagne, 2010)
410   (Huffington Post, 2011)
411   (Montonen, Jarvinen, Knekt, Heliovaara, & Reunanen, 2007)
412   (Chen, et al., 2010)
413   (Gross, Li, Ford, & Liu, 2004)
414   (Gross, Li, Ford, & Liu, 2004)
415   (Cordain L. , et al., 2005)
416   (Wolever & Jenkins, 1987)
417   (Jenkins, Wolever, & Collier, 1987)
418   (Ness, Zhao, & Wiggins, 1994)
419   (Ness & Chambers, 2000)
420   (Sir & Krauss, 2005)
421   (Cordain L. , et al., 2005)
422   (Reaven, The Insulin Resistance Syndrome: Definition and Dietary Approaches to Treatment, 2005)
423   (Liu, Manson, Buring, Stampfer, Willett, & Ridker, 2002)
424   (Cordain, Eades, & Eades, 2003)
425   (Roberts & Liu, 2009)
426   (Brand-Miller, Dickinson, Berkeley, & Allman-Farinelli,

           2009)
427   (Barclay, Petocz, & McMillan-Price, 2008)
428   (Last & Wilson, 2006)
429   (Jakobsen, Dethlefsen, & Joensen, 2010)
430   (Brand-Miller, Thomas, Swan, Ahmad, Petocz, & Colagiuri,
       2003)
431   (Wright J. D., 2010)
432   (Lui & Willett, 2002)
433   (Ludwig, 2002)
434   (Cordain, Eades, & Eades, 2003)
435   (Reaven, Pathophysiology of Insulin Resustance in Human
       Disease, 1995)
436   (Zhang, Zhang, Zhang, Karin, Bai, & Cai, 2008)
437   (Swithers, 2013)
438   (Feijó, et al., 2013)
439   (Cordain L. , et al., 2005)
440   (Ames, 2001)
441   (Escolar, et al., 2013)
442   (Guallar, Stranges, Mulrow, Appel, & Miller III, 2013)
443   (Denton, 1984)
444   (Freedman & Petitti, 2001)
445   (MacGregor & DeWardener, 1998)
446   (Bernstin & Willet, 2010)
447   (Fairfield, 2010)
448   (Centers for Disease Control and Prevention, 2013)
449   (Centers for Disease Control and Prevention, 2013)
450   (George, Majeed, Mackenzie, MacDonald, & Wei, 2013)
451   (Yang, et al., 2011)
452   (Micha, Wallace, & Mozaffarian, 2010)
453   (Rohrmann, et al., 2013)
454   (Larsson, Virtamo, & Wolk, 2011)
455   (Boughton, 2011)
456   (Larsson, Orsini, & Wolk, 28 July 2011.)
457   (O'Donnell, et al., 2014)
458   (Yang, et al., 2011)
459   (Fenster, Don't Pass on the Salt, 2013)
460   (Fenster, Don't Hold the Salt: Attempts to Curb Sodium Intake
       Are Misguided, 2012)
461   (Oparil, 2014)
462   (Centers for Disease Control and Prevention, 2011)

463   (Antonios & MacGregor, 1996)
464   (Massey & Whiting, 1995)
465   (Devine, Criddle, Dick, Kerr, & Prince, 1995)
466   (Gotshall, Mickleborough, & Cordain, 2000)
467   (Miller, 1945)
468   (Lindseth & Lindseth, 1995)
469   (Porcelli & Gugelchuk, 1995)
470   (Thai-Van, Bounaix, & Fraysse, 2001)
471   (Jansson, 1986)
472   (Tuyns, 1988)
473   (Carey, Locke, & Cookson, 1993)
474   (Taubes G. , 2007)
475   (Wright, 1991)
476   (Eaton, 1992)
477   (Storck & Teague, 1952)
478   (Burnett, 2005)
479   (JSTOR, 2013)
480   (Durtschi, 2001)
481   (Cordain L. , et al., 2005)
482   (Lindeberg, 2010)
483   (Alas-Salvado, Farres, & Luque, 2008)
484   (Tarini & Wolever, 2010)
485   (Trowell H. , 1985)
486   (Anderson, Smith, & Gustafson, 1994)
487   (Singh N. , 2010)
488   (Peng, Li, & Green, 2009)
489   (Lewis, Lutgendorff, & Phan, 2010)
490   (Cordain L. , The Nutritional Characteristics of a Contempo-
       rary Diet Based upon Paleolithic Food Groups, 2002)
491   (Baloch, 1999)
492   (Chrpova, Skorpik, Prasilova, & Sip, 2003)
493   (Vogel, Johnson, & Mattern, 1978)
494   (Shewry, 2009)
495   (Feldman, Wheats, 1995)
496   (Charles, 2013)
497   (Whole Grains Council, 2013)
498   (Sofi, et al., 2013)
499   (De Vincenzi, Vincentini, Di Nardo, Boirivant, Gazza, &
       Pogna, 2010)
500   (Sobel, 2007)

501   (Zhao, et al., 2009)
502   (Whole grains Council, 2012)
503   (Cordain L. , Cereal Grains: Humanity's Double Edge Sword, 1999)
504   (Vieth, 2006)
505   (Holick, 2007)
506   (Lee, O'Keefe, & Bell, 2008)
507   (Grant, 2009)
508   (Cordain L. , Cereal Grains: Humanity's Double Edge Sword, 1999)
509   (Bohn, Davidsson, Walczyk, & Hurrell, 2004)
510   (Cordain L. , Cereal Grains: Humanity's Double Edge Sword, 1999)
511   (Reichelt & Jensen, 2004)
512   (Pengiran-Tengah, Lock, Unsworth, & Wills, 2004)
513   (Barbeau, Bassaganya-Riere, & Hontacillas, 2007)
514   (Cordain, Toohey, Smith, & Hickey, 2000)
515   (Michaelsson, Gerden, & Hagforsen, 2000)
516   (Drago, El Asmar, & Pierro, 2006)
517   (Drago, El Asmar, & Pierro, 2006)
518   (Bernardo, Garrote, & Fernanadez-Salazar, 2007)
519   (Rakhimova, Esslinger, & Schulze-Krebs, 2009)
520   (Doherty & Barry, 1981)
521   (Karell, et al., 2003)
522   (Casteel, 2014)
523   (van den Broeck, et al., 2010)
524   (Spaenij-Dekking, et al., 2005)
525   (Van Herpen, et al., 2006)
526   (van den Broeck, et al., 2010)
527   (Lohi, et al., 2007)
528   (Cummins & Roberts-Thomson, 2009)
529   (De Vincenzi, Vincentini, Di Nardo, Boirivant, Gazza, & Pogna, 2010)
530   (Muskiet, 2010)
531   (Neel, 1999)
532   (Muskiet, 2010)
533   (Godfrey & Barker, 2000)
534   (Yajnik & Yudkin, 2004)
535   (Reaver, 2005)
536   (Frager et al, 2005)

537   (Cordain L. , et al., 2005)
538   (Ames, 2001)
539   (Frassetto, Todd, Morris, & Sebastian, 1998)
540   (Sebastian, Frassetto, Sellmeyer, Merriam, & Morris, 2002)
541   (Lemann, 1999)
542   (Sebastian, Frassetto, Sellmeyer, Merriam, & Morris, 2002)
543   (Sebastian, Harris, Ottaway, Todd, & Morris, 1994)
544   (Bushinsky, 1996)
545   (Frassetto, Morris, & Sebastian, 1997)
546   (Pak, Fuller, Sakhaee, Preminger, & Britton, 1985)
547   (Preminger, Sakhaee, Skurla, & Pak, 1985)
548   (Morris, Sebastian, Forman, Tanaka, & Schmidlin, 1999)
549   (Sharma, Kribben, Schattenfroh, Cetto, & Distler, 1990)
550   (Mickelborough, Gotshall, Kluka, Miller, & Cordain, 2001)
551   (Alpern & Sakhaee, 1997)
552   (Kankova, 2008)
553   (Singh, Barden, Mori, & Beilin, 2001)
554   (Wood, 2013)
555   (Escolar, et al., 2013)
556   (Muskiet, 2010)
557   (Pflughoeft & Versalovic, 2012)
558   (Tremaroli & Backhed, 2012)
559   (Cani, Bibiloni, & Knauf, 2008)
560   (Cordain, Toohey, Smith, & Hickey, 2000)
561   (HealthFinder.gov, 2013)
562   (Mason, 2013)
563   (Bakhed, Ley, Sonnenberg, Peterson, & Gordon, 2005)
564   (Ley, Turnbaugh, Klein, & Gordon, 2006)
565   (Ordovas, et al., 2002)
566   (Neufeld, et al., 2004)
567   (Samra, 2010)
568   (Ley, Turnbaugh, Klein, & Gordon, 2006)
569   (Dilli, Aydin, Zenciroglu, Ozyazici, Beken, & Okumus, 2013)
570   (Wang, et al., 2011)
571   (Koren, et al., 2011)
572   (Karlsson, et al., 2012)
573   (Wang, et al., 2011)
574   (Tang, et al., 2013)
575   (Loscalzo, 2013)
576   (Khaneja, et al., 2010)

577   (Perez-Fons, et al., 2011)
578   (Eaton, Cordain, & Lindeberg, 2002)

The Program
579   (Once-In-A-Lifetime, 1980)
580   (Warwick, Hall, Pappas, & Schiffman, 1993)
581   (Rolls, 2004)
582   (De Araujo & Rolls, 2004)
583   (The World's Healthiest Foods, 2013)
584   (Baranski, et al., 2014)
585   (Smith-Spangler, Brandeau, & Hunter, 2012)
586   (Fenster M. , I Want To Believe, 2014)
587   (Yan, 2013)
588   (Picard, Fioramonti, Francios, Robinson, Neant, & Matuchan-
        sky, 2005)
589   (Crislip, 2009)
590   (Anderson & Gilliland, 1999)
591   (Picard, Fioramonti, Francios, Robinson, Neant, & Matuchan-
        sky, 2005)
592   (National Center for Complementary and Alternative Medi-
        cine, 2013)
593   (National Center for Complementary and Alternative Medi-
        cine, 2013)
594   (Kelly, 2008)
595   (Fanaro, et al., 2005)
596   (Scholz-Ahrens, et al., 2007)
597   (Coudray, et al., 2005)
598   (Niness, 1999)
599   (Hsu, Liao, Chung, Hsieh, & Chan, 2004)
600   (Sheu, Lee, Chen, & Chan, 2008)
601   (Silk, Davis, Vulevic, Tzortzis, & Gibson, 2009)

Spiced for Life (AKA Step Ten)
602   (Wannabe, 1996)
603   (Penn State College of Agricultural Sciences, 2002)
604   (Oz, 2013)
605   (The Holy Bible, 1984)
606   (Chavalas, 1997)
607   (Steele & Cobley, 1976)
608   (McLaughlin, 2010)

609   (Casson, 1989)
610   (Turner, 2005)
611   (Turner, 2005)
612   (Turner, 2005)
613   (Nefzaoui, 1886)
614   (Nefzaoui, 1886)
615   (Hirsch & Gruss, 2010)
616   (Shah, Al-Shareef, Ageel, & Qureshi, 1988)
617   (Turner, 2005)
618   (Sherman & Billing, 1999)
619   (Rozin & Schiller, 1980)
620   (Sherman & Billing, 1999)
621   (Johri & Zutshi, 1992)
622   (Sherman & Billing, 1999)
623   (Calderón-Montaño, Burgos-Morón, Pérez-Guerrero, & López-Lázaro, 2011)
624   (Russell.Wendy. & Duthie, 2011)
625   (Masood, Chaudhry, & Tariq, 2006)
626   (Lai & Roy, 2004)

Moving Forward
627   (Samra, 2010)
628   (Kurlansky, 2002)
629   (Smilowitz, German, & Zivkovic, 2010)
630   (Smilowitz, German, & Zivkovic, 2010)
631   (Muskiet, 2010)
632   (Corella, et al., 2013)
633   (Brillat-Savarin, 2009)
634   (Winslow, 2013)
635   (OECD health data 2012, 2012)
636   (World Health Organization, 2012)
637   (Centers for Disease Control, 2003)
638   (Murray, et al., 2013)
639   (Carrera-Bastos, Fontes-Villalba, O'Keefe, Lindeberg, & Cordain, 2011)
640   (Cordain, Eades, & Eades, 2003)
641   (Reaven, Pathophysiology of Insulin Resustance in Human Disease, 1995)
642   (Cordain L. , Eaton, Brand-Miller, Lindeberg, & Jensen, 2002)
643   (Cordain, Lindeberg, Hurtado, Hill, Eaton, & Brand-Miller,

2002)
644   (United States Department Of Labor, 2012)
645   (Winslow, 2013)
646   (Cordain, et al., 2005)
647   (Leonard, Snodgrass, & Robertson, 2010)
648   (Cordain, Brand-Miller, Eaton, Mann, Holt, & Speth, 2000)
649   (Simopoulos, 2001)
650   (Renaud & de Lorgeril, 1992)
651   (Astorg, Arnault, Czernichow, Noisette, Galan, & Hercberg, 2004)
652   (German & Dillard, 2004)
653   (Cordain, et al., 2005)
654   (Mann, Shaffer, & Rich, 1965)
655   (Mann, Shaffer, Anderson, & Sandstead, 1964)
656   (Mann, Spoerry, Gray, & Jarashow, 1972)
657   (Jens, Hetfield, & Ulrich, 2003)
658   (Wells, 2013)

CPSIA information can be obtained
at www.ICGtesting.com
Printed in the USA
FSOW01n1011240316
18408FS

9 781940 192895